Trauma Therapy and Clinical Practice: Considerations of Neuroscience, Gestalt and the Body

Trauma Therapy and Clinical Practice: Considerations of Neuroscience, Gestalt and the Body

2nd Edition

Miriam Taylor

 Open University Press

Open University Press
McGraw Hill
Unit 4
Foundation Park
Roxborough Way
Maidenhead
SL6 3UD

Email: emea_uk_ireland@mheducation.com
World wide web: www.mheducation.co.uk

First published 2014
First published in this second edition 2025

Copyright © Open International Publishing Limited, 2025

Commissioning Editor: Hannah Church
Editorial Assistant: Phoebe Hills
Content Product Manager: Graham Jones

British Library Cataloguing in Publication Data
A catalogue record of this book is available from the British Library

ISBN-13: 9780335252473
ISBN-10: 0335252478
eISBN: 9780335252480

Typeset by Transforma Pvt. Ltd., Chennai, India

Praise page

"This book, now in its second edition, has become a classic in clinical studies of trauma. Its informed content, deeply humane style, numerous clinical examples, flowing narrative and ethical clarity make it an essential contribution to all contemporary clinicians and psychotherapists-in-training of any approach. Miriam integrates studies that respect the complexity of suffering resulting from trauma and recognise the crucial roles of both bodily processes and the therapeutic relationship. Yet she equally clearly draws a line between psychotherapy and techniques that promise modern, easy solutions. The complexity and depth of traumatic experiences require that the therapist be the main instrument of healing, with humility, compassion and trust. This book is a valuable companion for all contemporary clinicians."

Margherita Spagnuolo Lobb, Director of the Italian
Gestalt Therapy Institute, Italy

"In this second edition Miriam Taylor presents current thinking around the neuroscience of trauma with more emphasis on its relational aspects and relates it to Gestalt therapy theory. This book is relevant to both experienced practitioners and therapy students, providing counterpoints to the theory by using case studies, reflection points and experiential exercises offering the opportunity to assimilate learning in a holistic way."

Marc Williams, Gestalt Psychotherapist and Trainer, UK

"This well-written book is interesting and informative, acknowledging the changing ways that we think about the context of trauma. In this updated edition, Miriam Taylor presents a carefully considered approach to understanding and working with trauma, bringing the readers' attention to recent advancements gleaned from the field of neuroscience. In line with the Gestalt perspective, emphasis is placed on the subjectivity of the traumatic experience, with importance attributed to relationship and connection. I recommend this book as an asset for students and practitioners alike."

Dr Emma Bradshaw, Counselling Psychologist, UK

For the silent ones

Contents

Praise page   v

Acknowledgements   xiii

Preface to the second edition   xv

1   INTRODUCTION   1

    Defining trauma   2
    Contemporary trauma therapies   4
    The traumatized body   5
    The application of neuroscience   8
    Reductionism and technique   10
    Gestalt as a therapy for trauma   11
    About the book   15

PART 1 ENLARGING THE FIELD OF CHOICE   19

2   THE ORGANIZATION OF PARTS AND WHOLES   21

    A metaphor for the work   21
    Unformulated trauma   22
    Orienting to trauma   23
    Trauma figure, trauma ground – field, self and other   24
    Creative adjustments   28
    Polarities, balance and holism   30
    Rigidity, chaos and complexity   31
    Restructuring the ground   33
    Regaining control   36
    Immersion in the positive   37

3   MAKING CHANGE POSSIBLE   40

    Change from the viewpoint of the traumatized other   40
    Perspectives on change   41
    The Paradoxical Theory of Change and trauma   42
    Other factors in the change process   44
    Neuroscience, trauma and change   46
    Special functions of the brain   49
    The relational brain   50
    Creating the conditions for growth   50
    Towards an Integrated Model of Change   54

4   WORKING WITH AROUSAL   58

   Trauma as an arousal process   58
   Arousal and Gestalt   59
   The autonomic nervous system   60
   The polyvagal theory and social engagement   61
   The Window of Tolerance Model   63
   Clinical implications of the autonomic nervous system   66
   Working with arousal   68

5   THERE AND THEN, HERE AND NOW   74

   The timelessness of trauma   74
   Beyond the here and now   76
   Differentiating experience   77
   Repeating patterns   78
   Awareness of the here and now   79
   Awareness and the phenomenological method   79
   Phenomenology and the body   81
   Awareness, phenomenology and the process of change   83
   The role of mindfulness in trauma therapy   84

PART 2 AT THE LIMITS OF SELF   91

INTRODUCTION TO PART 2   93

6   FROM FEAR TOWARDS SAFETY   97

   Avoidance, triggers and phobias   98
   Responses to fear   100
   Orienting to danger   101
   The neurobiology of fear   102
   Survival-based defences   104
   Risky behaviour   106
   A secure base   107
   Establishing safety   108
   Case study: Part 1   111

7   FROM HELPLESSNESS TOWARDS AGENCY   115

   Helplessness and healthy process – a Gestalt perspective   115
   Two kinds of helplessness in the body   117
   The psychological impact of helplessness   119
   The shame of helplessness   120
   Locus of control shift   121
   Agency and choice   123
   Taking action   124
   Case study: Part 2   126

8   FROM DISSOCIATION TOWARDS CONTACT   129

    Theoretical perspectives on dissociation   129
    Depersonalization and derealization   131
    Making sense of dissociation   132
    Dissociation and the body   132
    The neuroscience of dissociation   134
    The fragmented self   134
    Collective dissociation   139
    Dissociation and relationship   140
    Supporting contact   142
    Case study: Part 3   144

9   FROM SHAME TOWARDS ACCEPTANCE   146

    Shame through the lens of trauma   147
    Attachment shame   149
    Shame, blame and responsibility   151
    Shame-full bodies   153
    The physiology of shame   155
    In an unreceptive world   155
    Working with shame   157
    Case study: Part 4   159

PART 3 A RELATIONAL HOME FOR TRAUMA   **163**

10   THE ROLE OF THE THERAPIST   165

    The therapist and change   165
    The therapist and emotional regulation   166
    Power and horizontalism   169
    Establishing the relationship   170
    Transference issues   171
    Therapist as (re)organizer   174
    The therapist and the here and now   175

11   THE WELL-RESOURCED THERAPIST   179

    Personal story 1: Gathering resources   179
    Mirror neurons   181
    Therapist vulnerability   182
    The embodied therapist   185
    Mindfulness as a resource   190
    Mutual healing   190

12   EMBODIED RELATIONSHIP   192

    Relational dilemmas   192
    What we already know   193

Mutual regulation   196
An experience beyond words: making sense together   199
Touch   202
Special considerations in tolerating relationship   204

13 TRANSFORMING RELATIONAL WOUNDS   206

Disorganized attachment and complex trauma   206
Rupture and repair in trauma therapy   208
What's going on? Trauma in the room   211
Acts of triumph   213
Integration, narrative and earned attachment   215
Case study: Part 5   217

Glossary   219
References   223
Index   234

Acknowledgements

Had it not been imperative for me to get to grips with my own trauma for the sake of my family, I would never have arrived where I am now. Ben, Rachael, Kat, Amelie, Ophelia, Erica and Sylvia will always come first.

People in my professional family are behind everything I do. Martin Capps has been faithfully at my right hand throughout the years of running the diploma in Contemporary Trauma Practice through Relational Change. I am deeply indebted to him as a colleague and friend. My colleagues on the Leadership Team – Lynda Osborne, Sally Denham-Vaughan, Marie-Anne Chidiac and Kate Glenholmes – also have a steady hand on my back. The commitment of Ed Fellows, Margaret Landale, Sonja Hookway, Jane Skinner and Nick Adlington forms a solid ground for this work. No less valued are my collaboration with Vienna Duff and the Relational Community of Practice that has grown around our Well Grounded Therapist residentials.

This book weaves together countless threads of conversations, reflections and questions arising from my teaching. To all participants, especially those in past contemporary trauma practice programmes, you inspire me and are reflected in these pages. Among those who have made workshops possible are: Margherita Spagnuolo Lobb, Ravi Kumar, Lena Grigoryeva, Sharon Grey, Igor Pogodin, Victoria Stephenson, Claude Charlier, Blagica Rizoska, Jorge Merino, Ania Maleka and Shelley Holland; to each I am grateful and honoured to have been invited. Those that I have not named individually are no less important, if you have been missed, the fault is mine alone.

My practice as therapist and supervisor of individuals and groups has also provided rich learning about trauma, relationship and healing. Threads of many personal stories and struggles come together in these pages. I cannot name them but I hope they know who I mean and their critical place in animating these pages; we change one another. Two more people have widened the edges of this book. Leah Manaema Avene does me the honour of calling me an elder, but her greater wisdom is not related to age. Darren McGarvey I thank for pushing me to continually revise my thinking.

The front-of-house team at McGraw-Hill Education have made this book real; they are Beth Summers, Bryony Walters, Tamara Haq, Graham Jones and Hannah Church, who have steered the development process. Behind the scenes is a group of skilled people who bring the book into being. Thank you hardly seems enough. Mark Howlett has added style to the images. In addition, Jim Kepner and Professor Larry Wald have both been gracious in allowing permission to reproduce their material. Emma Coonan and Emily Skye are both friends and have contributed to the index, for which I am relieved and grateful.

Other special people who have prevented me from drowning in trauma include Judith Armstrong, Sue Brock-Hollinshead, Sarah Buxton, Catherine Cook, Jan Cook, Ruth Dowley, Neil Jones, Jacqueline Ogden, Roshni Parmar-Hill, Sue Pitman, Karen Pounds, Sue Taylor, Mij Wilkinson, and sangha friends everywhere.

Together, we made this book.

Preface to the second edition

Hen, River, Otter

Those creatures I recognize as Two-Legs arrive onto the moor, holding their long sticks. I watch closely, alert to what they are doing. River is flying free, hunting for our brood, while I watch our nest with its new eggs. Two-Legs point their sticks upwards and there is a loud CRACK, a shriek of my name 'HEN!' and River falls clumsily, helplessly, to the ground. In panic I rise, heart wild with fear and distress, and fly towards the shelter of a tree as the creatures wave their torches and the moor lights with flame. Horror, sheer horror – my River, my clutch of eggs, my future, my life. I stay frozen very still for a long time, terrified of moving, terrified of what I might find when I do. This is beyond my endurance.

When I hear the Two-Legs leave it is dusk. I slowly open my wings and take flight, a silent flight, heart shattered, surveying the smoke-filled moor that has been my home and can be no longer. I don't recognize this place now, I can't get my bearings any more. I can't feel where I end and the world around me begins. There are no edges here. Nothing, nothing makes sense. I fly slowly to a beck and see Otter dipping in and out of the water, water I need for the fire in my soul. My hunter instinct kicks in and I swoop down towards Otter, but as I hit the water, I change and become Otter, lithe and free.

The persecution of hen harriers and the burning of moorland stand as a metaphor for the intersection of multiple traumas in modern times. In 2018, a ringed hen harrier known as River was found, having been shot (Thomas 2019). This bird of prey, an apex predator important for the ecology of parts of northern England, is now red listed, and yet subject to illegal persecution as part of 'management' of moorland for grouse shooting. This sport of the wealthy classes of England involves burning heather-covered moors to remove the habitats of voles and other small creatures – key prey of the hen harrier – and support the overstocking of grouse. This in turn has a devastating impact on the biodiversity of these areas. Under pressure, hen harriers have been known to take animals as large as rabbits or otters.

This we might see as a comprehensive dislocation and power play which underpins the experience of trauma – it is a profound loss of ground which plays out on multiple levels in contemporary society. It is not only a matter of loss for the hen harrier population; the consequences are many-layered, as is the case for much of the relational trauma in the world. Arguably, those consequences affect the perpetrators too, in terms of their loss of connectedness. Trauma radically alters our ways of being in the world, shapes our identity and underpins our future relationships. Polarities of alienation and identification come to the fore – in this case too much of the former and too little of the latter. Our capacity to join the dots and anticipate consequences, or to think of ourselves as part of an ecosystem (Taylor 2023) has been subsumed in a world of hyperindividualism which, I argue, comes at a cost to every one of us whether or not we have experienced identifiable trauma. It is not difficult to read these times as being marked by implicit trauma, which inevitably narrows our focus. There is a call here to hold some deeper themes in our current world and to face the challenge of doing so. More urgent than ever is the need for some ways of making sense of what's happening: the extent to which we have to adapt to a rapidly changing situation, so dissociation becomes a way of surviving. Trauma in many ways is a great unravelling (Macy 2009), a pivot on which the world as we know it turns. Such a world requires that we adapt and shape-shift as a means of survival, as does the hen harrier, and in these times we need to adapt at an ever-increasing pace.

In the ten years since the publication of the first edition of this book, trauma has entered our consciousness in new ways. I reflect here on those changes, some of which are developed later in this new edition. As a first overview observation, I notice how people seem hungry to understand themselves in this changing world in ways that circumvent traditional psychotherapy, and sometimes appropriate the language and concepts without ground, context or full understanding. I resonate with this longing for quick fixes in this increasingly complex world.

In popular psychology, the word 'trauma' is commonly applied to upsetting experiences. Truly, I saw a tweet that said 'OMG, I'm so traumatized to find that Boston is further north than New York'. That the writer may well have been aware of the irony isn't lost on me, but the incident touches a nerve for a therapist whose use of the word is quite specific and who needs a clinical language to convey the depths of suffering encountered in their work. How this might read, for example, for someone trafficked from Albania and working as a sex slave in the UK, struggling with immigration status, is altogether different. Of course context is increasingly important for those of us who seek the truth and to explain, and there are some thoughtful contributions to the world of trauma and of mental health in particular, that emphasize context. To this extent, the field of trauma is being repositioned as a social justice concern. In this volume, as I did in my second book (Taylor 2021), I attempt to redress the balance more to include contextual considerations and to attempt to decentre from westernized and medical mindsets. However, even as contextual thinking has come to the fore in the short time since my second book (and I am not alone now in taking this approach), criticisms are emerging at the time of this writing. The sheer enormity of the need for comprehensive systems change is turning back again on the individual who is left alone to cope.

I have touched on the polarizations that characterize modern life, and the worrying reluctance to think critically and to entertain other perspectives. This too is a change that therapists need to adapt to at the speed of light. Polarization, or splitting, is a phenomenon that accompanies traumatic experience, and in holding doggedly to a multiperspective position, I seek to find a point where integration and complexity replace reductionism and binary states. Ironically, this endeavour is in turn so infinitely complex that I am bound to fail comprehensively.

Nevertheless, some steps in that direction will, I hope, help. My work with trauma has always sought to achieve a degree of integration following fragmentation. Can we continue to hold that as a possibility in this fractured world?

There is a dominant narrative that is widely assumed to represent a gold standard of working in 'trauma-informed' ways, and I want to challenge this. Quite simply, I don't know what this means in practice. Teaching assistants, for example, may do three hours of training on trauma-informed approaches, while other professionals undergo lengthy training. Sometimes, being trauma-informed remains at policy level or as an organizational ideology, and I don't know how this translates for the traumatized individual who comes for help. It will, of course, mean different things in different places. However, at times this ideology can be used in ways that are clearly harmful, as the following quote describes:

> I couldn't move or breathe without being told I was doing so because of my trauma. It hurt, to be so completely defined by the most terrible moments of my life, especially when my attributes, the things I was proud of ... were also considered traumatic instalments.
>
> (Aves 2022)

In terms of the benefits of a trauma-informed approach, there is little evidence of real change. Implementation of policies has been found to be piecemeal, lacking shared vision and relying on top-down leadership (Emsley et al. 2022).

In a world of information overload, it is wise to be increasingly precise about the 'information' on which we base our practice. If we confine this to unspecified facts we remain in the mindset of scientific reductionism. However, no science can supply the ingredients of 'trauma informed practice', namely safety, trust, empowerment, collaboration and cultural sensitivity (Office for Health Improvement and Disparities Guidance, 2022). While we can create the conditions that support these states, we cannot provide the feeling that is desired. We are in danger of quantifying and commodifying trauma therapy. A more qualitative way of considering this might be to distinguish information from knowledge, leaning into a more implicit and integrated way of working. Here the capacity to favour process rather than content becomes relevant, and is consistent with trauma theory. All this needs to be more carefully and critically considered and discussed. I suggest that we need to be cautious about our use of this term until such time as a consensus about its meaning can be reached. Sweeney et al. differentiate a 'trauma-specific' approach: 'In trauma-specific services, the individual has a known history of trauma and interventions directly address its effects ... Conversely, trauma-informed approaches are founded on an understanding of the widespread exposure to trauma among service users and also among providers' (Sweeney et al. 2018). Of course, I cannot do the work I do without taking trauma into account, and I am not arguing against it, yet I *don't* claim to be trauma-informed. My preference is to move towards a *trauma-responsive* alternative.

A similar reductive mindset sometimes arises when the popular concept of ACEs comes into play. ACEs, or adverse childhood experiences, are a rule-of-thumb measure of the impact of childhood trauma. The simple scoring was only ever intended to convey information about the *epidemiological spread* of such experiences and not to be applied to individuals. However, the simplicity of the concept is attractive and is commonly misunderstood. The concept is deficit-based and assumes poor outcomes, failing to account for supportive resilience factors. There have been instances where ACEs scores have been applied as predictive, and thereby misused. Furthermore, the scores do not shed light on the severity or the duration of adverse experiences. The concept of ACEs is based on a westernized nuclear model of family and does not 'acknowledge more continuous, structural violence and neglect like the effects of racism, the fact of a prison system, capitalism, poverty etc.' (Fanen 2022: 219). Caution, therefore, is also advised in applying this concept to individuals. I am arguing for more precision in our thinking and not to fall into the temptation of assumptions about shared understanding and meaning, or simplistic thinking.

I suggest that the language we use to communicate about trauma matters for a number of reasons. Primarily, silence about trauma, particularly childhood sexual abuse, remains pervasive, and the move to break through that by campaigns such as #MeToo are still too often seen as radical. It is almost impossible to convey the felt, raw and visceral sense of traumatic experience in words – the hen harrier's story above being a case in point. 'It is excruciatingly difficult to put that feeling of no longer being yourself into words' (van der Kolk 2014: 237). Second, the language of 'disorder' and diagnosis has become the subject of heated debate, both among mental health professionals and the public seeking their assistance. The line I take is non-pathologizing, rejecting the imposition of the expert view which can replicate the power dynamics of traumatic experience. Nevertheless, as I have implied above, sometimes professionals do need a 'shorthand' to communicate to others. It is helpful when this emphasizes observable processes, rather than generalized labels. Further, language depends on a degree of self-knowledge, and that knowledge is sometimes hard to bear. It makes our experience real and relatable in a way that can't be taken back, however provisional our statements may be. Lastly for now, language begins to make a shape out of unformulated trauma, allowing us to conceptualize it and explain the ungraspable nature of what has happened. This is why I believe that accuracy in what we are saying is crucial, in a way that is too often ill-considered.

Another way in which language reflects the concepts that shape our contemporary life concerns self-identification. While we all have an inalienable right to identify as we choose – non-binary, neurodivergent, gender fluid, suffering from post-traumatic stress disorder (PTSD), minority aligned or whatever – I worry that in some cases these labels become fixed and unavailable for curiosity or possible change. This too, is language that is used to both define and separate, to exclude on grounds of difference, by and against those so defined. The degree of separation and alienation that arises from such differences can lead to trauma. There may not be right answers, but it seems to me that the questions that arise here are important.

If oversimplification is a reflection of an urgent yet ill-considered movement towards answers, the same can be said to be true of neuroscience. In the first edition of this book, the introduction of neuroscience to Gestalt psychotherapy and its application to trauma work was a key feature. To some extent I own that at the time this exciting new research felt like the 'magic bullet' that I and others so naturally sought. My position in relation to neuroscience has changed somewhat in the succeeding years. This is in part an easy assimilation of a set of principles that I have 'worn' like a familiar cloak for many years, so it has become second nature to ground my practice in them. But when I turn to other people I see yet again an enthusiastic but often simplistic and fragmented interpretation of neuroscience as a set of tools. There are advocates for polyvagal theory, or the role of the amygdala, or the significance of the freeze response. All of these are possible entry points into making sense of trauma, and none makes sense on its own. I don't think this does justice to the need for integration of complex and rich ideas and concepts that best support effective trauma practice. In reaching for answers, we risk missing the subjectivity of traumatic experience, make assumptions at risk of losing therapeutic curiosity, and may fail to listen deeply to those we work with. Having said this, one important development in neuroscience research in recent years reflects a greater complexity in approach, which is welcome. There is a current focus on the connections between different structures and functions of the brain – how the entire brain/body works together in synchrony to adapt, microsecond by microsecond, to our environmental and organismic needs (Abramson 2022). I find it exciting to see that far from confirming my fears about isolating structures and processes, the trend is towards relationship and connection.

I am frequently asked about the relationship between trauma and neurodiversity. The honest truth is that I don't know, but wonder if there is a 'chicken and egg' dilemma here. Clearly there are overlaps, in terms primarily of sensory overload or processing difficulties, emotional expressiveness and regulation, and of social engagement. Some who identify as neurodivergent find a trauma-specific approach helpful, and others are enraged by the implication that trauma is part of their make-up. Without doubt, to live a life with a minority identification, or to have your difficulties misattributed by teachers, for example, can be traumatic in itself. One thing we can say with some certainty is that early traumatic experiences change the wiring and structure of parts of the brain, and we can therefore allow that people with such a history are by definition neurodiverse. How this affects any individual is impossible to determine. However, in the case of traumatic experience we do also know that changes in brain wiring and function can take place over time with appropriate treatment, and this is unlikely to be the case for all those defined as neurodiverse.

Another question that sometimes comes my way is about the increasing interest in the use of psychedelics to treat trauma. Included in this category are MDMA, psilocybin, ayahuasca and ketamine. I cannot claim any of these to be within the scope of my experience, and yet I find the use of these substances to be both compelling and concerning. Maté came to the conclusion from his own use of ayahuasca that there are some principles of healing that can be available to anyone *without* the use of such mind-altering substances: 'the acceptance, the shedding of identity, the choosing to trust the inner guidance against the remonstrations of the conditioned mind, and the genuine agency that springs paradoxically from the willingness to give up rigid control' (Maté 2022: loc 7432). Maté cautions that 'Not everyone will, or ought to work with … psychotropic plants; relatively few people are likely to even have such an opportunity' (Maté 2022: loc 7432), and I am concerned that serious research is being done into 'treatments' that may not be accessible to those who are ordinarily oppressed and suffering. At the time of writing, legalization of psychedelics for treatment purposes is controversial and not universally endorsed. It remains to be decided whether these drugs are medicines or recreational. The interest in the subject has the flavour of a 'magic bullet' approach, of which I remain sceptical that such a singular remedy exists; it is a commodification of psychotherapeutic methods. Psychedelics also push against traditional understandings of the purpose and process of psychotherapy – we have always been interested in personal growth and accepted that the difficult and lengthy process of coming to terms with one's self cannot be circumvented. Usually the growth attributed to neuroplasticity evolves over numerous small iterations, rather than singular large events of note. Can psychedelics alter the structure and function of the brain in the long run? And how do you assess an individual's readiness to let go and tolerate potential recovered memories through the use of psychotropic substances? A further concern is about the potential appropriation of traditional healing methods removed from their cultural context and meaning.

On the other hand there are some extraordinary accounts of the healing potentials of such substances. As ever, working with trauma continues to challenge our traditional ways of working and conceptualizing therapy. 'It is intriguing to speculate that the pharmacological properties of MDMA, when combined with therapy, may produce a 'window of tolerance', in which participants are able to revisit and process traumatic content without becoming overwhelmed or encumbered by hyperarousal and dissociative symptoms' (Mitchell et al. 2021). We will look in more detail at the importance of this window of tolerance in Chapter 4 and elsewhere. For now, though, I think we have to give this possibility some credence, for the work of establishing the window of tolerance by other means is long and arduous. The experience of a more expansive and authentic sense of self, bringing a clearer understanding and meaning of vague memory, can also be seen as having real value. 'The ayahuasca did slowly open up a lot of those memories and all those things I had forgotten about as a child, and who I really am' (Maté 2022: loc 7337). I have had the privilege of witnessing people transcend trauma through hard work and determination, and yet accounts of the benefits of psychedelics often include a sense of transcendence, the language used verging on the spiritual: liberation, grace, surrender, mystery, 'entry into the realm of spirit' (Maté 2022: loc 7425). I conclude that there is something of interest happening in this area of research, but that it is too early to give it full endorsement.

The area of post-traumatic growth has also gained some traction in recent years. It calls into question what we mean by recovery from traumatic experience. I have witnessed enough times something that I can only call transformation following trauma to believe that profound, life-changing growth can be possible. To witness it takes my breath away. Note that I position transformation as a possibility and neither as an expectation nor a given; either of those alternatives is deeply unfair to those who do not have the conditions to make significant progress. A belief in the possibility of growth requires holding on to hope in the face of despair. I think it is contingent on the therapist to find such hope and to hold it for the other person who may feel that they are irrevocably broken. Indeed, my experience suggests that a powerful healing factor is when the therapist conveys implicitly that they believe in the person they work with. Growth, recovery, transformation – whatever you choose to call it – is contingent on so many factors coming together at the right time, some of which cannot be controlled. Typically, the course of trauma therapy is anything but linear, and this gives rise to some thoughts about markers of 'recovery'. Foremost are that setbacks become less frequent, less intense, and can be stabilized more quickly. It cannot ever be that trauma ceases to exist in someone's life, but my conviction is that one's *relationship* to the trauma does change over time. In new conditions that do not repeat or reflect the traumatic situation, traumatic memories can be accommodated into a revised sense of self. The trauma is no longer central to the shape of everyday life and can be assigned more effectively to the past. My primary interest, as ever, is in reducing the immense suffering that arises from traumatic experiences, rather than the individual's ability to function, which is a commodification of recovery.

With all these new ways of framing trauma in mind, I have attempted to reposition this new edition accordingly. To summarize, some key changes are in the precision of approach, the application of just enough complexity and the widening of the lens to include other perspectives and experiences. There are perhaps contradictions which more accurately reflect the human condition, thereby making the work more provisional. The limitations of space and my knowledge inevitably leave gaps and room for development of the reader's own thinking, and in that respect this is an incomplete work. My second book was written as a companion to the first edition of this one, and this present volume in turn comes even closer to *Deepening Trauma Practice*.

1 Introduction

> We all hover at different distances between knowing and not knowing about trauma, caught between the compulsion to complete the process of knowing and the inability or fear of doing so.
>
> (Laub and Auerhahn 1993)

Knowing and not knowing; self and other; before and after; body and mind; belonging and separation; control and letting go – trauma creates splits at multiple levels. Some of those splits run deep into the fibres of our being, some are so wide it can be hard to fathom that they might be bridged, others seem impossibly irreconcilable. Working with splits demands more attention to process than to content, and to consideration of the bridges between them.

Traumatic events are not isolated occurrences, and the inner experience of the traumatized individual becomes reflected in the wider world – and vice versa. Stolorow (2007: 13) accurately speaks of 'Traumatized people living in a discrepant world'. For the victim, splits occur in the continuity of their experience, in the coherence of **self**, and in the stability of the **ground**. Their experience is decontextualized. For those around them, there is often denial, disbelief, alignment with the perpetrator, blame or overprotectiveness. Trauma draws us personally to things we would rather not know about ourselves and the world we live in, and we respond by blotting them out. In the wider societal **field**, including the legal system, media and the political arena, similarly polarized positions exist. Traumatic reactions spill over from the individual to the collective in parallel processes which maintain and reinforce the trauma (Soth 2006: 74), and none of us is immune to them. The effects of this are profoundly deadening, and this book sets out to explore how to revitalize those individuals most affected, safely and effectively, without overwhelming or retraumatizing them.

To understand trauma we need to bring together the capacity to engage in complex thinking, the capacity to bear witness to random events and acts of extreme cruelty, and the ability to manage chaos, moral outrage and intense emotions. This is no mean feat as we seek to make new meanings out of utter destruction. It takes courage, honesty and integrity to do so. Personally and collectively, splitting becomes a natural response to managing the feeling of overwhelm; it makes trauma containable because it presents in small packages. To different degrees we dissociate from traumatic experiences, making them less personal and less real. According to Hillman (1996: 129) we engage in dichotomized thinking for comfort at the expense of clarity. Once trauma is embedded in the fibres of an individual or society, flexibility, choice and growth are hard to conceive of. Particular therapeutic challenges of integrating theory, selfhood and relationship are explored in each of the three parts of this book.

The integration which is widely accepted as a good outcome for trauma therapy is not simply a matter of reassembling the broken parts, as with a jigsaw puzzle. It is necessary to find a way of differentiating experience in order to make a new whole. We do so by understanding the organization of relationships and the connections between them. There is an appropriate metaphor for this process in human anatomy, where connective tissue throughout the physical **body** both forms partitions and connects: 'We cannot form connections unless we start at a place of separateness' (Stauffer 2010: 145). In trauma, the process of fragmentation is driven physiologically, psychologically and relationally. In recent years we have learnt much about the impaired connectivity in the brain which results from trauma (see for example Cozolino 2002: 257; Siegel 2003: 16). We can conclude that we need to rebuild a trauma victim's life from the cellular upwards, holding the dance between both micro (individual) and macro (field) dimensions together.

The process of differentiation is intrinsic to Gestalt psychotherapy and is one of its clear strengths. The phenomenological method is an excellent vehicle for specificity and precision. From a Gestalt perspective, splits describe the basic *conflict between* self and other which is inherent in trauma, while differentiation of experience is the *forming of self in relation* to other, by clarifying and strengthening. This then can give the trauma a new context and way of shaping and containing it. We need to gather a coherent theoretical, relational and phenomenological framework around the experience of trauma that embraces new insights and knowledge. It is this task the present volume seeks to fulfil, encompassing the integrative potential of Gestalt.

Defining trauma

Traumatic events are usually defined as being extreme enough to threaten life, exceeding the victim's normal resources. Put rather crudely, trauma is something that cannot be coped with. It is a moment in which everything is undone. There is usually an overwhelming sense of shock and an inability to escape in the face of unforeseen events. Witnesses to traumatic events are equally vulnerable to trauma reactions, becoming victims themselves. Trauma is so often bound up directly or indirectly with relationship. For people living in abusive or violent families, trauma is not an event but a relationship. The victim's instinctive cry for help underlines the importance of relationships for survival. The threat to life in this instance is of continuity of self. To complicate things further, according to Cozolino (2006: 229), this interpersonal trauma is 'more likely to be self-perpetuating and resistant to healing'. Trauma breaks the bonds of attachment and security which we understand to be the bedrock of a stable and coherent sense of self. Bromberg ([1998] 2001: 11) calls trauma a 'precipitous disruption of self-continuity'. To define trauma in Gestalt terms, it is a cata-strophic breakdown at the **contact boundary**, the point of meeting between interior self and the exterior world.

With this absolute breach between the individual and their known world, there are few resources to fall back on; there is no 'I' to alleviate this situation. Nothing – *but nothing* – is familiar, reliable, continuous or trustworthy. The traumatized exist in a strange country.

Stolorow, reflecting on a personal experience of trauma, writes:

> Massive deconstruction of the absolutisms of everyday life exposes the inescapable contingency of existence on a universe that is random and unpredictable and in which no safety or continuity of being can be assured.
>
> (Stolorow 2007: 16)

With the right support, most people who have experienced traumatic disor-ganizing events will recover and never come to the attention of therapists or psychiatrists for the symptoms of post-traumatic stress (PTS). It is estimated that between 25 and 30 per cent will go on to develop what is diagnosed as 'PTSD' (Herbert 2012: 511). Resilience factors differ from one individual to the next. Those who suffer a 'single event' trauma in adulthood often benefit from simple and brief interventions. They are not really the concern of this volume, because traditional ways of working seem to help.

Clinical practice suggests that when individuals do develop severe symptoms after a single traumatic event there is usually an underlying deficit, typically due to early relational factors. Bromberg observes that individuals who have suffered massive trauma as adults who also had a developmental history of disconfirmation were 'typically more debilitated by the later event than were victims of adult onset trauma who did not have such a developmental history' (Bromberg 2011: 58). The complexity of responses to trauma can be seen on a continuum, contingent upon the severity and duration of the trauma, the devel-opmental age of the victim and the level of social support available. Thus we arrive at the concept of complex trauma, now incorporated into ICD-11 (World Health Organization 2022), which is often less responsive to traditional ther-apy. Clients in this category need a more considered and informed approach to therapy, which is the subject of this book.

In line with some prevailing thinking, I avoid the use of the language of 'disorder' or 'PTSD' to explain trauma; the term 'disorder' translates more appropriately into 'What happened to you?' rather than 'What is wrong with you?' (see for example Perry and Winfrey 2021; Taylor 2021). It is rare to find a psychiatrist who considers trauma from the outset. It is common for peo-ple with complex trauma to arrive with a string of other diagnoses and failed treatments, from depression to anxiety, from bipolar 'disorder' to obsessive compulsive 'disorder' (OCD). They may also be treated for eating 'disorders', substance abuse and self-harm, or carry a personality 'disorder' label. This is not to say that these problems do not also exist; trauma clients who come for therapy often have multiple concurrent problems. In their own right, PTS symptoms as part of complex trauma are extremely debilitating, and these people suffer greatly. For these reasons, Davidson describes the 'all-too-heavy cost of PTSD, which, by any standards, must be viewed as among the most serious of all psychiatric illnesses' (Davidson 2000: 3). What the following pages will show is that this extraordinary suffering need not be a life sentence.

Contemporary trauma therapies

There is some overlap between approaches to trauma therapy, especially in relation to a phased approach to therapy and the need for a preliminary setting of the conditions in which the trauma can be processed. It has been understood for decades that trauma needs to be worked with in stages, the first stage usually being associated with stabilization before trauma can be processed (Herman 1992: 156). Cognitive behavioural therapy (CBT) for trauma, which is often presented as the therapy of choice, actually represents a 'broad class of therapies unified by a shared emphasis on observable outcomes, symptom amelioration, time-limited and goal-oriented intervention, and an expectation that patients will assume an active role in getting better' (Monson and Friedman 2006: 1). As we shall see in Chapter 3, this last point is extremely problematic for trauma victims. While CBT is effective for some people who have experienced trauma, it does not provide a cohesive theory of trauma. Herbert, originally a CBT therapist herself, makes a number of criticisms of this approach for trauma clients. She argues that a sole focus on protocols will not meet the complexity of these clients' needs, risking that clinicians will treat all trauma clients in similar ways (Herbert 2006: 148). CBT methods tend to rely on 'top-down' processing and pay less attention to the somatic dimensions of trauma as suggested above.

Furthermore, some CBT therapists promote exposure techniques with trauma victims (Riggs et al. 2006: 65), which clients may be unable to tolerate without becoming retraumatized. Van der Kolk et al. state that 'Flooding and exposure are by no means risk-free treatment techniques. Exposure to information consistent with traumatic memory can be expected to *increase* anxiety (thereby sensitizing and aggravating PTSD symptomatology)' (Van der Kolk et al. [1996] 2007a: 431, my italics). People with complex trauma *may already be suffering from too much exposure* in the form of flashbacks, nightmares and intrusive memories.

Dialectical behavioural therapy (DBT) (Linehan 1993) combines CBT techniques with skill training for mindfulness and emotional regulation. DBT was originally proposed as a combined individual and group therapy, but is rarely offered as both. Alongside the benefits, there seem to be some obvious problems with CBT approaches for trauma. According to Denham-Vaughan (2005: 10), cognitive approaches are predicated on both objective reality and on lack of **awareness** or inability to use reason to deal with that reality. This is a position incongruent with neurobiologically based trauma therapy, wherein the implicit traces of trauma are recognized as significant. 'Although cognitive approaches, including interpretation and verbal response to interpretation in therapy, are the left hemisphere's necessary contribution, they are never in themselves enough' (Schore 2007, cited in Wilkinson 2010: 10). Denham-Vaughan (2005: 8) observes further that '"Will-based" psychotherapies – such as CBT ... can inadvertently reinforce ... feelings of failure.' Having said this, the structure of CBT sessions and the brief time frame may be containing for some trauma victims in the early stages of therapy.

Eye movement desensitization and reprocessing (EMDR) was developed as a technique which helps to process difficult experiences, and is usually used with trauma victims. It involves the use of a protocol to provide successive short bursts of bilateral stimulation while the client focuses on a problem, interspersed with periods of reflection. It is a powerful and direct technique which brings the client rapidly in touch with charged material in carefully titrated doses. Figgess (2009) has provided an interesting integration of EMDR and Gestalt. CBT and EMDR approaches sometimes overlook the prolonged length of time it can take to help a client feel more stable. Clinical experience has provided many instances of people for whom either approach has failed or retraumatized them.

The same criticisms cannot be made, however, of sensorimotor trauma therapy (Ogden et al. 2006), which comes closest to Gestalt therapy and is the approach I most work with. Sensorimotor psychotherapy emerged from trauma research. It was developed in the 1990s by Pat Ogden, a collaborator of Kurtz. Ogden had been a body therapist and Rolfer, and she initially applied this to Kurtz's (2007) Hakomi method. Kurtz had been influenced by his work with Perls and others (Ogden, personal communication, 2011); Gestalt therapy can clearly be seen as one of the roots of Kurtz's approach. So sensorimotor psychotherapy holds the position of 'step-grandchild' to Gestalt. A number of the methodologies offered by sensorimotor work are derivatives of Gestalt, such as tracking, **contact** and **experimentation**. However, sensorimotor psychotherapy does not identify with any particular psychotherapeutic modality. While the theoretical base of sensorimotor work is different from Gestalt, being focused on trauma, there is much that is not only compatible with Gestalt, it also adds some valuable ideas (see Taylor 2013).

The traumatized body

Janet, as the forefather of trauma therapy, agreed with Freud on the significance of physiological reactions to trauma. He wrote that 'intense emotions are dissociated from consciousness and are stored as visceral sensations (anxiety and panic) or visual images (nightmares and flashbacks)' (Janet 1904, cited in van der Kolk et al. [1996] 2007b: 309). Kardiner, writing in 1941, noted that sufferers develop an enduring vigilance for, and sensitivity to, environmental threat, and described extreme physiological arousal in them, including sensitivity to temperature, pain and sudden tactile stimuli (cited in van der Kolk 2000). Later, van der Kolk's seminal paper on the neurobiology of trauma entitled 'The Body Keeps the Score' (van der Kolk 1994) brought together a series of interconnected neurobiological findings. Van der Kolk's early writing is highly technical, and provides much evidence of the changes to brain functioning that arise from traumatic events. This paper was the first to really point the way to working somatically with trauma. Van der Kolk (2014) states that psychological effects of trauma are expressed as changes in the biological stress response, ideas that he develops in his later volume of the same name, and which we will consider further in Chapter 4.

Apart from its psychological (loss of self) and relational impact (loss of secure connection), there is no doubt that trauma has significant effects on the victim's physiology. At the moment a trauma occurs a cascade of physiological changes takes over, preparing the victim to take instinctive defensive actions. Immediate alterations in heart rate, respiration, muscle tone, circulation, digestion and state of alert are supported by a flood of neurochemicals related to stress – adrenaline and cortisol in particular. The essence of panic and extreme fear is visceral. The stamp of that moment becomes embodied – terror, helplessness and disconnection are preserved in the tissues and cells of the victim. The body really does keep the score.

Clinical vignette

Francis went to an osteopath crippled by back pain. The treatment had limited benefit, and it was only when the osteopath commented 'It feels as though you've had a shock in the past' that the penny dropped. Fifteen years previously, Francis had an accident at work, falling from a ladder. His most serious injury was to his leg, and he had surgery to repair complex fractures. But he didn't connect his back pain with this event. The osteopath's comment triggered memories of falling, and a paralysing fear of landing on his back. Typical of many men raised to be stoical, Francis had dismissed the need for an ambulance and had got straight back onto his feet and tried to resume working. With the encouragement of his osteopath, Francis came into therapy.

Later, Francis was able to reflect on what happened. He told me, 'After my accident, everything felt like chaos, complete chaos, I couldn't handle it, I'd become someone different. That constant sense of urgency, telling myself "Do something, do something", but I couldn't. I just couldn't get away from those feelings. I can see it now, how it's been like my head pulling me forward ever since, all up in my head, still far away from the ground. Waiting, waiting, bracing myself for the thud, over and over, like living in free fall, nothing I could do. Now I'm a bit less afraid of feeling my back, I can go with it and not fight it. I know where the ground is, I feel completely different. It's not in my head now, I can think clearly ... and I can manage my pain.'

It is at the embodied level that victims remain most exposed to trauma, and many clients experience their bodies as the cause of their distress. Over long exposure, primarily through repeated early trauma, damage to structures in the brain takes place. The particular violation of bodily integrity as a result of physical or sexual assault radically alters the victim's relationship to life in the body. In adulthood, many victims of early trauma have physical health problems – digestive, endocrine, cardiac, respiratory, vascular and auto-immune systems all being potentially vulnerable (Maté 2022).

> The experience of trauma … calls into question our relation to 'having a body' and 'living in a body'… And yet it is undeniable that severe trauma is inscribed in and often on the bodies of survivors, leaving a mark that can perhaps be explained but never effaced.
> (Young 1992, cited by Armsworth et al. 1999: 139)

The enduring mark of trauma is borne out of what is initially an instinctive survival response to strikingly abnormal events. This is later maintained by the body's attempt to resolve the trauma. We will consider this in detail in Chapter 7. It is the body primarily that seeks recovery, but does so in vain. All the physiological processes involved continue inexorably regardless of the conscious intentions or wishes of the victim. It is no wonder then that trauma victims so frequently report feeling out of control. They are powerless over their own intense embodied reactions to what happened. When the body doesn't know how to repair itself it becomes alienated, split from its meaningful contribution to everyday life. Trauma victims can no longer feel the beat of their own heart or the stirrings of desire; it may even be dangerous to feel them. So the heart ails and desire contracts into the musculature. Gestalt body process work is predicated on trusting the body to know what it needs; following trauma this basic trust urgently needs to be restored.

In order to address these profound splits we need to understand the relationship between body and mind. If we change the body we heal the mind at the same time (Johnson 1995: 169). A cultural and linguistic split concerning body and mind persists. As van der Kolk (1994) observes: 'Brain, body and mind are inextricably linked, and it is only for heuristic reasons that we can still speak of them as if they constitute separate entities'. The brain is more than the matter within our heads; it is the entire nervous system, which distributes energy throughout the body. It is through the process of embodiment that we can access the deepest layers of our experience, including implicit relational knowing. This signifies the importance of non-verbal, subliminal, relational processes instead of hypothesized fantasy, unconscious process or drive theory.

Another body metaphor is indicated in Johnson (1995: 344): 'The indissoluble functional and somatic unity of the sensory-motor system is testified by the obvious structural and bodily unity that is built into the spinal column.' This is more than an individual function since we acknowledge the role of the nervous system in mediating our interactions with the outer world. Because it concerns the self in the world which is so compromised by trauma, we can claim that healing of the body is the essence of good trauma therapy. This is not as complicated as it sounds, for neuroscience has provided us with some clear indications of how this can be achieved which are described throughout this book.

The application of neuroscience

It is all too easy to pathologize that which we cannot explain, implicitly or directly blaming the individual for their suffering. What we learn from neuroscience gives us a new window on some of the difficulties encountered in traditional psychotherapy. Trauma has been intensively researched by neuroscientists. For a traumatized group of people, it may be harmful to ignore what neuroscience is telling us – hence the need for developing a trauma-specific approach. By providing explanations for lived experience, neuroscience represents a link between **phenomenology** and physiology. Most importantly for trauma therapy, it gives us insight into disconnections within the brain and processes that are not under voluntary control. This has huge implications for the way we understand the process of change and growth in psychotherapy, and informs the choices that may or may not be available to our clients. This is the subject of Chapter 3 in particular, but we return to it throughout Part 1. Neuroscience also shows us that recovery from trauma will not happen in the usual time frames proposed by health providers.

Learning some basic neuroscience has been the backbone of my practice for two decades. It has transformed my work and my understanding, and I have come to rely on what it has taught me. However, I have become far less interested in the facts and the accuracy of the details, and lean increasingly into some important principles neuroscience offers. The reasons for this are several, and, I think, important, so I present them here again (see also Taylor 2021).

First, neuroscience comes from the tradition of the medical model, intrinsically individualistic, and is founded on a Newtonian materialist paradigm. The brain is matter which can be studied, controlled and changed, determined by the opinion of the expert. Psyche or spirit play scant part in this, which disregards other ways of conceptualizing the human condition, or contextualizing distress. It makes meaning according to certain criteria only: a western mindset.

More specifically, in practice, considerations of neuroscience include the following:

- It has become possible to keep a focus on avoiding retraumatization through applying learning from neuroscience.
- Most traumatic reactions make sense when considered through the lens of their survival function.
- Neuroplasticity means that trauma responses are not a life sentence, even though this growth may take time.
- Reminders of traumatic material have a particular emotional intensity and speed of reaction that may bear little or no relation to current observable reality, and may therefore seem disproportionate.
- The emotional tone of traumatic reactions overrides the ability to think clearly or to process the situation. Therefore we need to intervene on a somatic level.

- The visceral involvement is a whole body experience, and long-term stress leads to long-term consequences.
- The availability of resources – especially relational support– is a determining factor in recovery.

How we interpret the findings of neuroscience is, in my opinion, questionable. We may study a finding and only be able to generalize from it, or be no wiser about how to respond in individual cases. One clear call in this book is for specificity which is not taken up in research or practice. The overemphasis on individual rewiring (Fanen 2022: 193) is a worry from the perspective of relationship and systems thinking, which I suggest is necessary for a fuller appreciation of trauma. My final concern is that too great a reliance on what we think we know will get in the way of listening deeply to people we work with. Having said that, let us now look at how neuroscience can begin to support our thinking about trauma.

Neuroscientific research focuses on different aspects of the nervous system. It has diverse branches of study, of which there are three that are of primary interest to trauma psychotherapists. First, a variety of neuroimaging techniques are used to investigate the structures of the brain, including neural circuits. The most commonly used of these techniques in trauma research is functional magnetic resonance imaging (fMRI), the 'f' referring to the function of different structures. This is done by observing blood flow to these areas, indicating changes in activity in them. Fogel (2009: 42) sees the notion of modularity in the brain as conceptually useful in attributing regions of the brain associated with particular activities – *all are always involved* – which may be helpful clinically, but not scientifically accurate. Wilkinson (2010: 191–2) helpfully points out that the 'time frames involved in fMRI studies are vastly different from the time frames of therapy'.

A much more detailed study of neural activity at a cellular level is provided by magnetoencephalography (MEG), which measures electrical activity. These studies point to particular deficits in brain functioning of trauma victims and suggest new ways of thinking about and working with them. One thing that we can learn from this is the concept of neuroplasticity, which demonstrates that even at microscopic levels in the brain, growth is possible. How to harness that growth is the challenge for trauma therapists, as we shall see. A more recent technique, the connectome, illustrates the vast, complex and lively activity of the brain as a whole, less reductive in scope.

A second branch of neuroscience is related to the study of neurochemicals, the substances that are secreted by the brain and other organs to maintain the balance of life. These include hormones, proteins, neuropeptides and neurotransmitters which influence the firing, growth and specific function of neurons. Some of these neurochemicals have a soothing function, while others are associated with states of stress and danger. For someone who has experienced severe trauma, there may be toxic levels of these stress-related chemicals, which eventually become exhausted and depleted and no longer serve to protect the individual. Dissociation is driven in part by a neurochemical reaction, and I will return to this in Chapter 8. 'The presence of high levels of chemicals produced by the endocrine system in the bloodstream may also suppress the immune system and account for increased physical illness in some chronically fearful clients' (Cozolino 2002: 251–2). Implicit in this is that trauma therapy will reverse the proportions of neurochemicals associated with stress and well-being. The relevance of this is discussed in Chapters 4 and 12.

Linked to this is the area known as affective neuroscience. This is the study of the neurology of emotion, mood and personality. Specific areas and networks in the brain seem to interact in individual emotional states. This has given rise to the understanding that there is a fear circuit involving certain areas of the brain under conditions that are traumatic, which gets reactivated whenever the victim is reminded of the traumatic event; I explore this further in Chapter 6. Because this branch of science is concerned with emotion, we can infer that it is also to do with relationship and connection with others. The implications of neuroscience reach far beyond the investigation of the brain as an organ in isolation.

Reductionism and technique

Essential though the new knowledge of neural processes is to trauma therapy, we have to be cautious about privileging science over relationship, subjective experience and the essence of human existence. The therapy room is not a laboratory, and the observations of the therapist do not stand in for the microscope or fMRI scanner. The science therefore can be seen as a valuable representation, or a metaphor for emergent subjective processes. It is a probability rather than a certainty about what underlies the phenomenological experience. We can also argue the case that to avoid phenomenological or 'subjective' evidence is unscientific.

It is an oversimplification to translate the science into techniques, although certain kinds of interventions have been shown to be beneficial. Yontef (2005: 94) argues that 'An accurate understanding of the phenomenological basis of these techniques protects against making the experiment into an instrument of directed change, as in behaviorism'. It is perhaps stating the obvious to say that *'techniques and interventions are relational'* (Boston Change Process Study Group (hereafter BCPSG) 2010: 196, my italics), however 'we should clearly distinguish between a merely technical attitude, focusing on *something* in terms of processes, mechanisms and dispositions, and a therapeutic attitude that uses techniques, but goes further, addressing *somebody* suffering, being impaired or injured' (Fulton et al. 2009: 28, original italics). There is a clear case for *skilful and knowledgeable* intervention in trauma therapy. 'Obviously, certain tasks, including many that involve an interaction with another person, require both individual mastery of some technical skill and that this skill be incorporated within relational spontaneity' (Bromberg 2011: 123). There is no formula that can be ethically or successfully applied to the delicate work of attending to people whose trauma has left them feeling broken. Therefore, where I offer suggestions of things you might say or do, they are illustrative rather than prescriptive in spirit. I encourage you to find your own words and your own style of being with the people you work with.

Gestalt as a therapy for trauma

From its inception, Gestalt therapy has taken an interest in making whole, a word derived from the Old English word for healing. The focus is on perceptual and experiential wholes and how they are related and organized. These relationships are discussed further in Chapter 2. Gestalt therapy has a unique understanding of holism, grounded in Lewin's (1997) field theory, providing a context for the experience of the individual client, including the organismic or physiological. For Gestalt therapists, self and other (also referred to as environment or field) are seen not as separate entities but indissoluble, self being a function of the field. These complex and sophisticated notions cannot be defined succinctly and are the subject of extensive literature (see for example Wheeler [1991] 1998; Philippson 2001, 2009). Parlett stresses the importance of this thinking, saying: 'Arguably, overcoming self-world dualism or the split between parts of the unitary field is one of Gestalt therapy's most radical contributions' (Parlett 2011: 54). At the heart of the self and other orientation lies the universal existential dilemma of who I am in the world.

The SOS model (Figure 1.1) developed by my colleagues Sally Denham-Vaughan and Marie Anne Chidiac (2013) captures succinctly the essence of what are known as the three pillars of Gestalt – phenomenology, dialogue and field theory. The Self relates to phenomenology, the subjective experience and meaning-making of the human; Other refers to the connections we make together; and Situation refers to the context or life space in which we operate. Together these three elements, in relative balance, provide a template for understanding our ability to be in the world which is of interest to us all and especially challenged for people who have experienced trauma. Trauma can be understood in terms of events affecting the individual such as assault

Figure 1.1 The SOS model

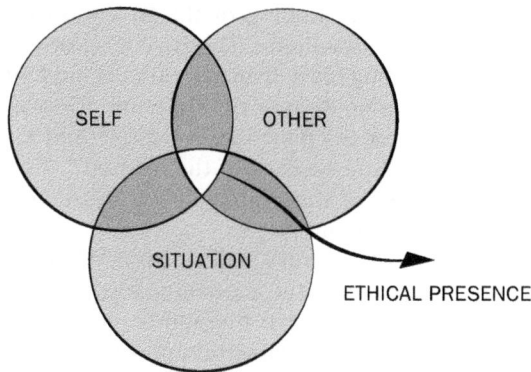

or accident; relationship and circumstances, each of which may be mapped onto the SOS model, and may also intersect with one another. So, for example, in the circumstance of the pandemic of 2020, there was an increase in domestic violence (relationship), within which specific assaults may have occurred. I have reconceptualized this model with regard to the breakdown at the contact boundary defined above, organized around what I call the black hole of trauma (Figure 1.2) is a representation of this breakdown, which alters our sense of being-in-the world, our relationships and ability to make contact that is definitional of trauma (see also Taylor 2021).

Figure 1.2 The SOS model revised

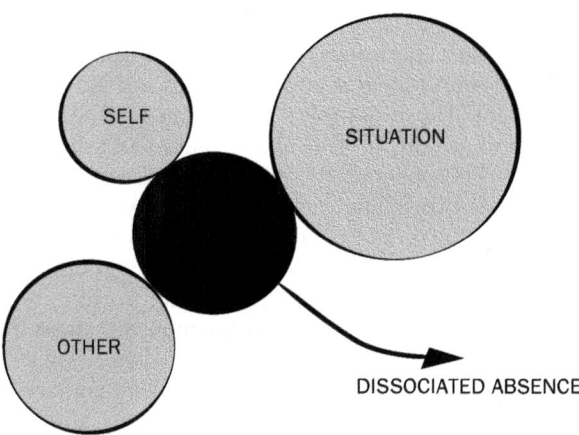

Perls' conceptualization of self and other was influenced by the year he spent early in his career as an assistant to neuropsychiatrist Kurt Goldstein. Far ahead of his time, Perls intuitively anticipated the findings of neuroscience research. 'In keeping with his holistic attitude, Perls valued human qualities and activities associated with both the left and right hemispheres of the brain' (Clarkson and Mackewn 1993: 36). He could not have foreseen that the accuracy of some of the central propositions of Gestalt theory would later be validated by neuroscience. A retrospective linking of the two and their application to trauma is made throughout this volume. The freshness of Perls' thinking has too often been overshadowed by his delivery of famous (and infamous) demonstrations of technique. As Elaine Kepner rightly put it: 'How is it that so many have mistaken the medium for the message in Gestalt, and have confused the techniques and gimmicks for the essence of the method?' (Kepner [1980] 2000: 6). Some Gestalt formulations of theory have been subsumed under different banners, which again dilutes the message.

The integrative capacity of Gestalt's holistic stance has nevertheless been understood by others from outside the modality. A psychoanalyst's (Tilmann Moser) view of the strengths of Gestalt therapy is recorded by Bocian (2009: 40): 'For the first time there are therapeutic approaches that offer different possibilities of making diagnostically visible and of enacting ... divergent parts of the self'. Similarly, Bromberg, in reference to Mayer, says 'the Gestaltists have shown us the key … to become adept at moving between one [coexisting anomalous part] and the other, holding the memory of [one] even as we see the [other]' (Bromberg 2011: 138–9). More specifically, Cozolino (2002: 60) regards Gestalt as being uniquely relevant to the notion of integration at the neuronal level. According to him, this is achieved by the focus in Gestalt on 'bringing to conscious awareness the automatic, non-verbal and unconscious processes organized in the right hemisphere and subcortical neural networks', maximizing awareness of all aspects of the self that supports the process of integration (Cozolino 2002: 61). These are helpful perspectives in positioning the value of Gestalt therapy in trauma work.

Contemporary Gestalt practice represents a qualitatively different paradigm from that of its founders. Although it was not obvious from Perls' demonstrations and verbatim accounts, Gestalt was distinctively primed as a relational therapy because of its theory of self. This book follows the relational turn in general psychotherapy, which in Gestalt was first articulated by Wheeler ([1991] 1998, 2000), Hycner (1993) and Hycner and Jacobs (1995). In my second book I extend the relational perspective to an ecological one (Taylor 2021).

Trauma is contextualized as part of the relational field which allows for integration, differentiation and processing. Take for example the empty chair technique, so often (and mistakenly) perceived as the main contribution of Gestalt. Classical Gestalt practice might use this in an overly provocative manner, assuming a certain robustness and voluntary control on the part of the client not usually available to traumatized individuals. Compare this to Spagnuolo Lobb's more relational version:

> The technique of the empty chair is replaced by saying *to the therapist* – instead of to the chair – what the patient would say to the person or part of her/ himself placed on the chair … This change enables us to bring … into the field of the present relationship, the relational block.
>
> (Spagnuolo Lobb 2009: 118, original italics)

Thus splits and conflicts are held within the therapeutic relationship.

Gestalt therapy continues to value the immediacy of the present moment, encouraging spontaneity and authenticity of contact. This permits reorganization of the experiential and relational field. The ways in which individuals adjust to trauma are treated in Gestalt as creative and the very best a person can do in difficult circumstances. Too often, however, they arise from a field of severely limited choice, and become incorporated into the structure of the personality as **fixed gestalts**. For Gestalt therapists, fluidity of response is a sign of healthy process; a sign of an expanded field of choice. As we shall see later, this marries beautifully with trauma theory and particularly with the theory of autonomic arousal.

Differentiation is supported by the phenomenological approach, replacing the 'Why?' with 'How, where and when?' (Perls [1947] 1992: 106). Gestalt does not propose a theory of causality and we cannot therefore claim that trauma has certain consequences. Rather we understand that the response to traumatic events is uniquely subjective and field-sensitive. Gestalt therapy has evolved as a sophisticated and finely nuanced approach, which by embracing a deep humanity and understanding of suffering has much to offer trauma victims.

Having said this, there are of course limitations in Gestalt. One in particular is relevant to the present discussion of splits between body and mind. Brownell describes 'residual' dualisms in Gestalt therapy: 'we need to understand how an immaterial "self" is related to the "conservative" and material physiology of the organism' (Brownell 2009: 72). Conceptually, body process is central to Gestalt thinking, as articulated by Kennedy (2005). The body is seen in Gestalt as valuable for heightening awareness, but this does not necessarily lead to a deep integrated embodiment. Many Gestalt therapists have not been sufficiently trained to know how to follow through with body awareness. Training institutes rarely teach students about the mechanics and systems of the body, leading to a pervasive lack of confidence in knowing what to do and how to apply it. A differentiated approach would seem to indicate this is necessary. Rather, we have at present to go outside Gestalt to other bodywork traditions in order to fill this gap. Chapter 11 includes a personal account of such development.

Because Gestalt addresses some of the essential dimensions of human functioning and of being in the world, it has traditionally been thought of as universally applicable regardless of an individual's presenting difficulties. Those who represent this line of thinking are concerned that the spirit and integrity of Gestalt is lost by changing its parameters. On the other hand, we can argue that certain large groups of people, including those who have experienced trauma, merit particular understanding of their difficulties. This view is represented by Yontef (1993) and his work on personality 'disorders', by Oaklander (2000) and McConville (1995) and their approach to working with children and adolescents, and by Kepner and his contribution to working with childhood abuse.

Kepner's model

Surprisingly, for many years there was only one significant work on trauma in the Gestalt literature, James Kepner's *Healing Tasks* (1995), specifically focusing on childhood abuse. James is the son of the aforementioned Elaine; he is hereafter referred to as Kepner. His important book is steeped in Gestalt values, and consistent with the spirit of the human potential movement. It is a foundation on which I build. Drawing on clinical experience, Kepner presents many creative ideas for interventions, but more often than not these are not defended theoretically. For this reason many of the interventions are difficult to translate into clinical practice. Published a year after van der Kolk's 'The Body Keeps the Score', the impact of neuroscience had not yet been felt. However, Kepner's message can be taken as being absolutely consistent with the principles of neuroscientifically informed trauma therapy. Therefore, while there remains much to commend in Kepner's work, it does need updating and grounding in a stronger theoretical base.

Kepner was among the pioneers of contemporary trauma therapy who advocated a phased approach to the work. His Healing Tasks Model is a stroke of genius, providing a hologrammatic, integrative and non-linear framework for the process of therapy (see Figure 1.3).

Figure 1.3 The Healing Tasks Model

Support phase	Self-functions phase	Undoing, redoing and mourning phase	Reconsolidation phase
Developing support	Developing support	Developing support	Developing support
Developing self-functions	Developing self-functions	Developing self-functions	Developing self-functions
Undoing, redoing and mourning	Undoing, redoing and mourning	Undoing, redoing and mourning	Undoing, redoing and mourning
Reconsolidation	Reconsolidation	Reconsolidation	Reconsolidation

Early	Middle	Late

Course of therapy

Source: Kepner 1995: 8 (Thanks to Jim Kepner for permission to reproduce this diagram)

This reflects accurately the recursive phenomenology of trauma clients, and defines the key therapeutic tasks within each overlapping phase. As Kepner explains, the four phases of his model are arrayed across the top of the diagram, and the four tasks are arrayed in the columns. Shaded boxes represent tasks that are more in the background during a particular phase, and clear boxes represent tasks that are more in the foreground and which thus tend to organize the field of therapy at a particular time.

The Healing Tasks Model is multilayered and iterative, maintaining a perspective on the whole of the therapeutic journey while attending to a particular element along the way. Importantly, '*all* the tasks are *always* present and being worked with in some fashion' (Kepner 1995: 8, original italics). Kepner's model has four phases of therapy, while most others have only three; the support and self-functions phases of Kepner's model roughly correspond to the first stabilization phase of other models.

About the book

In the pages that follow, readers will find an enquiry into the compatibility of neuroscience and Gestalt therapy theory, and their clinical application to psychological trauma. The book rests on the three pillars of Gestalt therapy outlined above, and draws on other sources, including trauma research, bodywork, social anthropology and relational psychoanalysis. The field orientation is voiced by Yontef (1993: 258), who says of Gestalt: 'We have always been an integrating framework … we take what we need from the total field'. While integration is to be encouraged, this application to Gestalt could begin to look as incoherent as other approaches. Brownell's more nuanced position is that a *modified* phenomenological, dialogic and field approach can be helpful (Brownell 2012: 124, my italics), and it is in this spirit that I embrace here the insights gained from neuroscience in respect of trauma clients. The intention is to create a coherent approach. We bear in mind that inherent tensions arise from integrating approaches with different philosophical foundations. Delisle suggests that integration between modalities should seek compatibility between them 'in such a way as to reduce their weaknesses and maximize their strengths' (Delisle 2013: 16).

This book is strongly influenced by three main sources relevant to Gestalt. Sensorimotor psychotherapy in many ways presents the necessary modification to the phenomenological method for trauma clients. Its derivation from Gestalt makes it a particularly compatible approach, and yet there are significant differences (Taylor 2013). Informed by neurobiology, sensorimotor therapy offers a number of theoretical maps that are invaluable in trauma work. Daniel Siegel is an interpersonal neurobiologist who is making a significant contribution to our understanding of the mind. Like Ogden et al., he brings together a range of findings and provides a multidimensional perspective on mind, trauma, emotion, regulation and mindfulness. Siegel writes a great deal about **body/mind**, rather than conceptualizing embodiment per se; for him, mind is body. This is implicit in his thinking about whole systems. Philip Bromberg is a relational psychoanalyst who offers important and rich understandings about trauma, focusing mainly on dissociation and the therapy process. Bromberg's wide definition of trauma includes early relational misattunement, unavailability and rupture.

The book has three parts. In the first, some of the foundations of Gestalt therapy are considered in the light of neuroscience and trauma theory. You will find some criticisms, particularly about the Gestalt understanding of the process of change, and also some ways of augmenting Gestalt practice with trauma victims. The intention is to inspire considered interventions which can enlarge the field of choice for these clients, taking into account the functional limitations as revealed by neuroscience research. A glossary is provided at the end for readers not familiar with Gestalt terminology; the first mention in the text of a term in the glossary is highlighted in bold. The second part focuses exclusively on the main phenomenological features of traumatized individuals, drawing the reader into a deeper understanding of their experience, and how to apply new thinking from neuroscience. Finally, the book brings the reader into the relational heart of trauma, considering the work from the point of view of both therapist and client. This part carries forward some of the thinking laid out earlier in the book, presenting it in a completely new light.

You will find many clinical vignettes throughout the book. To preserve anonymity, the stories about clients are largely fictitious, though based on facts about composite clients. The accounts of spoken and unspoken **dialogue** are more or less accurate examples capturing actual clinical moments. Because trauma therapy places considerable demands on us as therapists, as can reading about trauma, I offer a sequence of points at which you are invited to 'Drop In' to deepen your awareness of process and embodiment. To further support learning and integration, readers are encouraged to keep a written response to some of the Dropping In points offered. This rhythm of stepping in and out of intense material mirrors the theory and practice of effective trauma therapy.

Finally, a comment on terminology. For the most part, I have come to think of the people I work with simply as that – they are people, fellow human beings, and I tend to use this word in place of the more usual 'client', clumsy though it sometimes is (see also Taylor 2021). The word 'victim' is used sometimes in favour over the current convention of 'survivor'. 'Victim' too often has a pejorative overtone, whereas in this volume it is intended to convey the suffering of trauma, which 'survivor' does not encompass adequately. A victim is simply someone who has been hurt. There is also a relational aspect to my thinking about language: when you call someone a 'person' you reduce the power imbalance between you and reach more for your shared humanity; when you call someone a 'survivor' you move ahead of where they might feel themselves to be. It would be mistaken to suggest that where there is a victim there is also always a perpetrator. Accidents and natural disasters create victims without there being necessarily either individual or collective perpetrators. I also privilege the use of gender neutral terms such as 'they' and 'them'.

Part 1

Enlarging the field of choice

2 The organization of parts and wholes

This chapter explores the interplay of foreground and background known as the process of **figure** and ground formation, which is a foundational concept in Gestalt theory. We tend to pay attention to those aspects of our lives that most demand it, and let other aspects of our experience fall into the background. These are among the ways in which we organize and make meaning of our experiences. We will take a look at how this is of relevance to trauma victims whose attention is often consumed by managing the symptoms of PTS – the trauma figures. Very often, the experience of trauma leads to a polarized, and therefore unbalanced, view of oneself or of the world, and this restricts possibilities for growth and choice, and adjustments to the field reflect this.

Complexity theory sheds light in particular on stressed systems, and opens up new possibilities for conceptualizing the work of trauma therapy, and I will link this with Gestalt theory principles. In order to help trauma clients we need to pay more attention to the structure of the ground, enabling a wider and more nuanced perspective on their experience. I will conclude by presenting practical ways of building a repertoire of resources thereby widening the field of choice.

A metaphor for the work

I had the experience one day of feeling clogged up, not only in my thinking but also in my chest, back and lungs. I decided to go for a walk, and needing space and horizons I drove to the nearby downs. It was a brisk, bright midwinter afternoon. I gazed out over the landscape, the sweep and curl of hills reaching into the distance. I was aware of the sharp contrasts of dark trees and the glare of the low sun which impeded my vision. When I shielded my eyes from it I was able to make out the detail in a stand of trees about half a mile away, the quality of sunlight on the field beyond it and even the splashes of light breaking between the trees. It occurred to me that this was a good metaphor for trauma therapy, that when we take the glare off the trauma we can see more clearly the detail of the whole picture and new meanings and possibilities emerge.

Unformulated trauma

We start, as we should, with the suffering of the traumatized other. I say other, here, though I am not only referring to individuals but also to large groups of people and societies. The intersection between personal growth and systems change is an interesting one. From a relational field theoretical position I consider there to be a ripple effect, whereby changes in one part of the system create changes in all other parts too. The butterfly opening its wings in the Amazon creates a thunderstorm in Europe. We cannot but be in relationship in some way or other, an energetic reciprocal exchange in which we continuously affect and respond to one another. We are products of our environments. So the suffering of which I speak is both personal and collective, one being a reflection of the other. Therefore, what follows can be applied on increasingly large scales.

The traumatic breakdown at the contact boundary creates a profound level of disturbance at individual and collective levels, necessitating a massive reorganization of the sense of self and the entire experiential field. The two versions of the SOS model I presented in Chapter 1 illustrate the shift from organization or coherence of experience to relative disorganization or incoherence that follows traumatic experience. What follows is a kind of confusion, rather like the contents of a filing cabinet being thrown into the air, and not knowing how the papers will land. Moreover, as the papers swirl around, it is not possible to see what they are about, to read the contents. No themes are apparent. This is the experience of the black hole of trauma, disconnected and disorganized, in which therapists can also get caught, as I will describe later. All this assumes that we are talking about a discrete experience of trauma; however, more typically, there is no such event, but an ongoing background experience that weaves into a relationship. In this instance, experience may never have been organized with any coherence.

This incoherent experience can be understood as unformulated trauma – it lacks form. More particularly we can think of it as unprocessed trauma, carrying the implication that the trauma can potentially be processed. There is a lot of it in the world. The accompanying loss of meaning creates an existential position that is both overwhelming and terrifying. Alongside this, there may be an inability to account for yourself or your actions, or to foresee consequences. Mentalization, the taking into account of self or other, is compromised. Rather like trying to catch smoke in a net, the therapist too can be at a loss to know how to proceed. It is in the nature of trauma work to be messy and non-linear. Add to this the discontinuity of the sense of self and the complex adaptations that many people have to make to survive the trauma, the work becomes provisional and at times impenetrable. One major task of trauma therapy is to reorganize experience by means of *regaining control over the body*, about which I will say more shortly. The original use of the word 'sensorimotor' derives from Piaget's description of the increasing organization of movement in infants, from the involuntary and accidental to the deliberate and purposeful.

Orienting to trauma

We all tend to organize our lives automatically around our different dominant needs and interests. For most people, but especially those who have experienced trauma, the basic orientation is through the lens either of fear or of safety in the world. When we perceive our lives to be endangered, we automatically organize our behaviour for optimal survival. Self-organization may be goal-directed, but we also have ways of organizing our experience according to psychological needs, such as for intimacy or approval. These multiple layers of self-organization are not discrete: 'Human beings as living systems combine the organizational coherence of an ecological organization, i.e., the environment context, with a biological organization and with a psychological organization' (Sander 1991, cited in BCPSG 2010: 59, my italics). The different ways in which we organize our experience are typically out of awareness or implicit, and are dependent on the choices available to us. At each level of organization there is a search for wholeness and fullness of experience of self in relation to the environment.

Gestalt therapists understand such organization in relation to the satisfaction of dominant needs and interests as the basis for **gestalt** formation. One closely approximate way of translating the word 'gestalt' is as a 'meaningful organized whole' (Perls et al. [1951] 1998: ix). This is a rich concept embracing vitality, fluidity and growth, the antithesis of the experience of trauma, and provides us with another polarity to hold in the frame. Importantly the process of making dynamic and meaningful wholes is often interrupted, and for a myriad of possible reasons the opportunity for their realization becomes limited. We will consider this in relation to trauma shortly, but for now it is helpful to comment on the differentiating and unifying properties of the process of forming gestalts (Perls et al. [1951] 1998: 63). It is when we are able to distinguish clear gestalts that our organization of experience has the potential to becomes increasingly coherent or unified.

The concept of coherence of organization is also central to Sander's thinking, and he sees increasing coherence of psychological organization as a central overarching goal of development. For Sander (2000), increased coherence implies an increased inclusiveness of organization, so that more parts are integrated in more complex and adaptive ways into an overall wholeness. One way we can understand this increased coherence is as a restructuring from disorganized to secure attachment (see Chapter 13).

The ways we organize ourselves are related to how we orient ourselves in the world (Perls et al. [1951] 1998: 73) in line with our prior experiences, perceptions and the meanings that we make of them. It is relevant that Perls himself had a difficult childhood and a bullying and volatile father (Clarkson and Mackewn 1993: 2) and had to leave his homeland in a hurry as a political and Jewish refugee (Bocian 2009). These early experiences may have underpinned his interest in unfinished business and to the completion of gestalts. This orientation is particularly relevant to understanding trauma victims, perhaps like Perls, whose reactions to certain stimuli are organized according to meanings predetermined by their traumatic experience (Kepner 1995: 96). For example, the sound of screeching tyres may denote a very specific interpretation for someone who has been involved in a serious car accident, and their immediate and possibly lingering behavioural, emotional and physiological responses will be shaped by it. Traumatized people and groups tend to organize themselves in very fixed ways around trauma because their dominant need is to restore organismic equilibrium. This organization is what is known as the forming of fixed gestalts, as opposed to the free-flowing quality of emergent experience. Trauma is thus an overarching organizing principle in the lives of victims.

Trauma figure, trauma ground – field, self and other

Imagine standing before a large canvas in a gallery: you take in the whole and then begin to follow your attention to successive details of the image – figures, marks, objects, colour, texture – according to your personal interest; you stand back and take in the organization of the whole. At the same time you have emotions and thoughts and make associations and meanings from the experience, an ever-shifting interplay of figures emerging and receding from the ground. The figures you select for attention and the meanings you make of them in relation to the whole are entirely subjective. You will be drawn for similarly subjective reasons to some images in the gallery rather than to others which you may barely glance at. Theory of figure and ground relates therefore to which parts of our experience or environment we pay attention. It is also concerned with perception and meaning because we make more meaning of those parts we focus on and virtually discard those we do not. This is a key point in making sense of the trauma reactions we meet in our clients.

In classic Gestalt thinking, figures of interest emerge from and recede into an undifferentiated ground, like the relationship between a wave and water. The wave emerges from the water, is composed of it and recedes into it, is momentarily different from the water yet is never separate from it. We can see this in the image of Rubin's vase (Figure 2.1), in which the vase can only become a clear figure against the background of the two faces; one cannot exist without the other.

Figure 2.1 Rubin's vase

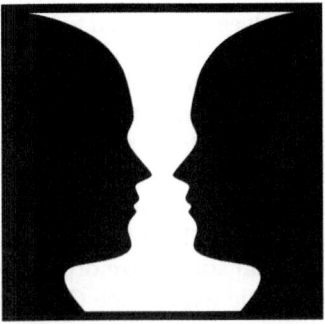

© Peter Hermes Furian/Shutterstock

Gestalt therapists are most interested in the particular ways in which figure and ground relate to one another and are organized; how does this figure emerge from this ground at this moment, and what are its energetic properties, associations and meanings? In the words of Perls et al. ([1951] 1998: 411), 'Energy is released for figure-formation when the chaotic environmental parts "meet" an instinctual excitation, define and transform it, and are themselves destroyed and transformed. Mounting excitement is the progressive leaving behind of the ground'. The model known as the **cycle of experience** traces the mounting excitement of figure formation through a number of stages, as well as the subsiding of excitement as the figure recedes (Figure 2.2). This cycle has been developed and revised by a number of writers (e.g. Zinker 1977; Wheeler [1991] 1998; Mackewn 1997).

Figure 2.2 The cycle of experience

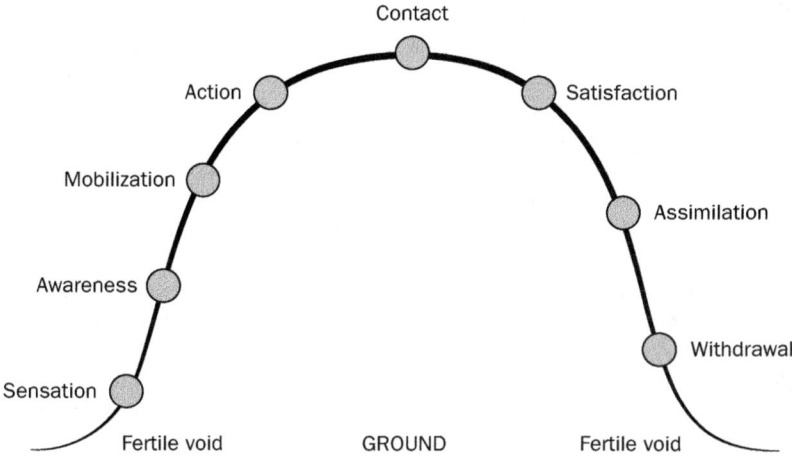

In a healthy process the relationship between a strong, clear figure and the ground from which it arises is constantly shifting and dynamic; when the process functions less well, figures are considered to be weak, stale or lacking energy. Yontef discusses further difficulties with figure formation that we can apply to trauma clients:

> Sometimes what is felt or needed is not allowed to become figural at all; sometimes it becomes figural only fleetingly, with the figure changing too rapidly for real insight to develop or activate new behavior; and sometimes a figure is kept in awareness and not allowed to recede to allow subsequent needed figures to emerge.
>
> (Yontef 2005: 90)

Set against this original formulation of Gestalt theory, Wheeler has postulated that the practice of Gestalt therapy is too figure bound, stating that this model depicts human life as 'impulsive, episodic, socially isolated, lacking in temporal continuity and overall organization' (Wheeler [1991] 1998: 86). In other words, it may be unformulated and meaningless. Taken from a field perspective, the impulses and excitements which we seek to promote can only be seen in relation to the ground, the two being indivisible Wheeler [1991] 1998: 87). With his articulation of the theory, Wheeler produced a more coherent framework and heralded a radical shift in emphasis from an individualistic paradigm to a system, dyadic or relational one. An implication of this is that we need to pay more attention to structure of the ground. By this I include the aspects of the situation and culture that influence us, often unseen: 'This is how things are' (see Taylor 2021). It is striking to recognize that Wheeler's proposition is only becoming more mainstream a generation later.

In my experience, it is characteristic of clients who have experienced trauma to have difficulties with figure formation. Generally these fall into one of two predominant styles; both have particular energetic qualities. There is the person who, with a sense of urgency, brings to our attention a number of rapidly changing figures within a single session. None is well supported; each feels dense and demanding. Rapid sequences of figures are not spacious enough to attend either to the early stages of sensation and awareness, nor to the later stages of **assimilation**, satisfaction and withdrawal, as though the curve of the cycle is too steep. This person tends to form figures that are *undifferentiated from one another*, and the therapeutic task is to slow down and work with one at a time. The second style is the person whose figure formation is so vague as to feel almost absent; they do not know what they want to work on, what is of interest and importance to them. For this person the curve of the cycle is too shallow and remains *undifferentiated from the ground* (Figure 2.3).

Perhaps they have learnt to defer to the dominant needs of others and will do so again with you. As a case in point, one person commented wryly: 'Perhaps we need to work on me knowing what to work on.' In either of these styles, there is little capacity to distinguish needs, to make choices, to allow emergence of spontaneity, or to bring appropriate energy to bear in the service of healthy satisfaction of needs. In addition, each style will have a physiological correlate, comprising too much or too little, charge, related to their trauma history.

If you look around you and take note of particular features of the space you are in you will notice things that stand out for you. If you look around again attending to things that you missed first time, your field of awareness

Figure 2.3 Variations of figure formation

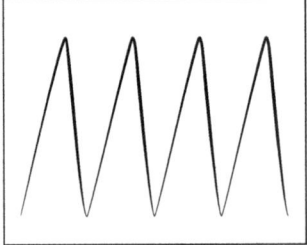
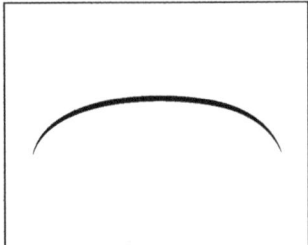

will expand. People with experience of trauma, orienting more instinctively towards threat, miss other figures that can enliven experience. Such is the impact of trauma that victims become preoccupied with figures associated with a concern about safety and threat, and which do not emerge with freshness and spontaneity from the ground or from an accurate appraisal of actual present circumstances. Change cannot occur in the usual ways for these people because of this preoccupation with symptoms which result in the recursive reliving of the trauma. This can be accounted for in two ways. First there is a need to complete the unfinished business – to restore wholeness – which is both biologically and psychologically driven, causing clients to 'rework' the figure; and second, intrusions of flashbacks, nightmares and somatic symptoms are interpreted as indicating the ongoing presence of threat. This means that trauma victims pay very particular and often exclusive attention to those parts of the field that are reminiscent of trauma.

As Kepner (1995: 94) comments, '[m]uch of the survivor's reaction and experience will be both theoretically and experientially groundless'. In so far as figure cannot be separated from ground, it is problematic to suggest that a figure can be 'groundless'; rather it is the *quality and the content of the ground* that defines the problem. Having said this, it is clear that trauma does radically change the ground from which the figures arise; it is a trauma-laden ground. Trauma-related figures are problems that cannot be solved by attending to those figures; the recursive nature of the client's attempts to do so have failed. We need instead to restructure, or reorganize, the ground.

Ground and field are not the same. Ground is more a phenomenological condition, formless and unbounded (Polster and Polster 1973: 30) which contains aspects of the field, both historical and contemporary. 'The ground consists of traces of experience, history and physiology contained in larger, deeper grooves out of which lively figures spring forth' (Melnick and Nevis 1997: 98; see also Taylor 2021: 26). I consider that the ground consists of traces of culture, ancestry and personal experience, bearing the imprint of transgenerational trauma via epigenetic expression and lived relationships. The Polsters comment that the main function of the ground 'is to provide a context which affords depth for the perception of the figure, giving it perspective but commanding little independent interest' (Polster and Polster 1973: 30). When traumatic experiences provide the context for the emerging figure, the victim's experiential world is restricted and terrifying.

We therefore need to question whether the statement that the ground is of 'little independent interest' is correct. Kepner (1995: 98) gives the all-too-common example of a client pushing to tell their story even when deteriorating, there being insufficient ground for a more supported figure. One person came into therapy having been retraumatized in hospital, including by the use of electroconvulsive therapy (ECT), physical restraint and being humiliated for their attempts to feel safe. They had been told that therapy had to make things worse before they could get better. With these historical fragments and introjects forming the ground of their experience, we needed to build a radically different context within which to work. According to Melnick and Nevis (1997: 98), 'Th[e] ground must ultimately be affected if a person is to experience a more permanent change.'

Creative adjustments

We develop new figures to enable us to deal with the emerging dominant needs, interests and challenges that life presents us with; these are new ways of making meaning which are called **creative adjustments**. Creative adjustments organize our experience in ways that are the best we can manage, in response to environmental demands, forming patterns, preferences and biases in particular dimensions. These adjustments are creative not because they are necessarily inspired – though they may be – but because they continually reshape our self at the contact boundary; Perls et al. ([1951] 1998: 247) consider that *the self is the system of creative adjustments*. Possibilities either expand or contract in response to a new perception of external 'reality', and it is this process of development which is creative.

For trauma victims, some of the typical adjustments that are necessary are extraordinarily creative, as in the case of dissociation, while others may appear to be self-destructive, such as self-harm. To these extents, creative adjustments may come at a considerable price. Creative adjustments emerge in a world in which choices are severely restricted, and trauma theory teaches us to honour them as the very best that the victim could do, under seriously compromised conditions. Some trauma clients experience unbearable levels of shame for the adjustments they have had to make, and find it difficult to understand and honour their creativity. When a creative adjustment is honoured, an opportunity for a new pattern to emerge is opened up, even if the new way isn't immediately available. Creative adjustments also represent hard-earned ways of managing which trauma clients may not relinquish easily because they have helped them survive in the past, and therapist and client need to come to a shared understanding of the subjective meaning and function of them.

Trauma theory gives us a context for better understanding creative adjustments. To do so compassionately, with sensitivity towards their meaning and functions, is a key to depathologizing some challenging behaviours. Self-regulation is a primary need that is served by making creative adjustments. For example, learning to freeze in order not to aggravate an aggressor is clearly adaptive and regulating. While this is true for anyone in any situation, it is a particularly urgent need for trauma victims, which we will look at in depth in Chapter 4.

One reason that traumatic events have the impact they do is that they are originally unanticipated, and there is a shock value. A common response to this is then to remain on constant alert for further possible traumas, in order to mitigate the potential for further shock and to maximize the chances of dealing with a threatening situation differently. The regulating function of this creative adjustment is clear, as is the cost for those whose energy is spent scanning the field for threats that don't exist and who may develop insomnia as the price for staying alert. A further cost is that the regulation achieved is not the result of a fluid and spontaneous process of figure formation and destruction leading to a coherent organization of the whole. I have found it more helpful, for many, to question how much vigilance is necessary at any given time: 'Do you have to be on highest alert all the time, or could you keep a part of you alert while you rest and recover?' Set this fixed attempt to regulate against a spontaneous **organismic self-regulation** 'based on acknowledging the complete array of sensory, mental and emotional data concerning both one's internal needs and the needs of the environment, and also the internal and environmental resources' (Yontef 1993: 214). In the right conditions in the moment, this will allow for differentiation, integration and assimilation.

Creative adjustments are part of the complex structure of the ground which influence the parts of the field we attend to. They inform our personal biases, prejudices, obsessions and assumptions, colouring our emotional range and tone, our relational style and **contact functions** together with the meanings we make of all of these. They also form a part of our physical being, the ways we move and our particular preferences for physicality. The biological organism adapts in response to trauma, engaging particular systems in the brain and nervous system in preference to others, and with the involvement of certain neurochemicals. At this invisible level these adaptations also become chronic, part of the make-up of the individual.

These interwoven dimensions of self-organization are not necessarily conscious or known to us unless we have the benefit of exploring them in therapy. Kepner ([1987] 1999: 49) confirms that 'A person's body structure is a total of the person's organismic adaptations to life' and therefore we look to the body to help us understand the subjective experience of the individual. When we, as therapists, focus on trauma, there are multiple other possible perspectives and presenting issues that we choose to ignore; they recede into the background. Exactly the same principle applies to our clients whose attention, even if they don't make the connections, is on trauma, and who thereby exclude other choices and possibilities from their awareness.

Dropping in

Look around the space you are in and become aware of what you notice. Are there things that catch your eye because you like them, or because they are irritating – something that needs tidying away or a window that needs cleaning? Does your attention rest in the interior space or out beyond the walls of your space? How do you position yourself in this space – the organization of your body and your proximity and relationship to the structures and objects that define the space? See if you can spot the patterns in what calls for your attention, a tendency towards pleasure or displeasure, towards inside or outside. Now ask yourself what you didn't notice the first time, what is calling your attention now. What do you discover about how you attend to place? How does this inform your sense of being in the world and of relationship to others?

Polarities, balance and holism

In ideal circumstances, all parts of the organism are in balance. Organismic self-regulation leads to integrating parts with one another and into a whole that encompasses the parts (Yontef 1993: 148). The maxim that 'the whole is more than the sum of the parts' designates the new organization of the parts when they are integrated and coherence is achieved.

The principle of **polarities** means that everything has its opposite and complementary equal, and that none could exist without the other. 'Day' is meaningless without its polar opposite of 'night', the personal requires the collective, and hope is irrelevant without the alternative of despair. All manner of qualities, functions and experiences of human existence can be viewed in this way. But in no case are these extremes set in opposition, for there are many shades between the two, such as dawn and dusk as stages along a continuum between day and night. A fluidity of movement along a continuum suggests that nothing is fixed and the individual is in a state of healthy process, with a maximal range of possibilities open to them. Joyce and Sills (2010: 126) observe that '[e]ach individual is a never-ending sequence of polarities', adding 'all parts of a continuum are potentially necessary' (Joyce and Sills 2010: 127). Traditional Chinese approaches to well-being include the concept of Yin and Yang, energetic (chi) forms which can be out of balance. This is not so very different from the contemporary western notion of traumatic arousal, of which I will say more in Chapter 4.

We naturally tend towards certain polarities and eschew others. For example, many people find it difficult to accept that their kindness can only exist against a ground of cruelty, and will likely disown this polarity. Joyce and Sills (2010: 127) suggest that some undesirable qualities are distortions of natural abilities. Cruelty could be a distortion of the ability to defend oneself or experience personal power and thereby restore regulation. Generally, polarities that are disowned are, for one reason or another, seen as unacceptable.

There is, however, a built in difficulty for those traumatized people whose biological functioning leads them towards polarities representing the perception of threat. Kepner considers that by disowning some polarities the trauma victim is able to preserve some sense of self-cohesiveness; under conditions of increased stress it is difficult to hold multiple perspectives on one's identity, and the cohesion of self becomes more binary and fixed. In the case of interpersonal trauma, the self may be defined in terms of reactions to either being unlike the perpetrator or identifying with them (Kepner 1995: 97), which leads to conclusions perhaps that one must never be weak, or must always find fault. In such instances, the split can be maintained by means of processes such as dissociation, shame, helplessness or fear (see Part 2). In any of these, aspects of self – often shadow aspects – are kept from view. Further, for these traumatized clients, it is often the body that becomes alienated from the sense of self, with implicit disowning of contact functions (Kepner [1987] 1999: 51). There is a disunity of body self, which I take to mean that, for example, someone might exercise excessively in order to stay strong, or dress provocatively in order to be 'looked after' by others. Polarities exist in the body, such as inhaling and exhaling, freezing or collapsing or contraction and expansion. In traumatized clients, polarities tend to become fixed and extreme. Evidence of polarization leads me inevitably to employ 180 degree shifts in my thinking which I have found to be invaluable in not getting stuck in narrow perspectives.

Splitting directs our attention more to process than to story. Splitting is a complicated process in psychoanalytic terms, but Gestalt writers have an accessible take on the issue which is helpful in regard to understanding trauma. Philippson (2009: 99–100) sees splitting as an alternative to choosing, perhaps between two seemingly irreconcilable polarities, which captures the dilemma associated with helplessness (see Chapter 7). For Yontef (1993: 262), splitting means being in touch with one part of the field and out of touch with another, perhaps polar opposites, and sometimes reversing this. Either way, splitting is a phenomenon common to trauma victims. Indeed, it is a necessary adaptation to massive threat – a way of managing overwhelming or unbearable aspects of experience. When we scale this up to the big themes of contemporary life, such as racism and climate trauma, the complexity of the field is even harder to bear (see Taylor 2021) and the splits can run so deep as to make it difficult to discern any middle ground. I believe that dialogue is an essential placeholder where there are splits, contingent upon a willingness of all parties to stay open and present. The pull in some trauma clients to one polarity of their experience is almost magnetic, and carries a great deal of shame – 'no one can ever persuade me that I deserved anything better' – and it can be a force which is not easy to resist.

It is tempting and sometimes harmful for therapists to align with a dichotomized process, for in so doing we too focus on one aspect of the field, limiting the therapeutic options. This inevitably has consequences for the therapy relationship. Furthermore, Yontef cautions against thinking that does not include the whole person *as agent*, the 'top dog' and 'underdog' being examples. In dissociative processes the self becomes fragmented into sometimes structurally distinct parts, of which usually only one is available or figural at any moment. However, by emphasizing experiential moments – the focus on figure or parts – we lose sight of the person who is experiencing (Yontef 1993: 266). *There is much therapeutic leverage in substituting the word 'and' for 'but'*.

The Polsters (1973) and Zinker (1977) are in agreement that polarities represent the inner struggles of the client, Zinker describing them as 'a conglomerate of polar forces, all of which intersect, but not necessarily at the center' (Zinker 1977: 196). In a traumatized system the intensity of these conflicts will mitigate against a cohesive and coherent sense of self. Zinker (1977: 200) goes on to say that '[t]here are massive holes in the awareness of a disturbed person. He has a rigid, stereotyped view of himself.'

Rigidity, chaos and complexity

The new science of complex adaptive systems has created a paradigm shift in our understanding of natural, biological and ecological processes, and can be applied across numerous fields of study, including human physiology, relationships and psychology. Complex adaptive systems are defined by their dynamic, self-organizing and emergent properties, which can be seen as ways of describing integrated healthy processes. These processes correlate to the notion of organismic self-regulation, because they are spontaneous and have 'no internal or external executive center that directs [their] functioning' (Grigsby and Osuch 2007: 40). Perhaps paradoxically, an outcome of complex integration allows the possibility of seeing the essence of a situation, person or experience without it being reductive.

Siegel (2012: 28-15) uses an analogy to illustrate self-organizing tendencies: 'If you just assemble choir singers, devoid of a plan or a conductor, they will generally find a way to sing together in a self-emergence that has vitality and a sense of life to it.' We have a natural tendency to move towards maximal complexity (Siegel 2010: 141), which is made possible by linking differentiated elements to one another and creates stability (Siegel 1999: 219). The degree of complexity demanded by certain contemporary life situations, such as the multiple perspectives of handling the threat of climate trauma (see Taylor 2021, 2023), can itself be too overwhelming, and there needs to be a midpoint which is more manageable – the right amount of complexity. There is, however, such a high level of convergence between the properties of complex adaptive systems and the principles underlying Gestalt therapy that it merits further consideration. For this discussion, however, I confine my thinking to the application of complexity theory to trauma.

When a system does not move towards complexity it can be seen as stressed. A stressed system or organism, of which trauma is an extreme and particular example, does not automatically organize towards complexity. Trauma tends to collapse complexity, or the possibility of integration (Table 2.1). Two polarities that result from stress, and which can define mental ill health (Siegel 2012: 16-3) are chaos (cacophony) and rigidity (monotony) (see also Siegel 1999: 220; 2007: 198). Such deviations move the system to either side of complexity. Either of these states limits the movement of the system as a whole from emerging complexity and adaptation to the environment (Siegel 1999: 220). Gestalt therapists will be familiar with a parallel concept of being underbounded or overbounded (Kepner [1987] 1999; McConville 1995). The more stressed a system becomes, the more likely it is that it will diverge from complexity by polarizing.

Many trauma symptoms can be understood as representations of chaos or rigidity. This is the hallmark of unresolved traumatic states. Identifying areas of chaos or rigidity in a person's life enables us to determine which structures of the ground need to be the focus of intervention. This thinking evolves from that of Perls et al. ([1951] 1998: 58), who saw chaos as undifferentiated ground. It is important to understand that in any individual system, both chaos and rigidity will coexist as polarized entities, and may occur as the push and pull of concurrent processes, neither of which is clearly differentiated. I am talking here about a process of integration of inner conflicts rather than the resolution of indecisiveness in external reality. It would be a mistake to believe that stressed systems are not self-organizing and adaptive to current experience. We cannot

Table 2.1 Illustrates the inherent complexity of Gestalt principles and its unique suitability to trauma work

Complex adaptive systems	Traumatized (stressed) systems
Continuous	Interrupted
Flexible	Chaotic, rigid
Holistic	Reductive
Non-linear	Linear
Probabilistic	Seeks predictability
Spontaneous	Habitual
Differentiated	Undifferentiated
Integration between parts	Discrete entities
Specificity	Generalization
Inter-relatedness	Self-preservation
Resilient	Unstable
Intangible	Reified
Energy modulated	Energy conserved or aggravated–

not organize and adapt, but under certain conditions do so in the direction of fragmentation and self-preservation, rather than in the direction of complexity and integration.

Complexity theory offers a further idea, known as the 'edge of chaos', which describes a system which is neither too orderly, stable and predictable, nor too fluid, chaotic and unpredictable (Piers 2007: 167). This condition of being on the edge of chaos relates closely to the Gestalt therapy notion of the **safe emergency**, the point at which intervention is most likely to be effective. I will return to this important point in Chapter 4. Being on the edge suggests a fine line, and it is true that complexity theory posits a tipping point or threshold which represents a transition between states. This can be compared to Siegel's proposition of a range of experience between states of rigidity and chaos, in which maximal complexity, fluidity, stability, resilience and integration are achievable.

It is at this 'tipping point' that a small intervention has a big effect. It is this threshold that we seek to find with our trauma clients, though it is never possible to predict what, how or when this will present. In keeping with this, Erv Polster (2012: 17) considers that fluidity is the very force which leverages change. These ideas will be explored further in the coming chapters.

Restructuring the ground

In Chapter 3, the argument that change can only happen within an enlarged field of choice will be presented, and the severe limitations on choice for trauma clients has been a theme of this chapter. It is clear that in order to support more vividly integrated self-processes we need to attend to the structure of the ground. Nevis (2001: 180) comments that 'It is possible that we can create new ways of enhancing figure possibilities through work to enhance the ground by addressing more fully levels of system greater than the intrapsychic world.' This indicates a relational and contextual perspective on recovery which is fundamental to this volume. Forming a reliable therapeutic relationship, while fraught with difficulties, is a resource in itself. Essential in this work, where interpersonal boundaries may have been absent or violated, is careful consideration of the containment of therapeutic boundaries. In itself, this provides a new foundation for someone whose relational experience is ungrounded and dangerous. The presence of an attuned witness cannot be underestimated, and I will address this in more depth in Part 3 of this volume. Developing resources is particularly apposite in trauma therapy, for which to do anything other would, to use Kepner's (2002) words, be 'like trying to repair a house whose foundation is faulty by reconstructing its second floor walls'. Kepner says elsewhere that '[w]e cannot expect the survivor to change ways of being that have worked so well for her in desperate conditions unless we have first helped her to develop new resources in the present' (Kepner 1995: 64). The availability of choice, or lack of it, may have contributed significantly to the development of trauma symptoms in the first place, and it is therefore potentially retraumatizing to face the 'task of remembering without any more choices than he had when the original abuse occurred' (Kepner 2002: 64). The field changes when more possibilities are allowed into it (O'Neill 2012: 145). Specifically applied to polarities of rigidity and chaos, Philippson (2009: 14) observes that: 'If the world is too ordered, there is no place for us to choose. If it becomes too disordered, choosing becomes mere randomness.'

First steps in reconfiguring unformulated experience come from the simplest of interventions. Many therapists are trained to enquire about immediate experience – 'What's happening now?' For those people who truly don't know, this is an impossible question. In my experience, a more effective entry point can be to ask 'As you tell me this, do you feel better or worse?' or 'When you imagine this, do you feel better or worse?' If it feels worse, you have the option of dropping the figure or changing it, at least taking a pause to settle before moving on. A second step can be to invite exploration of whether someone is thinking, feeling or sensing right here, right now. Both avenues of enquiry begin to differentiate experience and the one who experiences.

Organismically we solve problems – not by getting rid of them, but by incorporating new material (Perls et al. [1951] 1998: 249). As suggested earlier, we do this most effectively by taking the glare off the trauma. This can be achieved in a number of practical ways. Van der Kolk (2014: 253) stresses the importance of not getting drawn into the story. Cohen is among others who advise that clients learn to set aside their troubling thoughts, memories and feelings: 'Therapy should focus first on enabling the client to *turn away* from the traumatic figure' (Cohen 2003: 44, my italics), and pay attention to some alternative aspect of the field. I might, for example, enquire about better moments in someone's life, or what is working well for them. Immediately, the trauma figure enlarges to one of 'trauma and …'. This simple intervention presents clients with an immediate choice, one of which they are unlikely to have been aware. They thus become an agent in their own process; planting the seeds of realization that focus on the trauma is something they can take responsibility for. Inevitably, this intervention will need to be repeated over multiple iterations in order for it to be assimilated as a viable choice. This is not offered as a rote procedure, but as a response to the intensity of the trauma figure in the moment.

Attending to another part of the field begins to reorganize experience, by creating some distance between the trauma and the rest of the experiential field. Thus trauma is held in a reconfigured context, providing containment. Endless possible alternative figures can be suggested. Attention can be directed to embodied processes such as breath or posture; to orienting to present surroundings; to reminding the client about an experience of calm or safety – all are possible and relevant at different times. It can be helpful to offer the sound of a bell or the smell of an essential oil on a tissue. So long as the direction of the attention is towards something positive or neutral the polarity of the trauma is established. A neurobiological perspective would be to consider this as promoting the development of new neural pathways over time.

Alongside this capacity to turn away from the trauma, there needs to be a focus on building a range of positive resources that the client can come to rely on as part of the ground structure. The significance of resources is recognized in a number of contemporary approaches to working with trauma, including EMDR and sensorimotor psychotherapy. A resource can be defined simply, to use the phrase Lynne Jacobs (2006) attributes to Malcolm Parlett, as 'that which enables' the client to become more stable and strengthen resilience.

Resources need to focus on the capacity to regulate emotions, regain a sense of control, define boundaries, develop new perspectives and reflect on experience. There is an overlap between the idea of resources and Kepner's emphasis on self-functions, which he describes as 'the means by which the self organizes, manages and modulates the process of contact' (Kepner 1995: 59). With the support of the therapist, the client needs to be able to recognize and acknowledge existing resources, including current competence in adult life and 'survival' resources that enable them to cope with past traumatic challenges (Ogden et al. 2006: 207). Further new resources can be added in the spirit of creative experimentation as appropriate. It seems that a wide variety of resources is necessary, both to relieve the boredom of endless repetition, and to enhance access to them via different channels. It is not so much the content of the resource that matters as the state that it evokes.

Almost anything can become a resource so long as it leads the client into a positive state. The possibilities cover multiple realms of human existence, from the creative to the spiritual; from the relational to the skilful; from the imagined to the embodied; from the past to the future. Resources include creative adjustments in the past and disowned or unavailable polarities. By altering the structure of the ground and enlarging the field of choice, resources can be seen as new creative adjustments, and represent the beginnings of flow within a previously stagnant system, the emergence of vitality. While we need many resources, I caution against developing a self-centred indulgence. Resources may be developed throughout the duration of therapy, even after the therapeutic relationship has become a resource in its own right. Having said this, it is possible to overcompensate by leaning too far into the missing polarity; this indicates the need for pacing and grading in developing resources in order for them to be fully assimilated. Finding just the right amount of tension, for example, helps a client really differentiate their experience. The continual return to and repetition of resources strengthens and adds depth to the ground; a strong ground cannot be one-dimensional.

Regaining control

Valuable resources need to be assimilated as a felt sense. In addition, the body can be seen as a resource in its own right. Many people who have experienced trauma have a complex relationship to their body. It is a common experience to sense that the body has let them down in some way, by not being able to defend, by being vulnerable, by means of physical injury or arousal during sexual trauma. Later, the body becomes the container of overwhelming distress, memory and intrusive reminders of the event. It is characteristic to manage such experiences by shutting down sensation and the potential for aliveness and grounding based in the body. The body self comes to be seen as wholly negative, sometimes as an enemy to be attacked by misuse of substances, self-harm or distressed eating.

While Kepner (1995: 101) sees resources as a way of resensitizing the body, it is not adequate to use them as routes to feeling pain or distress; they have to involve pleasure and ease to become palatable. Furthermore, we need to approach resourcing via more than one mode/sense because integration does not result from one brain system alone (Grigsby and Osuch 2007: 49). The idea of somatic resources is common to body therapists, and more recently has come to attention via sensorimotor psychotherapy, and elsewhere.

Clinical vignette

Luke was a young man with a terrible past. He was born to parents who had both been in care as children, and his father had a prison record. What happened to Luke can be seen as a societal failure to provide adequate ongoing support for his vulnerable parents. Luke's physical presentation was impulsive and disorganized. He fiddled with objects in the room and moved around, distracted and with incomplete train of thought. The figures he formed were meaningless, and indicated a lack of regulation. My hunch was that to focus on one clear thing would represent danger for Luke – disorganization was his creative adjustment. One strand of our early work together involved Luke sitting on a large physio ball.

This automatically adds core strength, creating an embodied ground. I encouraged Luke to make both big and small bounces on the ball, learning to accelerate and slow down along a continuum, and everything in between. This practice, over some weeks, was one way of Luke gaining some voluntary control over his body. He went on to become an accomplished drummer, with all the fine degrees of co-ordination that involves. In both his use of the physio ball and his drumming, the rhythmicity of movement will have been important (Perry and Winfrey 2021: 197). Intentionality of purposeful movement is a good sign of access to somatic regulation.

Being positive about the role of the body is implied in the survival resources mentioned above. 'How did your body help you to survive?' is an enquiry that can reap rich results for trauma victims. Initially they may resist exploring this because it is difficult and contrary to their immediate felt experience. However, it is worth persisting with this line of exploration over time, because even a small recognition of the resourcefulness of the body can have significant meaning (see Chapter 13). Exploring physical prowess or successes as a child can be immensely helpful for clients traumatized as children. The loss of grounding function of the body leads to disastrous disconnection from the truth of one's own personal story (Goodwin and Attias 1999a: 5). Experiments to exaggerate a physical process, such as increasing tension, can help clients to find the more resourced polarity.

Immersion in the positive

Establishing a felt sense of being in a more resourced state cannot be stressed enough. A common question I hear is about the positive as a distraction or avoidance of the traumatic material. I suggest that this concerns therapists more than the people I have worked with. As we shall see in Chapter 4, resources become the foundation, or the scaffolding, around which the trauma narrative can later be constructed. Most trauma clients will admit that nothing changes for them unless they can feel into the new resource, knowing it through the body and not just as thoughts or ideas. Unless we work 'bottom up' we will not influence the structure of the ground. Equal attention needs to be paid to the subsiding of the figure as to the emergence of it – that is, the phases of satisfaction, assimilation and withdrawal.

Pertinent also is Bromberg's articulation of the extraordinary degree of growth that is possible by means of a 'controlled but consuming immersion by the patient in something positive' (Bromberg [1998] 2001: 89). This is an instance in which trauma therapy needs to be pleasurable: because of state dependent learning, the skills of recovery need to be established under new physiological conditions. An interesting corollary of complexity theory is that relatively small inputs can lead to large and unpredictable outcomes (Siegel 2010: 252), which is borne out in clinical practice.

Clinical vignette

Rich came into therapy after losing his job. He had been bullied by an executive in a corporate business, and was pursuing a claim for constructive dismissal after lodging a grievance. He felt both betrayed by his employers and a deep sense of personal failure, and was irritable with his partner and children, putting his relationships on the line. The more Rich felt he was falling apart, the more he was withdrawing into a solitary state, and drinking. When we followed his phenomenology of being around other people, Rich saw the association between sensations behind his eyes and his reactions to his former boss, and also with an experience of having been mugged in broad daylight on a busy high street some years beforehand. We explored together what had helped him get through this initial trauma, and he began by recognizing that he learnt to manage difficulties on his own and that he had been raised to believe that 'big boys don't cry'.

This did not produce an immediate positive experience for him, but when he stood back from this he could claim for himself that he had developed a certain bloody-mindedness. We paid attention to the positive value and meaning of Rich's bloody-mindedness, how he carried it in his body, and the thoughts and beliefs that accompanied it. In subsequent sessions, Rich reported a great improvement in his relationships at home, reconnection with social contacts, and a new understanding that his life did not depend on the outcome of his employment tribunal. Energy rose quickly around this new figure, his eyes and skin tone brightening, his shoulders and head more upright. This was a resource that we lingered with.

Rich's powerlessness in the face of a corporation that is defending its reputation repeats the bullying of his manager. Layered into this is a previous trauma and his socially constructed way of managing difficulty, which shaped his relationships. We found the value in his adaptation and by attending to that he felt less powerless. Therapy disrupted his pattern of cutting off and managing alone.

Summary

Gestalt therapy pays close attention to how we organize experience. One way of thinking about the organization of experience is to consider what is 'figural' in the foreground and demanding attention, and what is in the background. In respect of traumatized individuals we seek to understand how they include trauma in their organization of the field. It is characteristic of these people to pay focused attention to those aspects of their field that are associated with their traumatic experiences – these are their 'figures' that arise from a ground that contains the same experiences. For these clients, therefore, figures do not arise and recede with the spontaneity and vitality we would expect to see in a healthy process.

A further way we organize our experience is by means of creative adjustments, which are contextually responsive. Significant compromises have to be made to adjust to and accommodate trauma. Because traumatic events are so overwhelming, they cannot be organized into meaningful wholes, parts of them becoming split off or polarized. The study of complex adaptive systems provides a way of reconceptualizing the ways organisms self-organize in relation to stress, by diverging from complexity towards rigidity and chaos. It also offers the potential to intervene by finding a more fluid state between these polarities.

In order to work effectively with trauma it is necessary to pay more attention to the structure of the ground than to the compelling figures of distress contained in the story. By enlarging the experiential field to include additional aspects that may have previously been disavowed or unavailable, the figure of trauma is held in a more spacious way which reduces the intensity of the figures. Clients can be encouraged to develop a wide range of resources which represent disowned polarities and alternative healthy creative adjustments. Particular attention needs to be paid to embodied resources, harnessing the capacity of the body to integrate and organize experience. With an expanded field of choice, the client begins to reorganize their sense of self, to include the experience of self-as-agent.

Making change possible

For Gestalt therapists the principles of the **Paradoxical Theory of Change** lie at the heart of their existential and relational attitude, suggesting that change occurs only when we accept fully who we are. However, what we learn from neuroscience calls into question the assumptions on which the Paradoxical Theory of Change is based. This chapter looks at these assumptions and reconsiders this theory in the light of certain neurobiological features of trauma clients. Of particular interest is the model known as the triune brain, which shows how the fully integrated functioning of the brain and body/mind is compromised by traumatic experiences. This model points in the direction of creating the specific conditions for change that are needed in trauma therapy. A new Integrated Model of Change is introduced which is consistent with Kepner's phased approach to trauma therapy, and from which the conditions for the Paradoxical Theory of Change can later be applied.

Change from the viewpoint of the traumatized other

Traumatized people arrive at our doorsteps with memories, expectations and fears – or none. Some come with a story while others simply experience troubling trauma-related symptoms. There are those whose memory of trauma is intact, and others who have no comprehension that the difficulties that bring them into therapy are related to something in the past. Many simply seek relief for a particular symptom, such as panic attacks, and do not also connect their nightmares to them, for example. They may seek a return to their 'old self', the state they identified with before the trauma occurred, and for those abused in childhood the question may be more about seeking the self they would have been had their situation been different. In this there is inevitably deep loss. Some people arrive with very minimal expectations for change, while others have idealized and intense longings to be rescued; these polarized expectations reflect the splits that trauma generates. For many, change threatens the adaptations that have been made in the service of survival, making a complicated relationship with change. They want to feel better without losing the adaptations that have kept them functioning.

In an overmedicalized field there are people who come to therapy expecting to be made better by some means or any; they do not expect to take a collaborative role in their healing. There are those so terrified of intrusion and the unpredictable that they fear the therapist's interventions; the novel is for certain people a threat, and they make every effort to retain control over the process. One of the defining qualities of this group of people is that choice is very limited, and this affects their expectations for healing. It is common for traumatized people to have little understanding of what change is possible, the opening to new possibilities of which they are as yet unaware. One person told me: 'It doesn't help if you just focus on my experience, I need you to hold the bigger picture too, including a belief in who I can become', unable to do this for themselves yet. It was important to be able to meet them in their despair and not to get lost in it.

While, for too many, good trauma therapy is a last resort, they may also be deeply ambivalent about the process. People may come into therapy driven more by fear than by self care. They have a terrifying dilemma – the tension between their desperation for relief and their assumption that it will involve a reliving of their suffering. Overidentified with their trauma, they lose sight of their strengths and imagine being immersed in an agony they know they cannot bear. Therapy can therefore come to be perceived with more terror than hope.

Perspectives on change

Differences abound in the psychological professions about the nature of change. Traditional psychodynamic and psychoanalytic approaches favour development of self-awareness and the uncovering of the unconscious. Behavioural approaches may lean towards functionality as an outcome; the Diagnostic and Statistical Manual of Mental Disorders (DSM) uses the GAF Scale (Global Assessment of Functioning) as a way of determining 'health' or 'disorder' (APA 2000). Humanistic therapies may consider symptom relief a primary concern. However, 'What if the change that's needed is a change of heart rather than a ridding of a symptom, requiring the sufferer to listen to the symptom and respond to its message?' (Staunton 2022: 48). Potentially, symptom relief is a necessary step on the way to deeper structural change, as the Healing Tasks Model implies (Chapter 1). Integration is sometimes proposed as a desired outcome of trauma therapy, which makes sense in terms of the prevailing splits that define the condition. However, my intention to work towards increasing complexity takes things further. By this I mean a state of integration in which the component parts, as it were, are clearly differentiated and in awareness – a reorganization of the experience of self in relation to others.

Where the trauma 'symptom' can be located is worthy of discussion, for in postmodern times they may be individual expressions of a wider malaise. Trauma as a relational experience is inherently systemic and embedded in the structures of the societies in which we live (see Taylor 2021). Pressure to develop resilience to oppressive regimes and environments is common, and I never intend to suggest that this responsibility lies with the victim. It creates a power play that puts the onus on the individual, often repeating the dynamics of the original trauma. This becomes a fixed loop requiring a degree of opening in both parties. Nevertheless, we cannot avoid the need to do the work on a local level, whereby small and unremarkable changes can have profound effects. We might begin by looking at structures within mental health professions (see Taylor 2021).

> Does the need for change lie with the individual client, or is it possible that aspects of the therapy itself need to change in order for the profession to meet the collective danger that humans have manoeuvred themselves into: How do we widen our focus and allow the state of the world into the conversation?
>
> (Bednarek 2022: 143)

Conventional psychotherapy is not the only route to well-being. Western practitioners tend to privilege western approaches; other cultures will bring traditional wisdom and practices to inform their understanding of distress and healing. And, importantly, we might begin to think in terms of sustainable change, 'based on the assumption that we are an inseparable part of the web of life, of human and nonhuman communities and that enhancing the dignity and sustainability *of any one of these* will enhance all the others' (Capra and Luisi 2014: 371).

Advances in our understanding of trauma have been informed by neuroscience research and there is a proliferation of new approaches to this subject. It is tempting to look at any one of them as the 'magic bullet'; we prefer tidy solutions. Belief in a happy ending ties in with cultural denial and avoidance of suffering: make it all better and then the bad thing will go away – or never happened. As long as there is a solution, the problem doesn't exist in the same way. Often this is the fantasy of those we work with too, on entering therapy. While I aim to show that there is indeed much hope because change and growth are always possible, and that the most debilitating suffering of post-traumatic difficulties can be avoided, it is also true that individual victims of trauma are sometimes very damaged indeed.

Recovery is never something that we can make assumptions about. So there is a caveat which it is wise to bear in mind – trauma therapy may not represent a 'cure' for all; it may simply be enough to offer sufficient support to enable someone to take the next step (Perls 1992: 118), which may or may not turn out to be the first step towards breaking out of the cycle of trauma. Trauma therapy may not be about goals per se, but about taking one step at a time and seeing how far the journey takes you. Gestalt therapy values human potential; while change and growth are not synonymous because change can be for the worse, the spirit of potential and growth are implied in this book.

The Paradoxical Theory of Change and trauma

Beisser's (1970) Paradoxical Theory of Change has been a foundation of Gestalt practice for decades, reflecting the therapeutic principles of Perls and his colleagues, and it encapsulates many classic Gestalt values. The theory informs the process orientation, relational stance and creativity of Gestalt. The brilliance of the theory lies in its simplicity: change occurs not when someone tries to be other than they are – 'what he "should be" and what he thinks he "is"' (Beisser 1970: 89) – but instead when they enter fully into whatever they are experiencing in the moment. It is for this reason that Gestalt therapy is sometimes referred to as a therapy of the obvious. Being fully oneself, without effort to change, is the essence of Beisser's theory, hence the paradox. Here the 'personal therapeutic experience takes the shape of a refreshed, personal acceptance of [one's] troubles' (Davies 2022: 8). The theory rests on the premise of the client being able to '*stand in one place in order to have firm footing to move, and that it is difficult or impossible to move without that footing*' (Beisser 1970: 89, my italics) and it is this point that creates a difficulty when working with trauma. As a figure-bound experience with loss of ground, that necessary footing may be absent. The Paradoxical Theory of Change also has explicit implications for the way the therapist approaches the therapy, and this will be considered separately in Chapter 10.

There is an implicit assumption in Gestalt therapy that the people we work with have everything they need in order to grow. The Paradoxical Theory of Change is predicated on a number of assumptions about the client. The list includes the following abilities: to self-regulate; to make choices; to move forward with fluidity; to participate in healing; to bear pain; to trust in emergent process; to tolerate uncertainty; to reflect on, organize and integrate process; to stay with the here and now; and to be available for contact. These are among the absolutisms of everyday life that Stolorow (2007: 16) notes are lost in the aftermath of trauma. For such people none of these assumptions holds true.

From a Gestalt perspective growth becomes possible when organismic process is not interfered with. Beisser (1970: 89) states:

> The Gestalt therapist ... believes that the natural state of man is as a single, whole being – not fragmented into two or more opposing parts. In the natural state, there is constant change based on the dynamic transaction between the self and the environment.

While accepting this as an ideal and perhaps obvious situation, it has to be understood that this 'natural state' is far from the reality of trauma victims' lives. Trauma severely interrupts and fragments process, and the self tends to become much more rigid, the fixed gestalts being structurally embodied. Beisser is rightly interested in shifting the pillars of Freudian drive theory into processes, and in trauma work this needs to happen at a literal level rather than conceptually. The Paradoxical Theory of Change implies the here and now, whereas the concerns of the traumatized client are stuck in reliving a past that cannot be changed. The cyclical and repetitive nature of trauma is well recognized, while the Paradoxical Theory of Change needs a sense of forward movement to hold true. It implies 'experience-nearness', where trauma clients need first to find some *distance* from their experience. The Paradoxical Theory of Change is therefore somewhat at odds with trauma theory.

There are risks involved with adherence to the Paradoxical Theory of Change with trauma clients. We might suggest for example, that accepting fully that I feel out of control (as many trauma clients do) opens up a sense of control, or at least makes some choices available to me. We might reasonably assume that these choices would be 'top-down' (Ogden et al. 2006) decisions about how to restore some functional order to one's life. However, it wouldn't touch the *bodily* sense of feeling out of control, or address the 'bottom-up' need to be in control particularly of flashbacks, nightmares or other bodily based intrusions which so severely impact the lives of trauma clients. At best, keeping the client's difficulties figural in such a fashion would be unproductive. At worst, sharpening figures of distress can trigger a highly dysregulated state, perhaps inducing a reliving of the trauma in a state of utter terror. It is more helpful to gain some sense of being in control in order to fully realize what being *out* of control is. Turner et al. ([1996] 2007: 540) warn against revictimization by unscrupulous or poorly trained therapists. This not only risks retraumatizing people, which is highly questionable ethically; it may also result in some act of self-harm – picking a fight or going on a binge – following the session. I suggest that therapists who adhere too strictly to a particular method or philosophical position may also unwittingly increase the possibility of retraumatization. It is becoming clear that something different needs to happen to restore the client to a more natural state in which change can take place.

Other factors in the change process

The origins of Gestalt therapy lie in Fritz Perls' training in psychoanalysis, and while he deviated from many of its principles and practices, he maintained a belief in cathartic or expressive methods as a component of change. We can see this reflected in Beisser's subsequent theory of change, in which being fully oneself may require full expressive range of potentialities. The 'safe emergency' of the therapy setting allows for this, as do traditional creative techniques. Though most Gestalt therapists would agree with the philosophical and existential stance of becoming fully oneself, Gestalt psychotherapy has evolved since 1970 – the year Beisser's theory was published – into a rather less expressive and more explicitly relational, field-oriented paradigm. This is nothing new, for a clear relational position between therapist and client is espoused by Beisser, in which the therapist declines the role of change agent.

One implication of this is that the therapist should not interfere with anybody's natural growth. Contemporary Gestalt psychotherapy has become increasingly nuanced and sophisticated, with threads of both the experiential and the relational creating a fabric of different texture and quality. 'Any approach to change in psychotherapy that does not include both experimental phenomenological awareness work and a caring respectful dialogical attention to the relational contact is not complete' (Yontef 2005: 92). This emphasis on relationship and intersubjectivity begins to shift Gestalt away from the expressive and cathartic and align it with other therapeutic approaches with psychodynamic roots.

Stepping outside Gestalt for a moment, but in a way that is wholly compatible with it, we turn to address the issue of relationship as a catalyst for change. The BCPSG comprises eminent psychoanalysts, psychotherapists and researchers who together consider and deepen their understanding of the nature of change. Their thesis (BCPSG 2010) is founded on the dyadic properties of relationship, and 'moments of meeting' that happen within it. There is little difference between this and the Gestalt therapy notions of the I–Thou and of contact; it is perhaps unsurprising that this group has published in the *International Gestalt Journal* (see BCPSG 2002). Further, the BCPSG identify moments of meeting as moments of change because they create 'state shifts and organismic reorganization' (BCPSG 2010: 7).

The question of concern in trauma therapy is this: *how* do we meet with someone who is chaotic, fragmented, rigidified, dissociated or otherwise disorganized in order to create such shifts? The BCPSG describe what they term the 'local level', the minutiae of lived experience, similar to the Gestalt phenomenological method. For them, change occurs 'in the small, apparently unremarkable moments as well as in the "lit up" moments of more noticeable therapeutic change' (BCPSG 2010: 100). The small and unremarkable moments of being held in relationship matter more than we might know. Relational participation in therapy, however, can be a problem; traumatized people tend to bring with them a complicated relational history. I suggested above that clients need to be active participants in their healing, and this is a contradictory position for those who have experienced trauma and who may, for example, be compliant, overly self-reliant, or both. Furthermore, one way of defining trauma is that it is a denial or negation of self-determination (see Chapter 7), with implications for the change process. From a field perspective, relationship needs to be considered as a factor in supporting change, and we will look at some of these dynamics later in the book.

There is a link between self-agency in therapy and hope. If I have a sense that there is something that can be done about a situation, I may hope for a new outcome. Simply entering therapy evokes a sense of self-as-agent: 'I can seek help' is a new possibility, even where it is born out of desperation and hopelessness. It is a common expectation that the therapist will 'do' something to 'fix' the problem, especially in a contemporary field where difficulties are medicalized, and in which hope is placed in the 'powerful' other, rather than in a belief in one's own capacity for change.

Snyder et al. (2002: 16) suggest that a placebo effect may also contribute to change in therapy, which represents 'motivational expectancies for improvement'. Interestingly, Turner et al. ([1996] 2007: 541) suggest the placebo effect in trauma therapy to be as great as 40 per cent. A key point is made by the BCPSG: *'Not every direction that could be co-created would be healing or constructive for the patient'* (BCPSG 2010: 104, my italics). Bearing this in mind, there is a dilemma for the therapist working with trauma: does change come about as a result of the efforts of an expert practitioner, or by learning to heal oneself (Levin and Levine 2012: 6)?

The BCPSG writers make a further interesting point that change needs to occur in two separate domains of experience: the declarative, or conscious verbal, domain and the implicit procedural or relational domain (BCPSG 2010: 3). This is of particular relevance to working with trauma, for implicit relational knowing (how one is welcomed in the world for example) integrates emotional, cognitive, relational and behavioural dimensions. Additionally, the somatic or physiological level is also implicit: 'Implicit memories are best thought of as somatic and affective memory *states* that are not accompanied by an internal sense that something from the past is being remembered' (Ogden et al. 2006: 236, original italics).

This brings us directly to the experiential world of trauma clients whose lives are beset by incomprehensible and unbearable implicit knowing, and it is in this dimension that integration is crucial before processing can take place. It is common practice to spend some time reflecting on a novel experience, including Gestalt experiments, as part of 'processing' and assimilating it. Reflection can therefore be seen as a feature of change, a new knowing which completes the cycle of experience and allows for integration of unfinished business. Reflection is a useful self-function to develop as it provides a counter to the reactivity and sense of urgency of many trauma clients. This includes the more mindful awareness that I discuss in Chapter 5.

Dropping in

Recall an experience of personal change in therapy. What was it that helped facilitate this change – was it insight, something your therapist said or did, an experiment, making meaning or connections between different experiences, or something else? What had led up to the change – did you get stuck or blocked in any way or feel some conflict about moving forward? What part in the change did you attribute to your relationship with your therapist? What was your embodied sense of this change and how significant was that? Take some minutes to write about your experience, adding some reflections in hindsight.

Neuroscience, trauma and change

Neuroscience has changed the 'rules' about how we make choices, change and grow as human beings. It affords therapists the opportunity to be more considered in our choice of interventions by including an understanding of trauma in our thinking. The BCPSG (2010: 59) quote Weiss: '[the] "enduring co-ordinations" that constitute the organization of the organism environment system [rest] on the biological device of specificity'. I understand this specificity to be not only biological but experiential and relational, important for traumatized people whose experience of trauma is unformulated.

Traumatic experience which has not been completed and integrated becomes stuck, sedimented and embodied into rigidly fixed gestalts – those unending repetitions of fear, intrusions and avoidance which are so characteristic of trauma. As opposed to this stuckness, Gestalt therapy favours flexibility. Philippson (2012: 90) states: 'The paradoxical theory requires that the client has the neurological capacity to move flexibly into new perceptions and relations to the environment.' This flexibility is simply not available to trauma clients and the basis for this is neurological. Fortunately, we now understand that the brain is 'a dynamic process undergoing constant development and reconstruction across the lifespan' (Cozolino 2006: 50), changes which can be imagined as a process of pruning, maintenance and regrowth (Schore 2003c: 131). Included in our thinking and planning for trauma therapy, herein lies new hope for this group of clients.

A first principle of neuroscience is Hebb's axiom (Hebb 1949): neurons that fire together wire together. This means that the more we revisit or rehearse a particular situation, thought pattern, behaviour or feeling, the more strongly embedded it will become. Trying to complete the unfinished situation by going over and over the same problem, whether intentionally or not, is only going to reinforce it, hence the risks inherent in working from the Paradoxical Theory of Change. Clients' persistent efforts change nothing, for after trauma the natural fluidity of process has become blocked. However, in trauma therapy it is possible to take advantage of the plasticity of the brain to establish new neural pathways and networks to break out of the unresolved cycle. Siegel (2007: 291) summarizes this process using the acrostic SNAG – stimulate neuronal activity and growth. *This process appears to require conditions which are stress free, and so points to reducing stress as a precondition.* Neural pathways cannot develop under the original conditions, their growth being dependent on new experience: 'The experience-dependent plasticity of the mind-brain-body becomes key to understanding the possibility of changing minds and the learning that can take place in psychotherapy' (Wilkinson 2010: 2). Neuronal growth is stimulated by attention – where our attention goes so does increased blood supply – which supports the firing of neurons in a way that promotes integration between disparate regions of the brain (Siegel 2007: 291).

The triune brain

Treated as a metaphor rather than a fact, MacLean's (1990) theory of the triune brain is a very useful concept for understanding the regions of the brain that are implicated in trauma. Sometimes misunderstood as a model of brain structures that are anatomically distinct, and criticized for its evolutionary perspective, the theory does nevertheless propose usefully that there are three layers of the brain which operate together to a greater or lesser extent, under different circumstances (see Figure 3.1). I think that the model is nevertheless useful for trauma therapy because it has much to tell us about survival mechanisms.

Figure 3.1 The functions of the triune brain

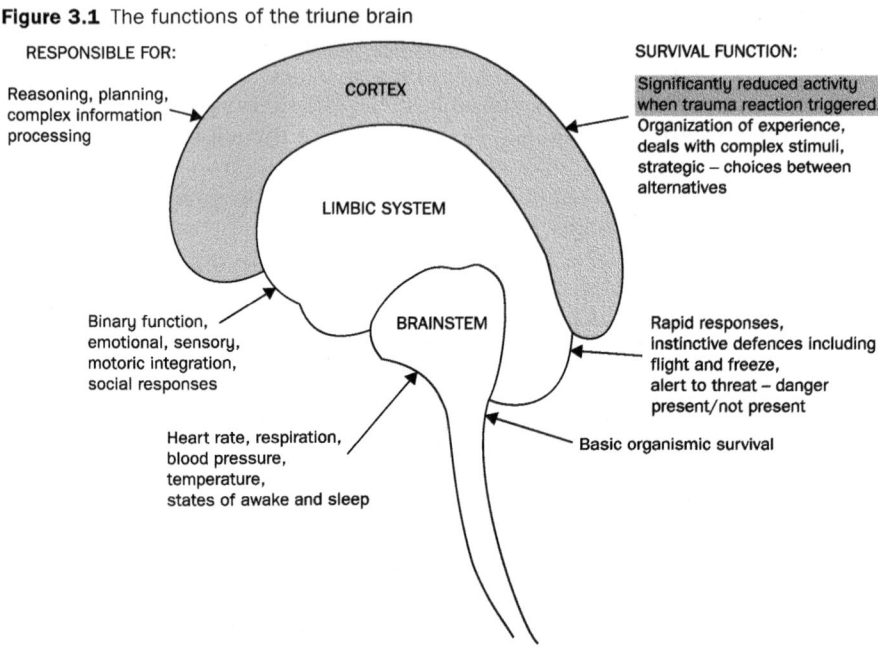

RESPONSIBLE FOR:

Reasoning, planning, complex information processing

CORTEX

LIMBIC SYSTEM

BRAINSTEM

Binary function, emotional, sensory, motoric integration, social responses

Heart rate, respiration, blood pressure, temperature, states of awake and sleep

SURVIVAL FUNCTION:

Significantly reduced activity when trauma reaction triggered. Organization of experience, deals with complex stimuli, strategic – choices between alternatives

Rapid responses, instinctive defences including flight and freeze, alert to threat – danger present/not present

Basic organismic survival

At the lowest, most primitive level is the brainstem, leading into the spinal column, concerned with basic physiological functions such as heart rate, blood pressure, temperature control, respiration and states of sleep and wakefulness. It is very much an on-or-off structure: when one or more of these functions is damaged by injury or disease, death of the organism will swiftly follow. Survival defences of freeze and collapse are associated with the brainstem. Sitting atop the brainstem is the limbic system. This level is more flexible, dealing with stimulus responses and sensory, emotional, non-verbal, social, and a range of reflexive defensive processes. It has been proposed that much of the circuitry of fear systems lies in the limbic brain. Reactions that are driven by the limbic system can flood throughout the body in as little as one twentieth of a microsecond – literally less than the blink of an eye. After all, in situations of danger speed is essential. Mobilized defences of fight and flight are probably mediated by this area. There is much debate about which precise structures constitute the limbic system, but as a functional concept for the seat of survival defences and emotionally charged states it remains useful (LeDoux 2002: 212). Lying over the whole, directly under the skull, is the cortex, largely translating material from the environment and the other two areas of the brain into verbal, reasoned, conscious thought. It is in this area that higher-order planning for defensive action may take place.

To counter this grossly oversimplified view, recent brain imaging techniques have revealed the complexity of connections occurring in any brain at any moment, as illustrated by the connectome (Figure 3.2).

Figure 3.2 The connectome

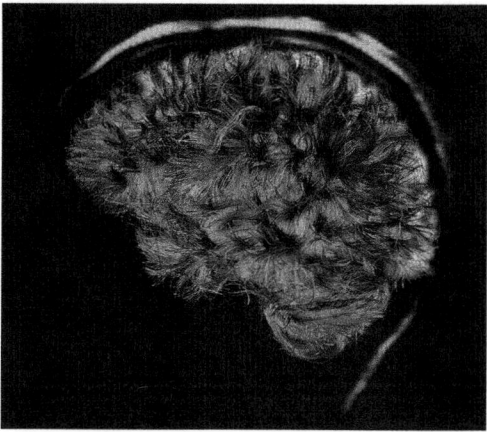

Source: An image of a brain from the Human Connectome Project. Courtesy of V.J. Wedeen and L.L. Wald, Martinos Center, Harvard University

Special functions of the brain

Of course the triune brain model is a grossly oversimplified representation of extremely complex specialist functions, none of which is wholly confined to a particular layer or structure of the brain; most functions are spread between areas throughout the brain. There are multiple bidirectional, dynamic and self-organizing connections between different structures and layers of the brain. It is interesting that much research into the neuroscience of trauma has focused on structures within the limbic system, particularly the amygdala, the hippocampus and the thalamus, and how they operate together in situations of fear and threat. Numerous studies have revealed that under conditions of threat, there is *increased* activity in these subcortical regions and *reduced* activity in the cortical regions of the brain. LeDoux (2002: 212) suggests that 'the argument that cognitive processes might involve other circuits, and might function relatively independent of emotional circuits, at least in some circumstances … seems correct'. It has been suggested that *under threat, the cortex simply goes 'off line'* (Ogden et al. 2006: 142; see also van der Kolk [1996] 2007: 233), which would account for the difficulty many traumatized people have in thinking or defining their process, and in working from a 'top-down' or cognitive basis. This has profound implications for how to intervene effectively in therapy with trauma victims.

Furthermore, in situations of chronic trauma, particularly during the stages of early childhood in which the brain matures rapidly, some structures may be unable to develop fully, including the hippocampus and the corpus callosum, the 'bridge' integrating the left and right hemispheres of the brain. Wilkinson (2010: 39) cites research by Teicher et al. (2003) showing as much as a 15–18 per cent reduction in the corpus callosum, with neglect being the strongest experiential factor associated with it. Schore (2003a: 259) reports that paralimbic areas of the right hemisphere are 'preferentially involved' in the storage of traumatic memories indicating that these are activated from this area. Once again we see that the brain thrives under the right conditions. 'The ongoing paradigm shift across all the sciences is from conscious, explicit, analytical, verbal, and rational left brain to unconscious, integrative, nonverbal, bodily-based emotional processes of the right brain' (Schore 2008, cited in Wilkinson 2010: 9).

The relational brain

Lest we go too far down a reductionistic unitary path in considering the adaptation of the brain to trauma, let us turn briefly to the relational aspect of brain development. Philippson reminds us that neurological development is relational, as evidenced by the work of Schore, Beebe and Lachman, Siegel and others, and he considers that the 'deficits can be worked with in a relational therapy which leads to *physical changes* in the functioning of the client's brain' (Philippson 2012: 89, my italics). *Neuroscience therefore has something to say about who determines the future for traumatized people*: 'Mind responds to the changes that occur in the brain as a result of mind-brain-body interactions with another mind-brain-body experience; brain is modified in response to mind, and so on' (Wilkinson 2010: 125).

The here-and-now focus, the phenomenological method and the experimental approach of Gestalt therapy usually offer a client 'a problem that cannot be solved in her habitual way' (Philippson 2005: 14), in order to introduce novel choices and possibilities. Without a neurobiological perspective, the field of choice is narrow; trauma remains a problem that cannot be solved. Stuckness and failure are familiar problems for therapists working with trauma. Psychotherapeutic concepts of resistance and impasse are challenged by insights from neuroscience. For people who have experienced trauma, there are aspects of their lives that they are no more able to change than walk a tightrope with a broken leg. This is not to say that psychological resistance or impasse are not also possible for these people as for anyone else, but that there are also processes over which they have no voluntary control at the outset. They come into therapy without the neurological connectivity to gain control and make the changes they desire. This client group requires something different from our customary ways of thinking about and enabling change.

Creating the conditions for growth

Beisser (1970) rather beautifully says that the goal of therapy is to be able to move with the times while maintaining some individual stability. I feel this in my body as I practice tai chi, which allows me to move without losing my balance. These two functions of movement and balance are precisely those that are impossible for trauma clients, who are both stuck in replays of the past and unstable. It is a tenet of Gestalt therapy that people are living organisms constantly in process, adapting and emerging in response to the internal and external field. Change is *always* happening, even if it is so slow that it appears static. Parlett's (1991) Principle of Contemporaneity shows that there will always be a degree of newness in each reliving of traumatic experience: this reliving is in this unrepeatable moment.

However, Yontef, aware of risk and unproductive therapy, raises a crucial issue:

> The central question is ... [how] do individuals and their societies, including psychotherapists, influence and support change in the direction of healing, growth and wholeness, and how do they *interfere* with healing, growth and wholeness – or even precipitate deterioration?
>
> (Yontef 2005: 82, my italics)

It is necessary to find ways of loosening the fixed gestalts in trauma without doing further damage. When '[the] person's brain cannot support different ways of being' (Philippson 2005: 16), the risk of deterioration is increased if we fail to attend to creating the right conditions for the emergence of novelty. Philippson (2005: 14) states further: 'The paradoxical theory cannot be simply applied in situations where the client is sensorily out of contact with where she is'. The need to bring the client more into sensory contact with 'where she is' is not at variance with Gestalt therapy values; the issue for trauma clients is rather about what we do and how we support their ability to be in contact. Stratford and Braillier's (1979) metaphor of glue and solvent in therapy is relevant here: 'What specific glue?' and 'Precisely how much solvent?' being key questions. Clients need both fluidity and stability.

Bearing in mind that 'The mechanisms that bring about change in psychotherapy are incompletely understood, at best' (BCPSG 2010: 38), and that 'traumatic threats to survival that produce extreme fear-based memories are more recalcitrant to change' (BCPSG 2010: 187), we turn now to consider some of the possibilities for trauma therapy that are opened up in the light of neuroscience. The glue and the solvent of trauma therapy need to include the building of self-functions that address some of the presumed neurological deficits. Earlier, a list of some of the self-functions upon which the Paradoxical Theory of Change is predicated was presented, all of them deficits for people with complex or developmental trauma. Trauma therapists need to embrace an *intentionality* of change as an active interference with the sedimented natural process which otherwise leads inexorably towards deterioration, emphasizing 'the sometimes very rational decision in favor of particular changes' (Fuhr 2005: 83). Much of the evidence for effective trauma therapy points towards working in particular ways with the body so as to facilitate the emergence of these self-functions.

Trauma clients need to be able to reorganize their fragmented, dissociated and implicit experience into a coherent, unified and differentiated gestalt.

To achieve fluidity and stability requires the resolution of polarized splits in functioning and increased integrative capacity. Problems concerning integration for trauma clients have already been touched on throughout this chapter. 'Without adequate integrative capacity, clients cannot maintain regulated arousal, resolve their memories, or lead productive satisfying lives' (Ogden et al. 2006: 182). It is the failure to integrate – or to metabolize – traumatic experience that is the substance of the unfinished business of victims' ongoing problems, and therapists need to use particular interventions to enable integration to take place. Importantly, if the disintegrated process is not reversed the sense of trauma for the client will worsen. This is because traumagenic neural pathways will only become more embedded. Kepner ([1987] 1999: 10) rightly points out the central role of the embodied self in the process of integration. It is only on this level that someone can fully comprehend their experience as their subjective truth, even in the absence of words. 'Emotion and the body are at the irreducible core of experience: they are not merely there to help out with cognition' (McGilchrist 2010: 185). Integration involves 'both differentiating and linking the separate components of internal experience and external events in order to create meaningful connections among them … This capacity facilitates the maintenance of an internal locus of control over one's body, emotions and thoughts' (Ogden et al. 2006: 182–3). The implicit can become explicit through the body.

Integration of splits has been positioned as a goal in trauma therapy. A dramatic split in brain function is that between cortical and subcortical regions during traumatic episodes.

> [The] goal … is to integrate and balance the various cortical and subcortical, left and right hemisphere, processing networks. This process requires a decrease in anxiety from high to moderate levels. High levels of emotion block thinking, whereas moderate levels can result in cognition *combined* with emotion.
>
> (Cozolino 2002: 58, my italics)

Anxiety and imbalance are prime consequences of disintegration. There is therefore much interest in those interventions that reduce stress, thereby promoting the *strengthening of neural linkage* between primitive responses and higher-order functioning. This requires more than a stress management approach. Goldstein (2007: 111) observes that 'the new order appears to arise out of the system's own internal resources when the right conditions are met rather than being imposed by external forces or factors', which concords with neurologically informed therapy. The body knows how to heal itself under the right conditions.

Sensorimotor therapy sees the body as a 'primary avenue in processing trauma' (Ogden et al. 2006: 166), creating the necessary internal resources and a sense of coherence. Fogel, reminding us that we can't impose change but can create the conditions for it, comments that:

> The more we actively practice opportunities for embodied self-awareness to emerge … the more we have the ability to stay longer in the subjective

emotional present ... neural learning is reflected in physiological changes in the nerve cells and their connections.

(Fogel 2009: 61)

Ogden et al. recommend a blend of top-down and bottom-up approaches to working with implicit memory. Top-down cognitive interventions are employed to foster regulation through meaning-making and observation by means of phenomenological tracking and are cortically mediated. In this mode language and story are 'entry points'. Bottom-up interventions start with the body, using sensation and movement to support emotional regulation and the processing of memory. 'Through bottom-up interventions, a shift in the somatic sense of self in turn affects the linguistic sense of self' (Ogden et al. 2006: 166).

'More directly associated with overall body processing sensorimotor processing includes physical changes in response to sensory input; the fixed action patterns seen in defenses; changes in breathing and muscular tone; and autonomic nervous system activation' (Ogden et al. 2006: 7). Gestalt body process work tends to be offered in the service of raising awareness; in trauma work we need to lean further towards embodied practice for integration and processing. A useful sensorimotor question is therefore to enquire of clients 'What goes with that thought/feeling/sensation?' which can link thoughts to somatic experience or vice versa.

Clinical vignette

Roseanna, for example, had been brutally raped by her partner, but for many years saw it simply as 'normal' unwanted sex. This was a defensive and dissociated fixed gestalt that carried with it much self-blame for not having said 'No'. She needed to feel the insult and violation in her nervous system in order to own it for herself as rape – being fully herself as the Paradoxical Theory of Change proposes. As a precondition for her acceptance of the unbearable knowledge of her rape, her capacity to tolerate the strong emotions and sensations that went with it needed to be strengthened. This was achieved over many months of detailed attention to building an internal sense of safety, repeatedly directing Roseanna away from her almost irresistible pull towards traumatic material – the figures she was not yet able to support. By learning to notice and identify body sensations and their accompanying thoughts without judgement Roseanna was able to make new meaning of them; through learning to track the flow of sensory experience she gained a sense of continuity.

*Over time, Roseanna learnt to regulate herself better and became able to stay more present. All this was offered through a respectful, dialogic and phenomenological focus, with interest and graded presence on my part as therapist, an experimental stance of discovering together what best supported Roseanna. At this early stage of therapy I had a clear goal in mind at all times, while maintaining a degree of **creative indifference** about how we reached it. Together we reflected a good deal on what was going on; there is nothing new in this for Gestalt therapists but I kept in mind that this was needed to allow for reorganization of Roseanna's experience. Although there was much 'technique' in this work,*

I knew that Roseanna would be quick to spot any interventions that were based only on technique; she needed authentic relating from me as her therapist.

It was only once she had reliably learnt to bear the pain – Beisser's condition of stability – that Roseanna could finally say, 'What he did to me was rape' and find her sense of 'No' in her body. This helped to reorganize her self-concept to include rape, making new meaning. Thus she could integrate her experience without dissociating, and the Paradoxical Theory of Change could apply. Of course neither Roseanna nor I ever knew what changes may, or may not, have taken place in her brain, and these were never part of my conscious thinking in our work. The very fact that I was standing on different philosophical and theoretical ground may have been enough to reorganize the field towards change. I was guided, however, by my understanding of the processes and principles of trauma theory, and always took my lead from phenomenological cues in Roseanna and myself.

Finally, I was conscious of how Roseanna's narrative about 'unwanted sex' reflects one of the enduring myths that surrounds sexual violence, rooted in a patriarchal social structure that minimizes and blames the female victim, in this case, which Scheper-Hughes and Bourgois (2004: 307) call 'The "symbolic violence of masculine domination" whereby victims actively misrecognize and thereby reproduce and naturalize the power relations destroying their lives.'

Towards an Integrated Model of Change

There is much of value to therapists in the Paradoxical Theory of Change. It is a fundamental philosophical position. However, it is very much a theory of its time, in accordance with the early view that Gestalt therapy could be effective for all client groups. Kepner's (1995) *Healing Tasks* looked at the specific issue of childhood trauma, and offered a phased approach to therapy. Within these phases Kepner identified a number of tasks, including the development of self-functions, that need to be fulfilled in order for recovery to take place. This is not entirely consistent with the essence of the Paradoxical Theory of Change, but *is* consistent with good trauma practice even though Kepner's writing came ahead of the emergence of neuroscience into the field.

Philippson is a contemporary Gestalt therapist who questions the usefulness of the Paradoxical Theory of Change for some clients, including those who have experienced trauma: 'It is only once the new functioning, allowing caring and being cared for, has "bedded in" neurologically that the paradoxical theory can function' (Philippson 2012: 90). He continues as perhaps many experienced therapists – including me – could:

In the past I have been guilty of trying to help create the conditions in the moment which would support growth, not knowing that the kind of relational growth I was trying to support was not possible for them at their present level of neurological functioning.

(Philippson 2012: 90)

Philippson (2005: 13) considers that we need something more subtle than keeping our clients within familiar responses, which is supported by a neuro-physiological perspective on trauma.

This subtlety can be found both in certain qualities of the therapeutic relation-ship (see Chapter 10) and in close attention to Kepner's phases. In particular we are interested in the early stages of Kepner's model, the support and self-functions stages, and of the relational element of that support. It is here that the Gestalt trauma therapist chooses deliberately to interfere with the processes that have caused the blocked completion of unfinished business, and here that they take a consciously different relational stance. These phases lay the relational and neuro-logical 'ground' for the processing and moving through of the trauma which take place in Kepner's undoing, redoing and mourning and final reconsolidation stages, which is where the Paradoxical Theory of Change finally prevails.

Philippson (2009: 137) argues for putting in place 'the prerequisites for the Paradoxical Theory of Change' for some clients who lack the neurological capacity to self-regulate. Consistent with the Healing Tasks Model, I propose a phased model of change for trauma work: an Integrated Model of Change. This can be expressed thus: *change happens under the optimal conditions in which one can be fully oneself.* The prerequisite is a preliminary phase of more directed and goal-oriented work, from which the Paradoxical Theory of Change can later emerge. Gestalt therapists might think of this in terms of an extended period of fore-contact (Mann 2010: 37). During the preliminary phase the therapist never loses sight of Beisser's theory; it is always an under-current, never trying to force change, waiting for the moment when the ability to tolerate being fully oneself becomes more possible. There may be goals towards which one directs the work, but growth is never linear: it is a 'trial-by-error pro-cess of moving in the general direction of goals' (BCPSG 2010: 9) in line with the hologrammatic perspective of Kepner's model. Thus the therapist is not being coercive, not seeking 'to change' the client in a disempowering manner, simply because 'the best we can do is to meet the other' (Lichtenberg 2012: 181).

We start where the client is, meeting their neurological challenges with attention, understanding and compassion. 'Where the client is' calls initially for more direction, more regulation and containment, more engagement with pres-ent reality. Yontef (2005: 83) says: 'The issue for me is whether goal-directed and planned change is done from a phenomenological and dialogic perspective consistent with the Paradoxical Theory of Change – or is merely behavior mod-ification based on a person's self-rejection.' This work is both attitudinal and intentional; some subtlety on the part of the therapist is needed to strike a bal-ance that includes the attitudinal stance and methodology of the Paradoxical Theory of Change alongside the intention to support particular changes. It is perhaps this attitudinal and intentional shift that most characterizes the change process for trauma that we need to embrace. Beisser's prerequisite is to have a firm footing in order to change, that it is 'difficult or impossible to move with-out that footing'; establishing that footing is therefore a prerequisite for those who have experienced trauma, as we shall see in Chapter 4. The same premise applies at all levels of a system – for the therapist, organizations, families and societies.

Summary

Trauma clients often have polarized expectations for change, on the one hand limited by a failure of imagination for what they can become, and on the other, an unrealistic expectation for rescue by the therapist. They also enter therapy beset with fears that their suffering will continue or worsen, or that they will confirm that they are truly broken. Sadly, it is true that some trauma clients bear deep wounds and their healing potential is limited by some of the constraints of therapy – time, money and boundaries, among other factors. And for many there is still hope that with new approaches to therapy, satisfactory and transformational change can take place.

The Gestalt therapy view of change is based on Beisser's Paradoxical Theory of Change, in which it is stated that 'Change occurs when one becomes what he is, not when he tries to become what he is not' (Beisser 1970: 88). This theory encompasses a number of core Gestalt principles, and is predicated on a number of assumptions about the client's inherent capacities, which can be summed up as the ability to make choices: **response-ability** in the here and now. However, for trauma clients the level of choice is impacted greatly by the involuntary neurological processes that maintain the cyclical trauma response, and there is a risk that by staying with these familiar responses the client will not recover, and at worst will be retraumatized. There is a growing awareness that something more than the Paradoxical Theory of Change is needed to facilitate healing for trauma clients. Beyond this theory, change can be influenced through a number of different factors, which include expressive techniques, relationship and hope. For trauma clients it is the neurological basis of change that is the most necessary to bear in mind.

There are two principal factors governing brain processes which need to be understood and taken into account in relation to trauma. The first is the phenomenon of neural plasticity, which shows that the brain is capable of development throughout the lifespan, by means of pruning, shaping and growth of new neural pathways. Repair of brain structures that have not developed fully after early trauma has been shown to take place after appropriate therapy. This opens up the possibility that the fixed gestalts of trauma can be loosened and choices made available. The second factor is related to disconnection in the architecture of the brain, presented as a hierarchical layering from primitive subcortical structures to higher-order cortical functions, all of which have a role to play in survival under threat.

This is represented by the metaphor shown in MacLean's triune brain. Neuroimaging techniques have demonstrated that the cortical areas of the brain are less active when traumatic memories are activated, the responses being driven by subcortical areas known as the limbic system. It is clear that interventions that increase the growth and integrative capacity of the brain are necessary in trauma therapy. Taking a neurobiological perspective of the brain and its capacities sheds new light on the issues of resistance and impasse in therapy, allowing for a more compassionate stance.

The repair of the brain, which supports change and the processing of the unfinished business of trauma, can only happen under the right conditions.

This includes enhancing the integrative capacity of the client by means of both top-down and bottom-up interventions (Ogden et al. 2006), which allow the client to differentiate and distinguish a range of elements of their experience, creating a more unified gestalt. The role of the body is therefore central in bringing about a more integrated experiential field, and trauma therapy cannot afford to ignore this. Something beyond the Paradoxical Theory of Change is needed, which includes the setting of some goals for therapy and a more directive stance on the part of the therapist. In line with the stages of Kepner's (1995) Healing Tasks Model it is proposed that a preliminary stage of change called the Integrated Model of Change be adopted. This model supports the neurological make-up of the client and sets the scene for the Paradoxical Theory of Change to operate when the client is ready to process their trauma. At the heart of effective trauma therapy lies a shift in attention towards particular figures and an intention to promote the integrative capacity of the brain.

4 Working with arousal

This chapter follows from the last in terms of complexity and resourced states. Here I explore how figure disturbances of trauma are accompanied by a physiological disturbance of arousal. This in turn activates instinctive organismic defences related to threat or the perception of threat. Explaining the mechanisms of arousal creates links to the Gestalt theory of arousal and figure formation. This provides some theoretical ground for understanding the ways of taking the glare off the trauma. The Window of Tolerance Model, which is a key to working with trauma and therefore central to this volume, is presented and explored at length and provides a coherent rationale for the clinical application of arousal theory. This model overlaps with the theories of complex systems and polarities addressed in the last chapter. The chapter also considers polyvagal theory as a supportive model for understanding trauma. Attention is paid to ways of working with states of dysregulated arousal.

Trauma as an arousal process

In his seminal paper 'The Body Keeps the Score', van der Kolk (1994) noted that the psychological effects of trauma are expressed as changes in the biological stress response. He describes a biphasic reaction: hyperreactivity to stimuli and traumatic re-experiencing which coexists with psychic numbing, avoidance and amnesia. This response is at the heart of his subsequent book of the same name (van der Kolk 2014). A typical pattern of numbing to the environment is punctuated by intermittent hyperarousal. Kepner (1995: 75) describes this in the language of polarities: stimulus is like a binary function, either off/ on, overwhelmed/numb. Loss of ability to modulate emotional experience is central to post-traumatic stress. Van der Kolk's paper also looked at the stress chemicals involved in PTS and the part they play in the maintenance of arousal: 'Chronic exposure to stress ... permanently alters how an organism deals with its environment on a day-to-day basis, and it interferes with how it copes with subsequent acute stress' (van der Kolk [1996] 2007c: 223).

Boadella emphasizes the capacity for emotion to either mobilize or paralyse the body (Boadella 1987: 4), and which way an individual responds will depend on their experiences and creative adjustments. Many creative adjustments serve to regulate emotional arousal. For example, 'aboutism' or intellectualizing often fulfil this function. Sapriel (2012: 107) observes that in the face of early trauma we learn that emotions, arousal and action are dangerous.

Self-harm, angry outbursts and destructive behaviours can also be understood as moderators of arousal, as can self-medicating behaviours involving abuse of alcohol or prescribed and non-prescribed drugs. Someone I worked with regularly had some sort of crisis a couple of days after a regulating therapy session and was unable to tolerate or sustain positive states. It is common early in therapy for traumatized people to have strong primitive affects but be unable to integrate them (Yontef 1993: 262), which underlines the importance of a phased approach to trauma therapy. Learning to manage stimulus is a self-function and a property of a self-organizing complex system. Gestalt therapists will recognize the relevance of the glue and solvent metaphor of Stratford and Braillier (1979).

Arousal and Gestalt

Arousal has been of interest to thinkers and writers in Gestalt theory since its inception, long before van der Kolk's published work on the physiology of arousal in trauma. So central are ideas associated with arousal that the 'bible' of Gestalt theory written by Perls, Hefferline and Goodman in 1951 uses the word 'excitement' in its subtitle. Arousal is implicit in two fundamental Gestalt concepts: organismic self-regulation and the cycle of experience – the process of figure formation. Contact is a valued and sometimes idealized notion in Gestalt. Spagnuolo Lobb (2009: 112) comments that 'the term "contact" implies consideration of physiology in the experience'.

Energy is required to support the development of a figure, and contact can be viewed as the turning point from which that energy subsides. The quality of contact is therefore contingent on the available energy that can be brought to it, or the ways in which that energetic emergence may become blocked. Gestalt therapists attend to the processes involved in contact and the ways in which it may be modified. While there is some debate about the validity and usefulness of individual moderations to contact which is beyond the scope of this discussion, it is, however, important to recognize that we *regulate the arousal of contact according to our ability to tolerate it.*

Other Gestalt writers link contact with regulation of the metabolism. Levin and Levine (2012: 3) state that organismic self-regulation occurs at the point of contact between the organism and the environment. This is the point at which we might moderate the arousal of contact. Philip Brownell in particular has explored the links between self-regulation, contact and neurobiology (Brownell 2009), coming to the position that Gestalt therapy is not merely concerned with holism but 'a literal understanding that physical functioning affects mental status' (Brownell 2009: 64). He says this: 'Physiology of the organism (its basic metabolism and sensori-motor functions) supports the psychology of contact at the boundary of the organism/environment field and is essential to its dynamic' (Brownell 2009: 65). Furthermore, he posits that 'What Gestalt therapists call self-regulation can be largely explained by the neurological construct of executive functions ... where the organization of a person's sense of self comes together' (Brownell 2009: 67). Although this is not mainstream Gestalt language, it tallies with the ideas of integrated functioning of the brain discussed in the last chapter.

These executive functions are associated with higher-order brain functions of the cortex. Recall that in Chapter 3 the compromised availability of higher-order functioning of the cortex under extreme duress was described. The implication of this is that when integrated brain function is disturbed by trauma, the client is less able to self-regulate. Thus, the organization of the layers of the brain is related to the capacity for self-organization or regulation. Executive functions are a subset of self-functions, including the ability to think before one acts, to manage emotions and to initiate purposeful action. Brownell (2009: 78) concludes: 'It must be recognized that self-regulation and executive functions are overlapping, if not synonymous.'

Perls et al. ([1951] 1998: 275) understood that there are situations in which self-regulation is fallible, determined by maturity and impulsivity. It would seem that *there is a threshold beyond which the organism is unable to self-regulate* according to prevailing field conditions, and requires help to do so. Trauma theory confirms this.

Further consideration of emotional regulation in relation to figure formation is provided by Delisle, who recognizes that:

> [t]he therapist has at his disposal a whole array of techniques designed to activate and heighten experience... unconsidered use of these techniques can put him in the position of the sorcerer's apprentice, capable of unblocking things without really knowing what to do with what has been unblocked.
>
> (Delisle 2011: 75)

This is a key point, identifying the problem that exists for those who understand the importance of physiological effects, but not necessarily what they are and how they work. The Window of Tolerance Model, to be described below, is one way of resolving these difficulties. But first we need to understand the physiological mechanisms that explain what's going on. After all, as Bowman (2012: 31) says: 'The domain of Gestalt psychology was clearly the scientific study of the nervous system.'

The autonomic nervous system

Central to understanding arousal is the role of the autonomic nervous system (ANS). This is 'part of the nervous system that deals with all the life processes that we cannot control with our conscious volition' (Stauffer 2010: 49). Physically separate in structure from the central nervous system which is organized in a specific segmental arrangement of the spinal cord, the ANS 'appears to be designed to broadly disperse any stimulation throughout its web-like network, *creating a general response*' (Juhan 2003: 292, my italics).

Thus the effects of the ANS are felt through many organs of the body. The ANS is responsible for modulating arousal; in Stauffer's (2010: 51) words, its role is to 'get our juices flowing'. This is because the ANS operates on smooth muscle, literally helping to move fluids around (Stauffer 2010: 51). Activation of the ANS is accompanied by a surge of neurochemicals throughout the body.

There are two branches of the ANS, respectively called the sympathetic and the parasympathetic nervous systems. The sympathetic branch mediates the fight-or-flight response associated with threat and anxiety; it also has qualities of spontaneity and vitality. One person described this as feeling as though 'all my senses are cranked up'. The parasympathetic branch is involved in states of shutdown, relaxation, recovery and assimilation. Further, the parasympathetic branch arises from deep cranial nerves, including the vagus nerve, to the extent that the two terms are sometimes used synonymously (Stauffer 2010: 51). The vagus nerve controls blood pressure and therefore heart rate, operating what is known as the 'vagal brake' to increase activation, having an immediate effect on states of activation and relaxation, with consequent alterations in breathing. 'The parasympathetic vagus nerve that can speed up (vagal inhibition) or slow down (vagal activation) heart rate interacts in the brainstem with the respiratory motor neurons of the phrenic and skeletal muscle nerves' (Fogel 2009: 232). Let us look at the polyvagal system, identified by Stephen Porges.

The polyvagal theory and social engagement

The idea that we are hardwired for contact has been prevalent in relational Gestalt thinking since about 1987 (Lynne Jacobs, personal communication, 2012). Neuroscience research has confirmed the existence of this process and the workings of it. One theory, part science and part concept, is the polyvagal theory developed by Stephen Porges in 1997. Polyvagal theory refers to the function of the vagus nerve. This is the tenth cranial nerve, whose fibres originate in the brainstem; it is the only nerve to derive from this deep emotional brain. It is also one of the longest nerves in the human body, the word vagus having a Latin root meaning 'wandering'. The vagus nerve has branches serving the head, face, throat, lungs, heart and stomach, and has a key regulatory action on these organs (Stauffer 2010: 51). This makes the vagus nerve essential for our survival (Stauffer 2010: 46).

The polyvagal theory elegantly makes clear the relationship between the brain and the body, and proposes a *bidirectional* communication between them. This is a theory of integration rather than dichotomy and links with states of arousal that are most pertinent to trauma work.

The regulatory function of the vagus nerve is associated with the ANS, which we know to be hugely important in managing states of safety and danger. Indeed, primary emotions are survival based and therefore have significance for the smooth function of cardiopulmonary regulation. Communication between the brainstem and the heart via the vagus nerve regulates blood pressure and therefore how relaxed we may feel (Stauffer 2010: 160). The poly-vagal theory proposes three distinct neurophysiological systems:

1 The ventral vagal state – the system of connection, meeting the demands of the day, connecting and communicating, going with the flow, engaging with life.
2 Sympathetic – the system of action, filled with chaotic energy, mobilized to attack or escape, anxious and angry.
3 Dorsal vagal – the system of shutdown, going through the motions, drained of energy, disconnected, giving up (Dana 2021: 6).

Porges conceptualizes each of these systems as being connected to the layers of the triune brain (see Chapter 3), and uses the metaphor of traffic lights to illustrate this. The green light indicates being in a safe environment, where we can engage socially, think, understand and play; this is a function of the cortex. This ventral vagal state or social engagement system, comparable to the Gestalt concept of contact functions. The amber light indicates the perception of danger which will not threaten our life, so we can mobilize and attend to the signs of danger. This shift in attention means that we are unable to connect well or to hear clearly; this is related to the limbic system and to defences of fight and flight. Third, the red light represents an immobilized state in the face of life threat, in which we shut down protective reflexes; this is known as the dorsal vagal state, associated with the brainstem and defences of freeze and collapse. Via the process Porges calls neuroception (2009: 45), we are able to distinguish sensory cues from the viscera as well as from the environment to help us to determine safety, threat and danger.

The impact on our ability to connect with others is clear in this model. The need for attachment and the proximity of others in establishing safety is an instinctive survival defence (see Chapter 6). Imagine for a moment that you are having a conversation with someone who suddenly turns away from you. How do you feel? Now imagine two people gazing softly at one another, and notice again how you feel. If we focus on the route of the vagus nerve via the muscles of the ears, eyes, face and larynx we can begin to get a clearer picture of the significance of this nerve in social interactions. The vagus nerve has a key part to play in contact functions. We tend to feel safer and more present when we seek eye contact, when we smile or speak gently, or when others non-verbally communicate approachability and safety.

Mediated by the vagus nerve is the slowing down of the heart rate and regulation of respiration that is associated with safe and calm states. This is the regulatory function of what is known as the vagal brake, bringing the right degree of energy needed to successfully navigate moment to moment (Dana 2021: 18), moving in a subtle pattern of release and re-engagement with every breath cycle. Taking something in from the environment or another person is keyed into this physiological process, the continual exchange of air on the inbreath and the outbreath. The impact the therapist has on the emotional and autonomic arousal of the client can be either regulatory or not, and I think the therapist's regulation of breathing has a significant effect in the co-regulatory process. Van der Kolk and McFarlane ([1996] 2007: 18) describe the case of a man whose wife had died while looking into his eyes and who could only recover when he took the risk of looking into the eyes of a female therapist who could tolerate his grief. This level of connection, primarily through gaze, also triggers a release of the hormone oxytocin, which is associated with bonding between mothers and infants and with a sense of well-being.

The Window of Tolerance Model

While increasingly popular, the language of polyvagal theory can be confusing. There are parallels between the polyvagal theory and the Window of Tolerance Model, also based in the arousal of the ANS, which I have found to be universally acceptable. Rather than speaking 'science' to people, this model addresses their felt sense. Trauma theory demonstrates that ANS activation takes the victim beyond the threshold at which their metabolism can automatically regain a regulated state. They need to learn to manage intensity as well as feelings in the middle range (Kepner 1995: 85), and in my experience the Window of Tolerance Model addresses this nicely, and provides a 'road map' for the trajectory of the therapy. 'Affect tolerance, which allows for the experience of emotion to enter into consciousness, is related to the capacity to bear pain' (Schore 2003a: 24). Clearly, in order for any trauma therapy to be effective we need to establish a condition in which the client learns to tolerate and process experiences, including increasingly strong primitive emotions of fear, anger, grief and joy, and is able to function well. To do so means nothing short of transforming the experience of trauma into the vitality and fullness of human existence.

Fortunately, on the continuum between the polarities of arousal there is a state that represents optimal arousal. Siegel proposes that we all have a '"window of tolerance" in which various intensities of emotional arousal can be processed *without disrupting the functioning of the system*' (Siegel 1999: 253, my italics). Sensorimotor trauma therapy, which was my own extensive trauma training, has adopted this model as a key to recovery (Ogden et al. 2006: 26ff). The window of tolerance does not have fixed parameters; constitutional and experiential factors determine these (Siegel 1999: 255). Furthermore, the window of tolerance varies for any individual in response to current conditions – it is state dependent. When we are tired or hungry we become rather less tolerant, and our field of attention is reduced; external factors such as being in a traffic jam or hearing a sudden loud noise affect us similarly (see Figure 4.1).

Not surprisingly, many trauma clients have a restricted window of tolerance. As one said to me after a stressful lead up to their session: 'My tolerance levels are paper thin'; this model speaks to the heart of their phenomenological experience of safety and danger. Because of this, I have found it is invariably supportive to clients to share a version of this model with them, and to help them identify those states that are most familiar to them. Doing so normalizes and provides a context for their experience, and gives us a shared language for understanding changes moment by moment, in addition to offering the possibility of something different.

Figure 4.1 The window of tolerance model

Cognitive: Racing thoughts anxiety, can't think, can't process intrusive images and thoughts	Emotional: Panic, overwhelm	Somatic: Agitation, impulsivity, increased respiration and heart rate, exaggerated startle	Relational: Clingy, controlling, lacking trust, abandonment, re-enactment

HYPERAROUSAL

Cognitive: Reflective, in perspective, oriented to the present	Emotional: Proportional to the situation, tolerable	Somatic: Calm, grounded, embodied	Relational: Present collaborative, flow, mentalize, shared experience and meaning, intersubjective

WINDOW OF TOLERANCE

Cognitive: Disconnected, disoriented, foggy	Emotional: Deadended, absent	Somatic: Desensitized numb, shut down, immobilized	Relational: Withdrawn, wordless, reduced contact functions, shame

HYPOAROUSAL

It is important to understand that this is not a linear either/or model, but represents the possible matrix of arousal suggested above. It is wise to be cautious about thinking that this model is merely reductionistic, because it is really a map of the degrees of human suffering. In Part 3 of this volume the Window of Tolerance Model is developed as an interactive systems model rather than a representation of unitary functioning and can be viewed as a model of connection. It is a theoretical and functional model which overlaps with complex adaptive systems theory of chaos, rigidity and the edge of chaos.

I think there is a risk of privileging regulated states as represented by the window of tolerance and ventral vagal activation, necessary though they are. My concern is partly that in an overmanualized approach to trauma treatment, some therapists become overcautious about working with charged emotional states, and I shall say more about this in Chapter 6. In working with this model the first task is usually to establish a point of stability and calm, which sits theoretically at the midpoint between hyper- and hypoarousal. For those clients who find *any* stimulation to be unbearable, it is necessary also to find neutral and apparently meaningless experiences. The stillness of the midzone may sometimes be experienced as boring or understimulating (see Figure 4.2). However, a state of repose lights up other parts of our brain, allowing uncertainty, fluidity and reorganization. As a state in which we can be more reflective it is a good antidote to states of traumatic activation, and leads us to being more able to be at home with ourselves (Dana 2021: 45). Just a moment of being with yourself without fear brings us to life in a less cluttered state. Additionally, Fanen (2022: 353) comments on the absence of stillness that is a

Figure 4.2 Within the window of tolerance

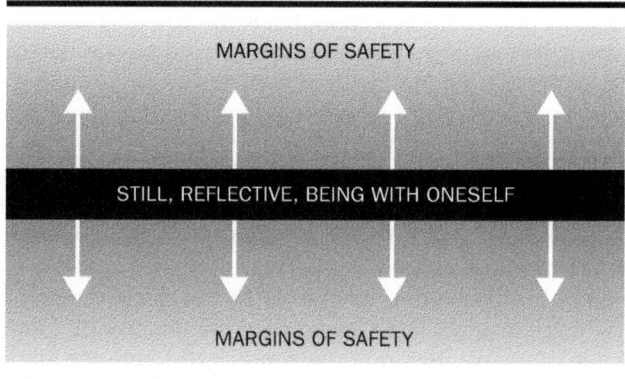

HYPERAROUSAL

MARGINS OF SAFETY

STILL, REFLECTIVE, BEING WITH ONESELF

MARGINS OF SAFETY

HYPOAROUSAL

marker of contemporary global capitalism: 'The culture functions in great part on the basis of rapid mania.' As a counterpoint to the need for stillness, for some people there can be creativity in a degree of chaos, and for others a sense of vitality can be found in states of hyperarousal.

Trauma therapists need to work extensively and thoroughly at the margins of the window of tolerance, learning collaboratively with the individual what takes them beyond their capacity to tolerate, and the subjective phenomenology of this process.

It is important for the therapist to be able to distinguish clearly the signs of both incipient hyper- and hypoarousal, in a moment-by-moment process of assessment. This allows for a finely balanced calibration of arousal: neither too much nor too little, but just enough. Someone's ability to stay in the window of tolerance or not informs the pacing and grading of the therapy on micro and macro levels, and is therefore an invaluable diagnostic tool.

Hovering near the thresholds of tolerance, finding the tipping point and the way back to the resources within the window of tolerance over and again, is by far the most time-consuming part of trauma therapy. It is also potentially the most rewarding for both the client and the therapist, because of the symptomatic relief it brings. Shub recommends (2000: 81) '[s]ystematic, repetitive, therapeutic experiences to loosen what is deeply lodged'. Incrementally, the trauma victim learns to be present to their aliveness, including their own suffering – the ability to tolerate more charged states. Of course we can never tell when or by what means they will find that tipping point which enables their recovery, either in the moment or over the course of therapy; we can only persist and be patient, trusting in the process and the body's innate ability to regulate. However, it is true that the body usually takes longer to enter a completely regulated state than the cognitive or emotional recognition that the conditions are favourable would suggest. This is good reason for lingering for extended periods of time within the window of tolerance.

Because so much time in trauma therapy is spent working with the window of tolerance it can come to look as though it is the whole of the therapy. This is not the case at all; it is an entry point and a means to an end. Learning to regulate arousal is a key self-function without which the others cannot develop. As the client becomes more able to access resources within the window of tolerance over the course of therapy they will begin to be able to sustain figures with increasing charge. It is as though the margins of the window expand. Powerful emotions are possible within the window of tolerance, the most salient consideration being someone's ability to remain present to these without becoming dysregulated or retraumatized.

Gestalt therapy proposes the concept of the 'safe emergency' (Perls et al. [1951] 1998), which can apply to the margins of the Window of Tolerance Model, at the very 'edge of chaos'. Being in the window of tolerance allows for depth and breadth of work consistent with complexity thinking, a space in which the client can come more into contact and in which trauma can ultimately be worked through and resolved. No longer is this a space where little happens, but one in which growth and healing can take place. Crucially, as the backbone of trauma therapy, the window of tolerance implies an increased sense of embodiment and points therapists towards attending to body process.

Clinical implications of the autonomic nervous system

The clinical implications of the ANS in relation to trauma merit being placed at the centre of our thinking. Stauffer (2010: 56) explains that trauma can be defined as a state of autonomic overwhelm that becomes unable to resolve naturally. Chronic arousal of the ANS means that trauma victims have difficulty tolerating stimuli and tend to shut down by desensitizing from their bodies or by moderating contact as an attempt to self-regulate. We might conclude that sympathetic activation is problematic and that induction of parasympathetic, ventral vagal states is to be encouraged. To a degree this is true, but because the parasympathetic activation causes a shutting down of major systems in the body, too much constitutes a threat to life.

The two branches of the ANS do not necessarily operate in a simple see-saw balancing action as we might imagine. Research suggests instead that there is a matrix 'consisting of a multiplicity of possible states of activation of the two branches' (Stauffer 2010: 51). This can result in states of high activation of *both* branches simultaneously, leading to the freeze response sometimes called 'tonic immobility' (Stauffer 2010: 51–2; see also Chapter 7). This explains why trauma victims may be in a perpetual condition of dysregulated arousal, either because of chronic activation of the sympathetic branch or because of concurrent high activation of both branches. In such a state the *person is unable to process anything*, even the therapy session, and it is necessary to intervene to support the calming effects of the parasympathetic branch (Stauffer 2010: 56). The operation of the vagal brake can be seen as the ANS trying to achieve some balance between sympathetic and parasympathetic arousal in the face of threat.

The ANS has many sensory nerves, and it is this that helps with the process of interoception – the feeling of internal states (Kepner 2002) – which is the process involved in resensitizing the body. Breathing is a particular way in which we can understand the role of the ANS, inhalation being in the domain of the sympathetic branch, and exhalation being in the realm of the parasympathetic; it is a self-regulatory function (interview with Speads, in Johnson 1995: 41). Most therapists will observe how their clients' breathing changes when they are upset or panicky, for example. It may be that by holding the breath we are able to limit the amount of stimuli to attend to, which modulates arousal, but it also holds a charge in the body and some people will need help to attend to their outbreath.

It is not surprising that many relaxation techniques involve attention to the breath in one way or another; the breath, like blinking, is under both voluntary and involuntary control. Observation of breathing is therefore a source of good information about arousal states. It is interesting to consider that by regulating the breath, changes in blood pressure may be communicated from the body to the deep emotional brain via the vagus nerve, an internal feedback loop. This kind of process is attracting considerable attention in the form of study into heart rate variability, the difference in time between heart beats, which indicates the balance between the two branches of the ANS (Gilbert 2010: 297). Gilbert (2010: 297) considers that people can be trained to improve their heart rate variability.

Dropping in

Take your right hand and place it about an inch away from your chest over your heart – close but not touching. Imagine compassion flowing into you and into this area through your hand. Notice if you feel any heat there. Maintain a soothing breathing rhythm as you do this exercise. Sometimes people like to associate a colour with compassion, so you could also imagine that colour flowing into your heart area, without condemnation.

Now, from this compassionate position, bring to mind the part of you that has had anxious, angry or upsetting experiences, and imagine this part in front of you. Look at your facial expressions and behaviour. Imagine what that part is feeling and thinking. Now simply send compassion to that part of yourself. Really feel this, if you can. Don't try to change anything – just sit looking at that part and feel compassion. Recognize that these fearful emotions are from the threat system.

As you stay with this experience, notice if anything changes in your muscle tone and your emotional state, and whether you have different thoughts or overall sense of experience.

(Adapted from Gilbert 2010: 298–9)

Working with arousal

It is impossible to work with traumatized people *without* them returning to states of dysregulated arousal many times over in therapy sessions. I contend that if you do not know how to recover from these moments, the therapy is bound to be ineffective and may be retraumatizing. However, the ways in which you support this recovery are crucial. You *both* need to learn about the phenomenology of these experiences in order to find a way out. There are some principles of working with arousal that apply to both extremes of the modulation scale. Perhaps it is stating the obvious, but the rule nevertheless needs to be stressed: *never work with a figure until you have gathered enough support.* This can do harm or even retraumatize the client: 'until feelings can be experienced without overwhelming the survivor and re-enacting the original trauma that created the need to dissociate or blunt the feelings, strong expression of feelings is damaging rather than healing' (Kepner 1995: 84). Tell the person that you will be checking with them repeatedly to ascertain their level of arousal by asking 'Can I just pause you there for a moment?', and suggest they monitor their changing arousal as well. Together you become 'stewards of arousal' which I will say more about in Chapter 10. Kepner (1995: 81) advises therapists to 'attend to signs of the client being "full"'. By putting in regular and fairly predictable 'stops', regulation will automatically increase because they permit more parasympathetic activation; Rothschild (2000: 79) speaks similarly of 'putting on the brakes', which lends support to the figure. This is a way for you both to learn to recognize when to back off a bit, return to a resource before continuing, or drop the subject for the time being. Another option is to work towards 'just the right amount' of activation, calibrating or titrating exposure to disturbing stimuli.

If you are working with someone who is coming closer to trauma-related memories, negotiate with them what support they need to help them stay as present as possible while also attending to the memory. By asking them to reflect in this way regulation will increase. The process of phenomenological description is a further way of supporting regulation, especially of body process that the client may be able to observe for themselves. Once regulation is established it is important to linger with it and to create new organizations of experience, joining and integrating how the rest of the body can be included in this, with the thought processes and felt emotional sense of this resourced state. One person commented: 'When I tried to manage this on my own it always escalated and went out of control. The way you bring me back and stop it going over the top means I can talk about it, I'm someone who can deal with what happened.'

Working with hyperarousal

Phenomenological observation that someone is moving out of their window of tolerance in the direction of hyperarousal may reveal agitation, shallow or quickened breathing, jumpiness, eyes darting or scanning, higher pitched voice, increased speed of speech and multiple figures being presented. You may also notice changes in skin tone or colour and dilation of the pupils. Some emotions are associated with sympathetic arousal, including anger, rage, fear and joy (Schiable 2009: 35). Learning to spot changes in the client's energy is helpful too; energy can have the quality of being higher or of flaring or blazing, and you may simply notice a sense of heat. The increase in muscle tone that often accompanies this constellation of signs is different from that associated with hypoarousal. Try the following experiment to help you get a felt sense of this.

Dropping in

Tighten your muscles as though you were frightened, anxious or panicky. This is tension associated with preparation to move – to hit or kick or run. Notice what this feels like. Now tighten your muscles like the proverbial rabbit in the car headlights. This is tension associated with staying extremely still; freezing. Compare the difference.

Once you can distinguish between the two for yourself, you are more likely to be able to spot what is happening in someone else. In addition to these observations of the other person, you will be likely to pick up similar experiences in your own body and perceptions.

As a rule of thumb, it is most helpful to find a way to slow down someone who is becoming hyperaroused. Delisle (2011: 81) observes that 'One of the best ways to maintain the client's affect is to use interventions that slow them down or that stop at times of emotion, and to do this the instant that emotion becomes present, even very slightly.' This provides not only the needed regulation but a sense of being able to contain and manage the emotion differently. People who are hyperaroused are overloaded by excessive stimulation and need to limit the amount that they are processing in the moment. Most writers agree that attention to sensations is the most effective way of reducing stimulus and thereby calming. You can suggest that the person you are working with attend simply to the physical features of their experience at this moment – tight, tingly, churning – directing them to drop any associations or meanings that they attach to them. The pace and tone of your voice are also important in helping to slow things down.

Use of deliberate rhythmic movement can help regulate and offer some sense of control over bodily reactions (Perry and Winfrey 2021: 197). Some people like to stand and rock gently from foot to foot, or to sit and rock their upper body from their pelvis. Swinging the arms around the body is another variation of this. In either case, finding the slowest possible movement or a gradual transition from fast-to-slow-to-still is often beneficial, and similar experiments can be created using a physio ball, which is grounding. Mostly, an experimental attitude in which you find out together what is helpful and what isn't remains the best approach.

Another way of helping to contain is to frame a single figure, among others that may be competing for attention: 'Which of these things do we most need to focus on now? Can you put everything else to one side for the moment and just stay with that?' Sometimes it is helpful to ask just for the 'headline' of what's happening and to take note of accompanying changes in arousal. Similarly, asking someone to tell you something in the fewest possible words, like a single bullet point, can help to frame a figure, and reduce stimulus.

You may want to remind the person you are with about a resource or creative adjustment, or choose to work with the polarity of the current figure. 'You feel a lot of distress in your chest at the moment; could you find somewhere else in your body that is not in such distress? Maybe just a tiny area…'. It usually helps to tell someone to take their time over a regulating process, especially close to the end of a session; by saying 'We've just got a couple of minutes left today…'. they may leave in a dysregulated state. The use of images can help to increase body awareness, both those elicited from the client and those suggested by the therapist, such as 'Can you think of a calm colour/scene/piece of music and notice the effect on your body?' Romanyshyn (2007: 81) comments that 'the imaginal world is by its essence the intermediate world between the intellectual and the sensible' and is therefore a route to sensation. The sense of smell is functionally related to the ANS, and you might offer aromatherapy oils, asking the client to choose the ones they prefer. People can also be encouraged to develop and practise a variety of self-soothing strategies outside of sessions, especially for 'emergency' situations (Fisher n.d.).

Clinical vignette

Susannah became distressed by a painful body memory in her pelvis during a session. Her breathing was shallow and staccato, her inbreath shorter than her outbreath. She said she felt panicky and she tightened the front of her torso. I invited her to slowly explore the experience of the pain, making a slowly paced series of enquiries about it. I was curious about the qualities of it, the colour, the dimensions, the temperature, the volume. I also asked her to think about any energy in it, any sense of movement and direction. Susannah reported that it was a jagged, dark pain, cold, and solid at the bottom, that went through her right side and disappeared near her spine. I became curious about her sense of the pain disappearing in that way and Susannah was able to get a sense of it dissolving away through a point.

I suggested Susannah explore the edges of the pain: were they clear and sharp or diffuse, how did they relate to the surrounding tissue? I wanted her to get a sense of how the pain was held in her body, how the rest of her body cooperated with this pain. She then reported that the edges of the pain were clear, but softening as she studied them, and that outside the tissue was red and pulsing and tight and angry. 'Oh, that's me, that's where I can feel myself', she said with surprise, and then 'the pain's going now'. During this process of several minutes Susannah's breathing had steadied and she was quiet and focused. Notice that I did not ask her to consider the intensity of the pain because that could have increased her arousal again, nor was the story necessary here.

Working with hypoarousal

Parasympathetic states are generally more difficult to work with than sympathetic ones, because of the degree of shutting down involved. So little happens in this state that the work can hold negligible interest for the therapist. Hypoarousal and dissociation are almost synonymous. The 'drop' from hyperarousal to hypoarousal can be quite sudden and dramatic, the client reaching a point at which they can no longer sustain the charge of the arousal.

Signs of hypoarousal therefore include a stilling of the body and breathing, and dilation of the pupils or aversion of the eyes. Muscle tone is often tightly held, sometimes over extended periods that would in other circumstances be painful, but it may also be collapsed. There is an analgesic effect in hypoaroused or dissociated states which makes this possible (see also Chapters 7 and 8). The person's reactions may become slower, and their speech flatter and deeper in tone. There may be increasing silence as they withdraw from contact. For such a person, available energy is minimal and everything appears to be much more of an effort. Indeed, the amount of effort a hypoaroused client needs to summon in order to become more present is considerable and must not be underestimated. In this state, the quality of the energy present is thick rather than heated. Emotions of sadness, depression and despair are consequent to the parasympathetic dominance of hypoaroused states (Schiable 2009: 35).

Working with hypoarousal is not the converse of working with hyperarousal. There is risk involved in trying to enliven things too quickly because the client might dissociate further or become hyperaroused again. In this instance the work needs to *gradually* restore the available energy and contact. First, try suggesting the individual orient themselves to the present surroundings (see Chapter 6) by asking them to look at particular objects. It is a good idea to identify something in the room that can remind them of where they are, a familiar resource that can help them feel grounded (Boon et al. 2011: 19). Naming four red objects or three shiny objects is another common way to begin to bring the person more into the present, and sometimes elicits a state shift. It can also help to encourage the client to look at things to either side or in different parts of the room, because this requires some movement of the eyes and head. Techniques from sensorimotor psychotherapy are to try pressing the feet into the ground or to lengthen the spine a little as though being pulled from the top of the head. Both of these interventions begin with the periphery of the body but involve the core muscles around the pelvis, spine and abdomen, achieving a sense of stability. Simply standing up together can help enormously.

It can also help to ask someone if they notice any impulse to move, usually in the arms or the legs, or can imagine making a movement that would help. 'Frozen' muscles are part of a movement pattern related to aborted defensive actions in situations where escape is impossible, so there is often a **retroflected** action such as fight or flight that is already known in the body. It is helpful to think about a muscle tightening in preparation for movement, such as an arm drawing backwards before throwing a ball. It is this process that we hope to capitalize on with hypoaroused clients.

The contraction and flexion of any muscle will begin to increase regulation, particularly when done mindfully. Ideally the person will imagine a potential movement and be able to tell you, even if it's not possible to do yet. In such a case the therapist can demonstrate that movement, or suggest another in order to mobilize them through engagement of their mirror neuron system (Chapter 11). The fundamental movement patterns concerned with push, pull, reach, yield and grasp described by Ruella Frank (2001) are useful in thinking about how to build movements slowly with the intention of supporting regulation. Most implicit and unintended movements, no matter how small, fall into one of these patterns. Working with the smallest amount of energy that is available or possible is sometimes the best that can be tolerated.

Clinical vignette

Quite suddenly Lina goes still and looks down. The muscles in her upper arms and chest tighten as do her legs, lifting her feet off the floor. I ask, 'What's happening?'

In a low voice she replies, 'Nothing, I'm alright.'

I tell her, 'I'm sure you know how to be alright by tightening up; did you notice something change just now?' A small pause.

'Don't know', she says in the same voice, not moving.

'Can you open your eyes and look at the plant over here that helps you know where you are?' I ask her, thinking that contact with me might be too much at the moment. No response. 'It looks like you've gone to that scary shut off place where you remember things', I suggest, keeping up the contact. Lina shrugs slightly; she's listening. 'Perhaps we can find a place where you can be quiet and have some space without taking yourself away. Would you be interested in that?'

My thinking here is to invite a more integrated state without taking away her survival resource of shutting down. 'Maybe, I don't know', she says. I sense that she's engaging with me, we are in dialogue. 'I wonder what would make this a tiny bit better just now?' Another pause. 'May I make a suggestion? How would it be if I moved a bit closer to you?', I offer, knowing that this has helped in the past. Another pause. 'Whatever', she says. I take this as permission, and move so that I can place my toes against hers, offering some contact and grounding. I tell Lina that I will stop if she tells me to. She moves one foot away. Her breathing deepens and the muscles in her arms soften. I ask her to let her attention rest on her feet. She opens her eyes and looks into the room. We begin to discuss being in a better place where she can access resources.

Summary

The process of physiological arousal was intuitively understood by the fathers of Gestalt therapy because it is implicit in the energy required to form clear figures, support good contact and self-regulate. Because Gestalt therapists value spontaneity and liveliness, assumptions and expectations were made about the centrality of these processes. However, there was also some early recognition that there are limits to the ability to regulate in some situations. Trauma is an example of this, because a key feature of trauma clients is their inability to maintain a sufficiently regulated state to support contact.

Typically, two phases of dysregulated arousal form part of the trauma response, and these accord with the two branches of ANS arousal. The sympathetic branch is linked to escalating arousal and the parasympathetic branch is associated with decreasing arousal. A reasonably balanced process between the two is sometimes thought to be the ideal; however, there is more often a mesh of different states in trauma clients who may be constantly shifting between either hyperaroused (sympathetic activation) or both hypoaroused (sympathetic and parasympathetic activation). The former leads to states of agitation and overwhelm, the latter leads to shutting down and 'freezing'. Each of these states is triggered by trauma-related memories, and therefore in neither space is contact possible.

Two theories associated with the ANS are helpful in trauma therapy. In both cases, following the state of the ANS moment by moment is called for. The first is polyvagal theory, which is concerned with the activity of the vagus nerve in mediating states of connection and danger, with corresponding sympathetic and parasympathetic arousal. Secondly, it has been postulated that there is a window of optimal arousal, called the window of tolerance, conceptualized as sitting between hyper- and hypoarousal. This roughly correlates to the concept of the 'edge of chaos', in which integration can take place. For many trauma victims, it is access to this zone that is severely compromised. Therefore working to strengthen this zone is central to successful trauma therapy. If we imagine a line across the centre of this zone, the client is able to feel safe, calm and in contact. Both client and therapist need to know that such a state can be attained, and have ways of reaching it. However, it is at the margins of the window of tolerance that much of the work of trauma therapy takes place. In order to provide regulating experiences for the client the therapist and client both need to pay much attention to the transition between this and dysregulated states. This is similar to the Gestalt therapy concept of working with the safe emergency.

Finding ways to interrupt the therapy process and check on states of arousal is important, providing breaks in which some regulation may take place. In addition, there are particular approaches to both hyper- and hypoarousal which can be effective. Hyperaroused clients in general need help to slow down and settle, because their physiological, emotional and cognitive processes have become overwhelmed. This involves avoiding particular figures associated with trauma and developing those associated with calm. Attention to sensation brings them quickly into their bodies and restores the possibility of contact within the window of tolerance. For hypoaroused clients the slow development of movement, coupled with encouraging orientation to present surroundings, is recommended. This work needs to attend to the impulse to move which may be retroflected, imagining the possibility of doing something different.

5 There and then, here and now

Gestalt concepts of unfinished business and the fixed gestalt underpin this chapter. The seemingly unresolvable nature of trauma has a clear time perspective, in which the client continues to live as though the trauma was ongoing. Gestalt therapy naturally orients towards working in the here and now, which is invaluable in trauma work, helping, under the right conditions, to consign the traumatic events to the past, for which current awareness and the phenomenological approach apply. Neuroscience shows us that an integrated state of mind can bring us into a more mindful and embodied sense of the present moment. Trauma clients tend to generalize associations from everyday situations to their trauma, and these linkages are uncoupled by means of using curiosity to differentiate experience in the here and now. Reference is made to the Integrated Model of Change, organization of experience and self-regulation, bringing together the themes of the previous three chapters, and provides a methodology for taking the glare off the trauma.

The timelessness of trauma

Although many trauma victims have found ways of functioning more or less successfully in everyday life, for others there is a never-ending background of terror that breaks through unpredictably as flashbacks, nightmares and other intrusive reminders. Their fear hovers at the edge of their awareness almost constantly, leading to an increased alert to perceptions of danger – hypervigilance. Such experiences are quite outside the influence of conscious or voluntary control. Without doubt, these phenomena have very visceral qualities, bringing with them intense emotions and reactive escalation of ANS arousal beyond the window of tolerance. There is an immediacy in these reactions that brings the memory of past events tangibly into the present; they are re-experienced not as trauma-related symptoms but as part of current reality.

To experience an event that leaves you traumatized is dreadful enough; to relive elements of that event over and over again, across decades, with feelings and sensations at least as vivid as the original event, is truly horrific.

This explains why the avoidance of retraumatization is a first principle of trauma therapy; retraumatization does more than repeat or amplify the experience, it multiplies it. At the moment of a traumatic event there may be such an element of shock and confusion that there is a degree of numbing to the intensity; when that event is re-experienced sometime in the future, the accompanying feelings can be stronger than before. In my experience, people have an implicit knowledge that this is going to be the case and it adds to their fear of therapy and 'reliving' what happened. For these people, the trauma has not stopped; the gestalt is unfinished and the past is all too present. It is as though the interval between the traumatic event and the present never existed. Perls ([1947] 1992: 104) noted that '[memories] are not subject to change as long as they remain in a system isolated from the rest of the personality'. This is the characteristic of unprocessed trauma: the continual reliving is never truly about memory until it can be assigned to the past.

Clinical vignette

Hilary was 48 when she came into therapy. She had been raped almost three decades earlier by a university lecturer while on a field trip. Sexual abuse has been recognized as rife in education, sports, religious and youth groups, and in many other organizational settings. After some time in therapy, during which we had numerous times focused on current experience, she was feeling more stable and felt better about her day-to-day life, but still had times when she was badly affected by her memories of that evening. One day she was flooded by fears that her perpetrator would track her down through social media. I commented: 'You give a lot of power to an old man.' Hilary looked momentarily taken aback. I followed on: 'How old was he at the time he raped you?', to which Hilary replied, 'Oh, I've always thought of him as being the same age as when it happened, but of course he isn't... he'd be in his 70s I suppose ... if he's still alive ... it's so obvious but I never realized it... [her energy rising] I'm stronger than an old man ... I could knock him over, I could kick him, I could really hurt him, show him what he did to me...'. For Hilary, being able to update her memory by separating past from present completely changed her relationship to what happened and to her sense of self, and this became a turning point in her therapy.

Stolorow (2007: 17) evocatively says that 'trauma destroys time'. This has clinical significance:

> Trauma, in altering the structure of temporality, also disrupts one's understanding of one's being; it fractures one's sense of lunitary selfhood ... clinical features typically explained as dissociation and multiplicity can additionally be comprehended in terms of contexts of trauma in disorganizing and reorganizing one's sense of being-in-time.
>
> (Stolorow 2007: 20)

Fragments of the past re-emerge in seemingly random fashion. 'In trauma-related disorders [*sic*] fragments of memory take on a life of their own, able to intrude at any moment, thereby fuelling hyper- and hypoarousal states that are beyond cognitive control' (Ogden et al. 2006: 155). The need to find some control may be one explanation for why victims become fixated on the past, endeavouring to close the gestalt that seeks completion. Trauma clients' preoccupation with things that have passed is often counterbalanced by a foreshortened sense of the future. I suggest that this may go some way to explaining the common response to the climate emergency where, as if frozen in time, the future cannot be imagined for the trauma it contains.

Through the lens of trauma, the present moment takes on a particular meaning. Bromberg ([1998] 2001: 214) observes that: 'For certain people, here-and-now experience – the living present – cannot be ... mentally represented without the felt danger of traumatization.' A client declared: 'I don't *want* to be in the present, it's *too awful!*' This presents both a warning and a conundrum for Gestalt therapists whose orientation is to work in the here and now. Fortunately, the Window of Tolerance Model contains a temporal dimension. The window of tolerance is a zone in which it is possible to be in the here and now, and anything outside of it can be understood as being in a different time frame. Trauma clients become locked in time physiologically because of their dysregulated ANS arousal.

Beyond the here and now

Because he considers that the here and now espoused by Perls is not enough, Yontef refers to four time spaces which we need to take account of in therapy. First, '[w]e center on here-and-now moments of experienced contact, but that is not the end of our horizons' (1993: 260). Second is the 'there-and-now' frame – the person's life space outside the therapy room. This includes all the social conditions and implicit traumas of past generations that constellate in the present. Next is the 'here and then', the therapy context, meaning 'that which happened here in the therapy room, but not at this very moment' – for example, the development of the therapeutic relationship over time. A client said of therapy: 'This is where the past and present come together', acknowledging the ways in which I played a part. Finally comes the 'there and then', by which is meant the person's life story (Yontef 1993: 260–1), or the chronological sense of biographical self. Yontef's perspective opens the possibility of honouring the client's past, their current concerns for safety and creative adjustments over time. I think that there are, in turn, some things that Yontef has missed. He offers no sense of the future, which arguably the Window of Tolerance Model provides. He also does not have a way of accounting for what psychoanalysts call enactments, in which the therapist's role as part of the enactment in current time is working with both the past and the here and now.

More recently, Delisle (2011: 21) has expanded these four fields of time to include internal and external levels for each. His thinking can be applied directly to trauma: 'it is not the historic past that is at stake but the past as it acts upon the configuration of the present field' (Delisle 2011: 20) – or, in other words, how it is enacted in the present, which frames the gap in Yontef's formulation. For clients such as Hilary above, whose trauma occurred decades ago, we are not simply dealing with an event in the distant past but one that has been *ongoing* over those decades. In arguing for the distinction between external (observable) and internal (experiential) time fields, Delisle places the distress of the recurring trauma on the internal level and the historical event on the external. In learning to recognize these multiple time frames the client is able to reduce the 'experiential dissonance' between them. We might frame this as 'I feel this now when I remember that experience in the past'. This supports differentiation as opposed to generalization.

All this is predicated on the assumption of linear time, which is not a concept shared by all peoples. Yunkaporta, for example, is one indigenous writer who explains an alternative view on linearity, cause and effect: 'One man tried going in a straight line many thousands of years ago and was called wamba (crazy) and punished by being thrown up into the sky' (Yunkaporta 2020: loc 228). Time in an indigenous cosmology is seen as circular, whereby one's children can become one's grandparents. This creates new multiperspective solutions to complex problems, and positions human life in a time frame that is cosmological. In my article, 'The ecological self', I have considered the position of humans in the context of deep time (Taylor 2023).

Differentiating experience

Traumatized people have a tendency to generalization which needs to be addressed in therapy. When life is organized through the lens of trauma the nuance of differentiation is not possible, and the sense of self is diminished. By excluding parts of the field other than those related to trauma, awareness becomes either diffuse or fixated on a single piece of 'evidence'. The ability to differentiate aspects of experience, and therefore of self, is prized in Gestalt therapy, which offers many ways of approaching it. For the Gestalt therapist, this differentiation happens most clearly at moments of good contact, in the meeting between self and other at the contact boundary. This involves forming clear and well-supported figures.

In addition, Gestalt therapists work to enrich the experiential field of the client by attending to three zones of awareness (Perls 1969). The outer zone includes aspects of the current field, both concrete and abstract. The inner zone relates to sensations, physiology, movement and impulse. The middle zone is that of thoughts, imagination, representation and dreams which mediate the inner and the outer zones. We can learn much about how clients organize their experience by studying their zones of awareness. Trauma clients tend to overemphasize the inner zone of awareness, which keeps them on the alert for signals of danger; their middle zone is full of ruminations, intrusive memories and trauma-related conclusions about themselves and others, while they tend to have difficulty turning their awareness to the outer zone *as it is now*.

Dropping in

Let your attention settle on anything in your outer zone of awareness, becoming aware of its features and qualities. Now bring your attention to whatever inner experience it is drawn to – a sensation or posture, perhaps. Taking your attention back to your outer zone of awareness, begin to shuttle between the two zones. Try doing this for some minutes. Notice, perhaps, the reflective quality of interiority that accompanies the centre space of the window of tolerance, and the state shifts as you shuttle. Then ask yourself, 'What thoughts or images go with these different zones of awareness?' They may or may not be related; it is more important to notice them as they are than to try and make connections between them.

Repeating patterns

Relating to the wiring of the ANS that has conditioned the person to orient to the past, the notion of unfinished business is core to making sense of the often slow process of trauma therapy. We can consider that unresolved trauma, as experienced in states of immobilized freeze and collapse, are fixed repetitions of traumatic experience that have not been able to move through to completion. We see, then, a pattern of habituated response as an attempt to complete the active defence that was not available at the time. Jacobs (2003) distinguishes between repetitive and recursive patterns. The repetitive pattern is stuck in time and nothing changes, while the recursive pattern has a more fluid time element: it is now that I recall the past. Trauma theory helps therapists to recognize clients' recurring trauma-related symptoms as memories belonging to the past. It is much more difficult for clients to recognize this than it is for their therapists. Kepner (1995: 89) underlines the necessity for traumatized people to differentiate the present from the past. In particular, these people need to understand their sensations, body memories, flashbacks and other intrusions as *memories and not as actual current experience*. From the client's perspective, triggers occur in present time and create a bridge to the past.

A similar position can be taken in relation to time frames as to zones of awareness. By developing what Rothschild (2000: 129) has named 'dual awareness', clients can begin to shuttle their awareness between different fields of time. This act of differentiation can open the experiential space enough to allow for the processing of the trauma, because it is no longer so immediate and experience-near. As opposed to triggering escalating trauma-related thoughts, sensations and emotions about impending danger 'the act of mindful exploration facilitates dual processing' (Ogden et al. 2006: 169). In order to counter the natural tendency of trauma clients to become fixated on the past, therapists need to favour working with here-and-now awareness.

Awareness of the here and now

Gestalt therapy takes a clear philosophical and existential position in relation to the here and now. In a reimagining of Zen philosophy, Perls states that '*There is no other reality than the present*' (Perls [1947] 1992: 104, original italics). This underpins an understanding that everything we need to work with is present in the room. Parlett's (1991) Principle of Contemporaneity is consistent with this: we can only turn towards the past from the viewpoint of each unrepeatable and consecutive present moment. As Heraclitus said, we can never step into the same river twice. This important principle is embedded in Kepner's Healing Tasks Model (Kepner 1995: 8). The pressing needs of trauma clients, reworked over the course of therapy, are always approached from the here and now.

As Perls et al. ([1951] 1998: 416) propose, awareness is a figure against a ground, specifically our perception of a singular figure and its ground. Wheeler ([1991] 1998: 87) considers awareness to be an act of organization, and as such has potential to be integrative. 'Awareness is ... an emergent pattern of neural integration across all the levels of the interoceptive network' (Fogel 2009: 59).

In the here and now of the therapy setting, we can help to increase clients' awareness of the present moment, and the rich processes and meanings that it contains. We may do this multiple times in a session. When we base our work on the establishment of resources and regulation, however, *we must avoid developing awareness of trauma-related content*. Awareness involves a temporal component, an experiential fragment and an 'I' who is experiencing. The gradual accretion of aware experiential moments thereby supports a growing sense of self that is not possible in unaware states. However, it is also valuable for trauma clients to restore a sense of the continuity of their experience over time. The concept of the **awareness continuum** comes to our aid, whereby one experience flows into the next and the next and the next, in an unending sequence of the flow of life: a state of optimal arousal. Clarkson argues that following the awareness continuum is one of the most important skills a client can acquire: 'It may appear a very simple process, yet in many ways may take a lifetime to learn' (Clarkson 1989: 79). The phenomenological approach, which puts the experiencing self of the client at the centre of the work, is ideally suited to this purpose.

Awareness and the phenomenological method

Mackewn (1997: 34) speaks of the 'development of awareness through a sustained enquiry into clients' subjective experience'. The term used for the subjective component of awareness is 'phenomenology'. This refers to the investigation of phenomena – units of personal experience – drawn from Husserl's existential philosophy. From phenomenological reasoning, Husserl derived a methodology for working therapeutically (Spinelli [1989] 1998: 2) which supports the development of awareness. Phenomenology is one of the cornerstones of Gestalt theory and practice. This approach eschews interpretation in favour of observation – by either client, or therapist, or both.

The advantages of the phenomenological approach are numerous. There is a rightness in privileging subjective experience over imposed perspectives for those who have been objectified during trauma or by medical diagnosis. Of particular relevance to these clients is the neutral and non-judgemental stance it fosters, the containment of being held in a discrete moment of time and the fact that the amount of stimulus calling for attention is limited. Learning to tolerate small moments of experience is invaluable. The phenomenological approach is also an entry point into direct, lived and embodied experience. Gestalt therapists usually refer to the felt sense, as opposed to talking about something in cognitive process. As Romanyshyn (2007: 89) comments, 'the task of phenomenology is to loosen the grasp of the pre-conceived'. By means of the phenomenological method, implicit learning and assumptions are challenged and made explicit. There is a shift from the known to knowing, the formation of self-in-process.

There are three strands to the phenomenological method: bracketing (sometimes referred to as epoché), horizontalism and description, which I will describe in turn. Each of these denotes a therapeutic attitude, and it is useful to recognize how, through the modelling of the therapist, trauma clients might learn to use these elements of phenomenology on their own behalf; we will return to this point shortly. Bracketing refers to the ability to set aside prior assumptions and knowledge in order to meet the client and their concerns afresh in the here and now. In seeking to regulate arousal and to reorganize the experiential field, the need is for the client to 'drop' trauma-related material and turn to other aspects of their experience; this is bracketing. It involves the *deliberate and choiceful redirection of attention to other possibilities in the field*. Horizontalism means paying equal and even attention to phenomena as they arise, without attributing particular significance to any one. A position of neutrality can be achieved, taking some of the heat out of charged material. The use of this for uncoupling of trauma-related associations and generalizations by means of here-and-now awareness is evident. Description is a therapeutic account of what is observed, the act of noticing without judgement or interpretation. For clients, this can offer the possibility of being with discrete elements of their experience.

Description has an important role in the development of an observing self which is so often difficult for those immersed in the immediacy of re-experiencing. The capacity to stand back from experience in order to reflect rather than react is crucial, creating some therapeutic distance from the event. This is rather at odds with the Gestalt phenomenological precept to keep the focus 'experience-near'. I am arguing here for healthy **egotism** in the service of reorganizing experience, of regulation within the window of tolerance and being more present to current reality as opposed to the past. However, Philippson (2001: 98) cautions against awareness that creates understanding that remains on a verbal rather than a 'gut' level, involving a mere 'verbalization of the sensation'. These two positions describe the tension between the Paradoxical Theory of Change and the step that needs to be taken by trauma clients in preparation for this to be effective. Consistent with the Integrated

Model of Change proposed in Chapter 3, both positions are relevant in working with trauma at different stages of the work – taking a step back from direct experience first in order to be able to later step towards it in a more organized and supported fashion. Phenomenological description, tracking and enquiry are necessary for both steps.

Phenomenology and the body

For example, how do individuals inhabit their sadness, longing, satisfaction or their attachments? How do values and beliefs take their place in our being? What is the shape of shame, the quality of helplessness, the energy of 'Stop that!'? How much of our embodied core supports our posture and movement? These deeply personal questions exemplify the essence of the phenomenological approach, and point directly to the lived body. Kepner (2002) suggests that early trauma disturbs 'the process of fusing consciousness to matter', meaning that we must reconnect awareness with the body. Developing this theme, Merleau-Ponty ([1945] 2009) distinguishes between 'having a body' and 'being a body'. Kennedy calls the lived body *'the body that is me ... my total self as I respond to the world which is with me in unending dialogue'* (Kennedy 2005: 110, original italics). Further, he considers that the 'layer of living experience ... is the level of perception [that is] subverted in trauma' (Kennedy 2005: 109).

Because of the physiological impact of trauma, it is through embodied life that trauma becomes timeless. Our histories are encoded in our tissues, skeletons and nervous systems. Maté (2022) suggests that illnesses are representations of our life stories and of the context in which we live, the past presenting through suffering. Bodywork therapists intervene by directly affecting those tissues; however, their interest is not in the self of their clients as psychotherapists understand it. Just as we cannot heal trauma without integrating the body, psychotherapists cannot do integrative holistic body work without a phenomenological approach, by including the self.

Supporting an individual's increasing awareness affects their entire organism. Conscious awareness has energetic properties (Kepner 2002). We can take this thinking literally. Empirical evidence shows that skin temperature rises from the moment attention is directed to a particular area (interview with Alexander, in Johnson 1995: 286). Blood flow is increased and nerve endings are enlivened over time, supporting awareness of sensation and fluidity of process. For trauma clients we do not just seek to support awareness of sensation as a stage in figure formation, although this is important: 'One role of the senses in our daily lives is to wake us up, to pull us away from automaticity, to sharpen the acuity of awareness so that life is both richer and more present in the moment' (Siegel 2007: 77).

Related to the awareness continuum, phenomenological tracking is a method of following subjective experience as it emerges over time. In tracking experience the trauma client is enabled to develop their awareness of their experiencing self, including repeating patterns, and to make links such as 'when

I remember this I also feel this way and it is accompanied by these thoughts'. The technique of tight therapeutic sequencing (Polster 1991) supports the ability to 'stay with' a figure over a expanded period of time, allowing the client the opportunity to dwell in an experience and assimilate it, rather than move away from it too quickly. Gestalt therapists understand this as experimenting with 'directed awareness'. Sensorimotor trauma therapy adds an edge to this approach by encouraging the client to *attend to the smallest possible units of experience over the longest possible stretch of time.*

According to Stern (2004: 41), the present moment has a duration of between 1 and 10 seconds, the unit of time needed to reorganize experience and make it conscious. It takes longer than this – much longer – for experience to be incorporated into an individual's being. Thus the phenomenological approach can be employed in the service of the finest possible calibration of arousal at the margins of the window of tolerance. 'How do you know when you are about to tip over into a more upsetting state?' can lead to an enquiry about how to catch it earlier in the process of escalation: 'What happens in the instant before that, can you tell?' Many trauma clients already know how to do this, for their sensitivity to danger keeps them acutely alert to changes in their inner zone of awareness. The observational skill of hypervigilance can be more healthily transformed into the ability to track and stay with a wider range of possibilities.

Furthermore, a sensorimotor-informed approach is interested in developing trauma clients' phenomenological awareness of particular sensations which are the precursors to movement, those impulses to **aggress** in the sense Perls intended, which are so often retroflected or held in the body's relationship to the past.

Dropping in

Standing up, start in the middle zone of your awareness by thinking about your feet. What attitudes do you hold towards them? Perhaps you will want to look at them. Do any memories or images come to you as you do so? Now, in the inner zone of your awareness, let your attention come to your feet. Become aware of the feel of your sock or shoe and the contact of your feet with the ground. Direct your awareness to investigate whatever sensations you notice – heat or cold, pressure or tingling, pulsing or aching. What are the qualities of the tissue in your feet – airy or dense or weak? Try to become aware of the dimensions and volume of any sensation you notice. Notice also any differences between your left foot and your right, which may not feel the same. Does anything change as you pay attention in this way? Really try to get a felt sense of each foot. Having done this, 'let your feet themselves be aware'. This is quite different from directing awareness into a part of the body. What do your aware feet experience? You can repeat this experiment by bringing your attention to different parts of your body. Write about the differences you noticed.

Awareness, phenomenology and the process of change

The emphasis in Gestalt therapy is on using awareness and the phenomenological approach to establish a full sense of 'what is' in current time, without effort to judge or to change. The Paradoxical Theory of Change is exactly this: change follows when we do not try to be different but instead fully accept how we are. Let us reconsider the Integrated Model of Change proposed in Chapter 3. There it was argued that for trauma clients the Paradoxical Theory of Change cannot apply without some preliminary steps being taken. It is important to understand the sequence of steps that are necessary to support the Paradoxical Theory of Change.

The steps are specifically about the journey into deep embodiment. The problem for trauma clients is that they may not yet have developed a reliable sense of inner safety to be able to claim their embodied existence in present time. Orange (2010: 65) uses a helpful metaphor: 'It is ... like finding oneself in a strange house that is supposed to be one's home'. The task of trauma therapy is to help relocate clients into their current embodied experience of self. There is no clear point at which the Integrated Model of Change gives way to the Paradoxical Theory of Change; they are meshed together (see Table 5.1). In keeping with Kepner's Healing Tasks Model, there will be times when one paradigm for change is emphasized more than the other. In a non-linear process there is a gradually growing capacity for most trauma clients to learn to tolerate their current lived experience.

Table 5.1 Matrix of concepts

Stage of embodiment	Process of change	Kepner's healing tasks	ANS arousal
Functional body Desensitized body Thinking about body	Integrated Model of Change	Support and self-functions	Dysregulated arousal – hyper- and hypoaroused; fixed gestalts; polarization and limited choice
Awareness of body Body as possession (I have a body)	Shuttling between Integrated Model and Paradoxical Theory of Change		Moments of dyadic regulation; some choice Moments of self-regulation; loosening of gestalts; expansion of choice; increasing differentiation
Felt sense of body Body as self	Paradoxical Theory of Change	Undoing, redoing and mourning	Reliable dyadic and self-regulation; reliable resources; spontaneous gestalt formation; integration
Lived body		Reconsolidation	

The inherent paradox is that the phenomenological method of raising self-awareness is both the means and the end result of this sequence of steps. We cannot do something without learning to do it. According to Kennedy (2003: 78), the phenomenological approach can be learnt: 'phenomenology is only learned by doing', and it is not just the domain of the therapist, though the therapist is a necessary teacher of the method. This is what is implied in the first steps of the Integrated Model of Change.

Just as the body needs exercise and training to become fit and healthy, so does the mind. Posner takes this analogy further by suggesting that attentional training can strengthen the psychological 'immune system' (in Fulton et al. 2009: 14). By this we can infer that a degree of resilience accompanies the optimal arousal of the window of tolerance. This point is of crucial significance in working with traumatized clients: that working phenomenologically needs to be *very repetitive and very consistent*. Requiring intensive and sustained attention to the minutiae of the client's experience, it is in addition *painstaking and demanding of infinite patience* in the therapist.

The role of mindfulness in trauma therapy

In recent years there has been an upsurge of interest in the benefits of mindfulness in helping people with a range of difficulties, from depression to 'OCD' to working with chronic pain. Research programmes, courses and apps abound. The concept of mindfulness is difficult to distinguish from that of awareness: a simple definition of mindfulness is 'awareness of the present moment'. Mindfulness is a modern derivation of the ancient spiritual practice of meditation, typically but not exclusively Buddhist. Perls was influenced by Eastern religions, which probably informed his view of present awareness (Clarkson and Mackewn 1993: 18). The word mindfulness implies simple yet profound ideas. It is a particular kind of awareness, usually referring to a meditative state of open and alert attention. To some extent the differentiation between the concepts of mindfulness and awareness is a matter of semantics, but not entirely (Fulton et al. 2009). While it is true that these are nested concepts, there are also some differences that are worth considering.

Let us suppose that you become aware of having a dry mouth. You might make an evaluation of this as being mildly unpleasant and decide to take action and make a cup of tea. We can track this process using the cycle of experience (Chapter 2). In mindfulness, however, you notice the dryness of your mouth and sit simply with the direct experience of what is, without judgement, 'I notice that I am thirsty'. Here there is an acceptance of the sensation, and the capacity to be present in the fullness of the experience. It is possible to put some space around the sensation, which eases the discomfort – that is, until it becomes the more urgent sensation of being dehydrated. Sooner or later, another sensation emerges as a new figure for mindful attention. Mindfulness invariably brings you into contact with the body at the level of sensation in the here and now. The important point here is that, unlike awareness, mindfulness is a quality of attention, and concentration on a single figure, one moment at a time. Perls ([1947] 1992) called Gestalt a 'concentration' therapy, and a level of concentration can be learnt. In addition, I think what is known as the awareness continuum in Gestalt could be more accurately be called the mindfulness continuum.

Now clearly, for some people who have experienced trauma, this focus on sensation may be dysregulating, creating an aversion to mindfulness, especially where other ways of grounding and self-regulation are not well established. Mindfulness is an advanced skill of being open to experience. Paradoxically, while it involves a state of mind that is present and alert, this altered state can for some increase the sense of dissociation. My concern is that mindfulness may be suggested as something to do alone, or for prescribed periods of time, without the support of the mindful practitioner who is attentive to signs of dysregulation and knows how to stop the process after just the optimal amount of time. In my experience, it is a very different matter to weave in and out of mindful moments together, in the wider context of a therapy process, than to follow a protocol. I will say more about that shortly.

At its best, an important relational component to mindfulness in trauma therapy can be understood as mutual regulation between the therapist and client in staying with a figure and accompanied phenomenological enquiry. This relates to what Harris (2011) terms the 'shared mindful field'. The mindfulness of the therapist will influence and model, moment by moment, the state for the person they are working with. To be clear, mindfulness is already a property of the field and needs to be brought to the fore. *How* it is done is a crucial consideration, so it not imposed in a top-down fashion, but created together.

Mindfulness can comprise properties of micro-attention as well as meta-perspectives. Siegel considers that this metacognitive function is important, because it offers multiple perspectives on experience (Siegel 2007: 242) that enables the loosening of fixed gestalts. Fonagy (2002: 79) further links this metacognitive perspective to safe relationships and to the development of resilience. Compare this to the important process of (simple) awareness in figure formation; in mindfulness we are not concerned with processes, actions or figures per se, but with a state of being. Mindfulness is always embodied; the knowing that derives from mindfulness involves neither insight nor any mental processes, unlike awareness or attention. A further distinction is that simple awareness does not necessarily involve the settling of arousal – indeed it may be disturbing – while mindful awareness is more commonly calming and requires a sense of letting go.

Fulton argues that the most transformative and liberating feature of mindfulness is that it changes 'our *relationship* to experience' (Fulton et al. 2009: 16, original italics), which I have confirmed numerous times. The relevance of this to trauma therapy is implied by Kolodny:

> To the degree that the meditative practitioner can be successfully mindful – present for the exact experience of each succeeding moment and not lost in thought of past or future – then for that interval there is no suffering ... So *being present* provides a sanctuary from mental afflictions.
>
> (Kolodny 2004: 94, original italics)

This is not always the case, but is an important possibility. Once a trauma victim has reliably learnt mindfulness as a means of taking the edge off their suffering a further development opens up.

A sense of compassion frequently results from repeated and sustained mindfulness practice. Buddhist meditation practice includes mindfulness of suffering which seems to naturally evoke compassion for the suffering and the self who suffers, leading to a sense of compassion for others. Mindfulness practice brings with it a deep sense of connection, consistent with a self/other orientation. 'Concentration, the mindful immersion into the given moment, ultimately leads to an expansion of the self, to opening and connection' (Bocian 2009: 54). It is therefore unsurprising that Brownell (2012: 99) considers mindfulness to be ripe for assimilation into Gestalt therapy because it is so similar.

Mindfulness and the brain

One important finding of research into mindfulness is that it has profound effects on the function of the brain.

> An understanding of the roles of nonfocal attention and focal attention in the differential encoding of implicit and explicit memory can not only help to understand the impact of trauma on the mind, but also can lead to new strategies for clinical intervention.
>
> (Siegel 2012: 7-4)

In Chapter 3, I described the role of the limbic system of the brain in the heightened responses of trauma. Neuroimaging techniques have demonstrated how fearful conditions alter the activation of the prefrontal cortex in particular, which Ogden et al. (2006: 149) consider is partly responsible for the 'timeless' nature of traumatic memories. They suggest that the significant contribution of mindfulness to trauma therapy is that it *re-engages the prefrontal cortex* 'in support of observing sensorimotor experiences, rather than allowing these bottom-up trauma-related processes to escalate and "hijack" higher level information processing' (Ogden et al. 2006: 194).

This thinking is consistent with Siegel's, who proposes that simple awareness does not involve the same regions of the cortex that are concerned with mindful awareness (Siegel 2007: 144). It is suggested that the *medial* prefrontal cortex is activated by simple awareness, not necessarily involving other regions. Siegel argues that regions located in the more integrative *mid* prefrontal cortex are 'likely active during mindful practice and grow and strengthen their connections as a consequence' (Siegel 2007: 213–14). By this token, we can conclude that simple awareness is not enough to create a state of integration in the brain. Through training in mindful awareness it is presumed that '[r]etraumatization is minimized because the pre-frontal cortex remains "online" to observe inner experience, thus inhibiting escalation of subcortical activation' (Ogden et al. 2006: 195). Mindfulness appears to have a generally *associative function in the brain, rather than dissociative.*

Thus mindfulness of the present moment has an important part to play in regulation of the ANS. Perhaps not surprisingly, the regulation of sympathetic and parasympathetic activity of the ANS is located in the mid of the prefrontal cortex, bringing about a state of 'nonreactivity' (Siegel 2007: 213). Access to feelings of well-being is also made through mindfulness, because it increases activity in 'areas of the brain associated with positive affect' (Davidson et al. 2003, cited in Ogden et al. 2006: 169), and facilitates the observation of the mind by the mind.

> Through a process of internal attunement the observing self attunes to or focuses attention in an open and receptive manner, on the experiencing self. This internal attunement creates and amplifies states of neural integration.
>
> (Siegel 2010: 41–5)

One reason for this is that myelin, the protein sheath that permits smooth and rapid transmission of impulses through nerves, is increased by the practice of deep awareness – the energetic properties of awareness change the body.

Introducing mindfulness to therapy

The discussion below comes with a caveat. Mindfulness is not always tolerated by people who have experienced trauma, and I caution against leaving them alone to practise. Part of the problem may lie in the decontextualization of mindfulness from its spiritual roots, resulting in only part of a 'solution'. Mindfulness practice may also fail those whose expectations are of achieving calm or blissful state, when it is a means of getting in touch with reality safely but sometimes difficult to tolerate. My proposition is that mindfulness is best introduced to therapy as an informal, titrated and shared experience, a property of the therapeutic field rather than a 'tool'. Mindfulness training can include specific structured exercises, spontaneous emergent experiments and exposure to nature (Posner, in Fulton et al. 2009: 14). Certainly, access to nature and immersion in positive resources outside the therapy setting is to be encouraged, while mindfulness is supported *within* the therapy session. There will be countless opportunities to respond to emergent process with the use of mindful interventions. A first principle is to avoid mindfulness of unpleasant sensations; finding what is pleasurable or neutral will probably be tolerated better at the beginning. And because it is less frightening, applying mindfulness to the ordinary and everyday makes a lot of sense.

Dropping in: Making a cup of tea

We are so accustomed to making a cup of tea that we probably do it on some sort of autopilot, without being mindful of the process. We may even multitask, buttering the toast or packing a lunch box while the kettle boils. Try instead to make a cup of tea in full mindfulness, as though it is the most interesting thing you have ever done.

Which hand do you pick up the kettle with? How do you move to the sink to fill it? What is the sound of the water as you fill the kettle, that changes when you have filled it enough? Which hand reaches for the cup, the tea bag?

Feel the movement as you do it. Listen to the bubbling as the water comes to the boil. Try pouring the water slowly onto the tea bag, watching as it changes colour. You can fill in more details of micro-movements and sensations for yourself as you proceed.

According to Ogden et al. (2006: 194), mindfulness questions are those which 'discourage discussion, ordinary conversation, and brooding about past or future experiences'. A principal therapeutic stance is of maintaining curiosity about current experience. I have found a useful starting point for those that cannot differentiate their experience is to enquire 'Are you thinking, feeling or sensing as you say that?', or 'As you say that, does it feel better or worse?'. Strangely, the ubiquitous Gestalt intervention 'What's happening now?' may not be very helpful because the question is too open and the person concerned may not yet know. Our enquiries can be made more relational by asking 'Would you be interested in exploring what happened just now?' Phenomenological observation, naming a change that has been noticed, can be used to increase the client's self-observational skills: 'Did you notice how you did that? There's no need to change it, just stay with it and notice what happens next.'

Gestalt therapists are trained to facilitate awareness of processes that lie beneath the content of a story or talking 'about' something. They might comment, 'As you are telling me about your father, I notice that you become very still', or ask 'What feeling goes with that thought?' directing awareness towards something specific. Ogden et al. helpfully describe this as studying 'the effects of our speaking on internal experience' (Ogden et al. 2006: 194, original italics). Clients can be asked to 'drop' a level of awareness, from observing to the felt sense. These are all entry points to states of mindful awareness, which can be expanded and deepened. This is done through sustained enquiry and observation over time and immersion into the microscopic phenomenological experiences that comprise ongoing moment-to-moment existence. As one client observed: 'It's a skill – to sit and wait and watch, to not jump up and drive myself into action, it's clearer to me what to do.'

Summary

For many trauma victims time does not heal. Trauma severs a sense of continuity and of self over time. The past breaks through into their present experience not as capsules of ordinary memory but as vivid, visceral and recurrent intrusions outside the window of tolerance. These are fragmentary and discontinuous reminders of events that destroyed the victim's world view; they feel as real and present as though time had not moved on. These are bodily imprints of the past, even where clients are unable to differentiate the somatic elements of their current reality. Gestalt therapy focuses on here-and-now process, however we cannot ordinarily separate the past from the present – we look back from where we are now. We work to help clients understand that their bodily reminders are not present reality, a process known as dual awareness. This can only be considered from within the window of tolerance.

Awareness of the present moment is a key feature of Gestalt therapy. This is the process by which a reorganization of figure and ground can take place, and a sense of self emerges. By stretching awareness over consecutive 'present moments', continuity and fluidity replace the fixity and fragmentation of experience. The phenomenological method enables the study of embodied subjective experience in ways that are safe and tolerable for trauma clients. Simple awareness can give rise to mindful awareness, a state of being that can help to change the client's relationship to their experience, including the past. It also permits the sense of being able to inhabit the embodied self. Research into mindfulness suggests that it helps to create necessary changes in the brain which can reverse the impact of trauma. Developing mindful awareness within the therapy setting is an important route to change, consistent with the Integrated Model of Change.

Part **2**

At the limits of self

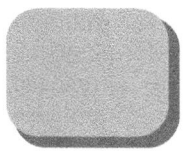

Introduction to Part 2

The four chapters that comprise Part 2 of this book focus on the subjective experience of trauma, the phenomena of fear, helplessness, dissociation and shame, each considered with its polarity. None of these experiences is discrete or stands alone; they are enmeshed with one another. I present each through the lens of lived experience, neurobiology, relationship and the polarities that can guide the work of trauma therapy. I stress that the polarities are offered as points on a continuum of experience to guide the direction of travel, as it were, and not as goals, ideals or potential 'outcomes' of therapy. Without wishing to be prescriptive, I offer at the end of each chapter, some thoughts about how to find a counterpoint to the distressing and fixed phenomena in question. These are not intended to be comprehensive guidance, merely starting points from which you are encouraged to find your own words and develop your own ideas. There are a number of salient considerations to point out, in no particular order.

I have chosen these four headings because they seem to relate to many people's experience, acknowledging that the language is not helpful for everyone. As in so much of contemporary trauma practice, understanding context is paramount. We could look at trauma through multiple lenses, including spiritual and collective ones. It would be a mistake to consider that these phenomena are universal, part of the hardwired human instinct to survive threat. 'By isolating trauma as a malfunction of the mind … cultural narratives are erased' (Watters 2010). Other cultures set more store by collective than personal experience, and their approaches to healing are not focused on the individual. By the same token, fear and its polarity, safety, for example, have different meanings in different cultures and for diverse demographics. Experience can be transmitted across generations and may not be 'located' in an individual's story. I have made much in previous chapters of personal and subjective experience, and own that this thinking is rooted in a dominant western and medicalized field. Thinking through a wider lens challenges some of our existing theories, or our interpretation of them (Taylor 2023).

A first question pertains to the concept of the self, specifically the individualist self, which is not a universally accepted construct. An Indian perspective, as one example, is of self embedded in community (Fanen 2022: 308). In many traditional and indigenous cultures self is inextricably associated with place and the beyond human (Yunkaporta 2020; Taylor 2023). This is not such a big step away from the Gestalt definition of self, which is formed, moment by moment, at the boundary between human organism and the entire environment, which we are for ever in relationship with (see Taylor 2021), but which we sometimes exclude from our thinking. A broader perspective on self 'is dynamic and situational, a perspective we can choose to adopt according to context and need' (Macy 2009: 244), which leads me to think in terms of the ecosystem of which we are a part. Naess suggests that 'the self to be realized extends further and further beyond the separate ego and includes more and more of phenomenal world' (quoted by Macy 2009: 244).

A contemporary view of self as increasingly conflicted, anxious and ambivalent is indicated, in which 'individual concerns are overridden by societal and contextual factors' (Crompton 2013: 221). Broader factors – social, political and global challenges – create an escalating sense of the helpless self. This trajectory, from overwhelming stress to helplessness, can be mapped onto the Window of Tolerance Model at ever-increasing scales. The forces of culture and the phenomenal world reshape our sense of who we are, and are not separate from who we can become. So much of our potential is also predicated upon privilege, including access to resources (Taylor 2021), which might lift us out of the helpless state and are entirely situational. They delimit the possibilities of therapy particularly for those already significantly disadvantaged or enduring systemic oppression. Sheldrake describes how when we track the chain of connected and interdependent matter, tracing the links from a single node, we discover that 'To talk about individuals [makes] no sense anymore ... We are ecosystems that span boundaries and transgress categories' (Sheldrake 2021: 39). In questioning how we can grow the concept of ourselves by studying the interconnected webs in the natural world, he wonders whether our sense of self might be more an assumption than a fact. 'What more are we capable of? What would happen if we made individuality and selfhood a question rather than an answer known in advance? Where would this leave "us" ?' (Sheldrake 2021: 40). This is not to suggest that we privilege contextual factors over the individual, but that we hold *both* paradigms in the therapeutic frame, with their inherent tensions and contradictions. How do we account, in our therapy practice, for these perspectives and what we mean by working with 'self'? This leads to a further question: can we continue to think in terms of a subjective phenomenology without *simultaneously* accounting for the idea of a collective phenomenology?

If potential growth is helped or hindered by forces beyond the control of the individual or the therapeutic dyad, how may we be realistic about 'outcomes' of trauma therapy? This may pull on the rescuer within the therapist, unable to control the uncontrollable, and their own co-transference concerns. Naturally we hope for the best and need to sit with the tensions inherent in the field. A third question, therefore, relates to our assumptions about recovery and healing. The notion of 'recovery' rests in medical and social institutions, by which interventions aim to restore an individual back into 'damaging and lacking social systems' (Fanen 2022: 300), and shifts responsibility from supportive service provision to an emphasis on personal recovery. Healing, however, a concept shared by many traditional communities and practices, has more nuanced meanings which may be helpful in thinking about outcome. The roots of the word 'healing', meaning health or wholeness, is something very different from functionality. Health can be seen as a state in which the personal, social and ecological are interconnected (Fanen 2022: 242). Connectedness calls to mind a sense of integration and the reduction of the distress created by fragmentation. Reduction of personal distress is a different notion to being able to 'function' according to societal norms, which may reinforce or exacerbate distress.

Finally, we might be open-minded about the validity of different approaches to healing. In the developed West, we naturally make assumptions about what is helpful based on prevailing wisdom, generally informed by science. A shocking instance of cultural imperialism is provided by Watters (2010) who gives many examples of well-meaning, but culturally insensitive, attempts to bring western trauma interventions to Sri Lanka in the aftermath of the 2004 tsunami. These interventions overlooked traditional community approaches to working with the distress that 'we' in the West, deem to be trauma. In some cases this created different expectations based on the assumed and perceived power of white aid workers. This was not the help that was needed and a mismatch of expectations resulted. Uncritical assumptions of the dominance of western ideas and practices ignore the science of other traditions and cultures. Traditional Chinese medicine, for example, is one approach that considers the imbalance of energies in the body, and seeks to release blockages and restore flow. We might consider the Window of Tolerance Model to be a 'scientific' western perspective on the same energies. What brings about healing for some communities may include ritual, trance, remedies, storytelling, community and anticipatory joy (Avene, personal communication, 2023), practices that are embedded in the communal self.

We would do well, therefore, to listen closely to the collective voices of the traumatized, perhaps as articulated by the #MeToo movement, Black Lives Matter or Fridays for Future, to name a very small number of the rising tide of actions pushing back against oppressive western and consumerist ideologies and systems. Perhaps this resistance, the naming of experience and the expression of rage, is healing in and of itself. Without falling into the trap of appropriation, what healing practices might we embrace and encourage with the people we work with? How might we restore the wholeness of the deeply wounded – those who have suffered soul wounding or soul murder – by calling the soul back into the body (Fanen 2022: 206)?

6 From fear towards safety

This chapter explores the phenomenon of fear which for most people suffering severe trauma is a foreground experience. It considers how fear is present in the triggers to unresolved traumatic states, avoidance, intrusions, and hypervigilance to danger. The chapter goes on to explain the neurobiological basis of fear systems, and links are made to the instinctive survival defences that operate under conditions of extreme threat. I will consider the meaning of safety in a wider context, and conclude the chapter by describing ways of working to establish internal and external safety, illustrated by the first part of an extended case study.

Fear dominates the lives of many of those who have experienced trauma. We have seen in Chapter 2 how this experience can result in creative adjustments that are more or less predictable, rigidifying or loosening structures within individuals. Familiar features of PTS reflect the fear of such individuals, evidenced by hypervigilance and avoidance. It is through these behaviours that fear becomes an organizing principle for trauma victims. For many, it is not simply a recurring fear of bad things happening in the external field that is a cause of massive anxiety. Their internal world, somatic experience and felt sense also become a source of terror. Mental images, flashbacks, nightmares, intrusive ruminations and inability to discriminate between past and present all add to the picture of fear that feels global.

It is perhaps stating the obvious, but as a corrective to the narrative that all bad things lead to trauma, Bromberg ([1998] 2001: 169) points out the difference between a 'danger situation and a situation that actually becomes traumatic'. Bromberg considers fear to be a natural response to danger distinct from the experience of psychological shock which, containing 'a generalized flooding' of feeling is definitive of trauma. I suggest that we consider terror rather than fear as a primary feeling, though some will resist the language as being too vivid. Historically, one of the first ways of describing what we now call 'PTSD' was 'shell shock' (van der Kolk et al. [1996] 2007c: 48). We might well call it 'post-traumatic shock disorder', or in a less pathologizing tone, 'post-traumatic shock'. Closely aligned to fear is a sense of panic. To experience fear under threat is adaptive because it elicits alertness and caution (Soloman et al. [1996] 2007: 107).

The contemporary assumption that we can or should remove fear and restore enduring calm is problematic because our survival depends on the capacity to respond to danger, which is present in our day-to-day lives. The key issue here, I suggest, is the extent to which our immediate response to actual danger is shaped by past trauma. When the sense of threat and horror become embedded in memory, fear is not proportionate to the current situation and contributes to the development of PTSD (McFarlane [1996] 2007: 172). The experience of chronic fear brings with it an abiding sense of vulnerability and reduced capacity to cope.

Avoidance, triggers and phobias

Put most simply, a trigger can be anything that evokes a lingering change of state. Imagine you are sitting in a garden or park reading this book when a butterfly lands on the page. That moment of delight which redirects your attention is a change of state elicited by the butterfly. If, however, you have a phobia of butterflies, your reaction will be rather different. Either way, the butterfly has caused your attention, and with it your emotional and physiological state, to shift momentarily. If you are delighted by the visit from the butterfly, you will settle more quickly than if you are activated by it. State changes can be positive as well as negative, and what for one person is pleasant or neutral may for another be a source of terror; it is this last condition that we can rightly call a trigger. Triggers are problematic according to the meaning we make of them, and are highly subjective. Underlying any triggering experience is the linkage, or association, that is made to a traumatic event or situation. Clients will associate the trigger with a perceived present danger and not with an event that has already passed. We know from Gestalt studies of perception that danger is perceptually vivid and paramount (Jacobs 2012: 65).

Trauma clients live in a world of triggers; some are related to personal history and others may be cultural or environmental. I have referred already to our sense of fit in the world (Chapter 1); if your appearance in some way makes you 'different', perhaps because of your skin colour, age or visible disability, you are more likely to be alert to the threat of discrimination, oppression or micro-aggressions on a daily basis. These are important therapeutic considerations, in addition to whatever presenting issues may call for our attention; indeed, they may give ground to the most pressing figures that arise which we ignore at our peril.

Generally, triggers elicit dysregulated arousal, an automatic defensive response, or both. It is characteristic for people to avoid returning to the scene of a traumatic event, sometimes going to great lengths to circumnavigate particular places. They come to believe that the scene of an accident, for example, is dangerous, when it simply *represents* past danger. In the recursive, unfinished situation of the trauma response, the location becomes feared.

Others will avoid representations of violence for example, in films, on television or in print. While for most people weapons and unattended packages are rightly to be feared, countless objects which are intrinsically benign – almost anything in fact – can become linked in some way to a trauma and later avoided. Smells, sounds, facial expressions, times of day and accents are just a few among countless possible triggers.

Some cues are very subtle. One client came to a session on a sunny afternoon. He was already highly activated by a nightmare the previous night and had found the journey to the session particularly difficult. The sunshine emerged as a figure in the session, and the client made a link to his military service in Iraq. This client had not previously been distressed by sunshine and in this case the ground for the trigger was the nightmare. This is an example of how triggers are state dependent. Things experienced in one environment, or state, are recalled when that condition is repeated; this applies equally to 'internal' states as it does to 'external' environments (Eliotson 1835). State dependent memory may account for the common experience in which trauma clients are unable to remember the content of the previous session (Bromberg 2011: 77).

Reminders of trauma tend to be stored in implicit memory rather than consciously recognized as belonging in the past. More likely is that the individual most fears the internal state of intolerable arousal and not external stimulus. *The actual threat in the here and now is that of overwhelm to the autonomic nervous system.* Or, as Roosevelt said 'The only thing we have to fear is fear itself'. Viewed this way, avoidance has as much to do with psychological survival as it does with physical. When people have difficulty in knowing what sensations mean they may misattribute them, mistaking excitement for anxiety or calm for boredom. Fear of experiencing anything can be very intense, because *any* internal somatic activation, even positive, is traumatically linked: 'If I feel something I must be in danger'.

Out of this background of fear, specific phobias may arise. There is indeed much to be feared, and coming into therapy in itself may be triggering. Being in therapy carries with it risks of relationship, of contact, intimacy and of attachment, of reliving traumatic events, of vulnerability, of feeling feelings that have been disowned, of remembering what dare not be remembered, of knowing the unknowable, and speaking the unspeakable. Importantly, Kepner (2002) distinguishes *defensive* avoidance from the *incapacity* for felt experience. How might we, as therapists, learn to tell the difference as we sit with and experience the backdraft of fear in the consulting room? Many trauma clients have a great fear of reclaiming a body/mind that holds and mediates traumatic reactions; of loosening the defensive structures that have ensured survival and of changing boundary functions. Bromberg ([1998] 2001: 133) refers to Winnicott's concept of fear of the breakdown which has already happened. Clients sometimes indicate that they come into therapy because they 'can't go back there again' – to the place of collapse and disintegration. For others, talking makes 'it' – the traumatic past – more real, and while this is often experienced as helpful, it clearly has its downside.

Responses to fear

Dropping in

Imagine that you have just left a cinema in a lively town centre at night, and are making your way to a bus stop. Your attention is suddenly caught by a disturbance caused by a group of very angry young white people spilling onto the street from a nearby pub. Spotting a nearby group of Black youths, a fight develops quickly, and as some of them break into a run past you with others in pursuit, a shop window is smashed and bottles are thrown. You take cover in a shop doorway.

As you attend to the rapidly changing field conditions, what happens to your sense of embodiment? Take a moment to check if you are aware of how your body responds. Notice what happens in your arms and legs, to your breathing, to your heart rate. Does the temperature of your skin change; do you notice tingling or any other sensations? Do you have any other impulse to move? Do you notice any changes to your contact functions of sight and hearing in particular? What happens to your thought processes at this moment? Perhaps you notice a tendency towards chaos or rigidity, or both. Did you make a conscious decision to move into the doorway or did it 'just happen'?

Finally, it is relevant to think in terms of the following contextualization of the situation described: 'Any understanding of the violence of street culture in the inner city needs to be placed in its historical and structural context lest it serve to confirm racist stereotypes and psychological-reductionist interpretations that blame victims' (Scheper-Hughes and Bourgois 2004: 304). This context will include poverty, structural racism, poor education and lack of opportunity to work.

Fear has intense visceral qualities. Keenan describes it thus: 'I felt my own fear claw out and crawl over my flesh' (Keenan 1993: 46), adding '[It] will not let me go' (Keenan 1993: 64). First, there is an abrupt and unexpected change of figure, the shock element. The sense of outer reality redefines the contact boundary, and the sense of self/other becomes confused (see Figure 1.2). In situations like this many people recoil and become still, contracting muscles and making themselves smaller and narrower. It is interesting to note how completely the body corresponds to the situation. The drawing in and narrowing you probably noticed may be an evolutionarily based response creating a smaller or less visible 'target'.

Fear involves a retroflection of energy, suspending the easy flow of movement. In order to stay alert, the flow of fluids throughout the body is retarded (interview with Bainbridge Cohen, in Johnson 1995: 190). This outer stillness may be accompanied by an internal sense of high activation, while numbness is equally possible. There is a suspension of time. Other sensations you may have noticed in response to the above scenario would likely be signs of preparing to defend yourself either actively or through freezing, about which more will be said shortly. Individual responses will inevitably be shaped both by personal and societal history. As Scheper-Hughes observes: 'A constant self-mobilization for alarm, a state of constant hyperarousal is, perhaps, a reasonable response to [a] view of late modern history as a "chronic state of emergency"' (Scheper-Hughes and Bourgois 2004: 21). Any thoughts present are likely to be a variant of 'I'm not safe', 'I'm going to get hurt' or 'I'm not in control'.

Fear is a regulator or moderator of contact, reorganizing the contact boundary. Generally, attention to the field reduces the sense of embodiment, compromising contact, given that contact is a function of the bodily senses, perceptions, posture and movement. For example, Hesse and Main point out how lapses in reasoning or discourse may indicate unintegrated fear (cited in Siegel 1999: 111). What, then, about lack of reasoning in contemporary public discourse? Most contact functions are, however, non-verbal. In Chapter 8, we will look further at the changes in sensory perception that can accompany dissociation.

Because of the vivid reliving of trauma as though it were in the present, fear and its associated manifestations become an organizing principle in the victim's life (Cozolino 2002: 251). It is as though the victim has an internal smoke detector which goes off when the toast is burning. It signals 'Get out! Get out!' when there is no real emergency. Porges (2009: 46) states that 'some individuals experience a mismatch wherein the nervous system appraises the environment as dangerous, even when it is safe'. It is this mismatch that reinforces and maintains the hypervigilance of many trauma clients. There is clearly a perceptual difficulty here, usefully summarized as **False Evidence Alters Reality**. Perls et al. ([1951] 1998: 30) describe such chronic apprehensiveness as a 'misapprehension of actuality'.

Orienting to danger

Traumatized people are frequently on the alert for signs of danger, specifically to perceived danger rather than actual threat. You will notice an exaggerated startle response in some victims, who react to relatively low-key stimuli. Sensorimotor psychotherapy proposes the orienting response as a way of identifying how a client organizes their experience. The orienting response goes hand in hand with hypervigilance, keeping the perception of threat and the sense of danger in the foreground of the victim's experience.

The body anticipates posturally what is feared to happen, and this can be observed phenomenologically in the limbs as well as in the torso, leaning forward, pulling back or twisting away. 'What we turn our attention to, or orient to, determines not only our physical actions but our mental actions as well' (Ogden et al. 2006: 65). Hypervigilance comes in different guises; it can be generalized into health anxiety, restlessness, anticipatory anxiety or disproportionate impatience. Over time this response becomes reflexive (Cozolino 2002: 246), learnt from past experience. An example of this is illustrated by someone I will call Maria.

Clinical vignette

Maria lived much of her life with symptoms of severe dissociation. I noticed that she became particularly activated when her eyes moved towards the right. The first time I pointed this out to her and suggested that she tried turning towards the left, something small shifted, and she reported that her childhood bedroom door was on the right. The following session, when Maria was standing at the window alerted by noises outside, I noticed a similar state switch accompanied by looking towards the right. Again I suggested looking towards the left, which Maria did, but this time, because she was standing, she was able to shuffle her feet round to the left, while keeping her eyes on the same spot. This aligned her head and torso habitually again to the right.

Having repeated these dance steps a few more times, I then understood that it was not just Maria's eyes that oriented towards the perceived threat, but her whole body. The difficulty was not about looking – an external focus – but about the position of her head in relation to her shoulders. When Maria was sitting down again I suggested repeating the experiment, with a subtle differ-ence. Instead of asking her to look towards the left, I asked her to turn her head towards the left. Because in the sitting position she could not move her feet, this movement helped reorganize the familiar relationship of head to shoulders and torso. Maria immediately responded, 'Oh, I feel calm now, more stable'. (This story appears also in Taylor 2013.)

This vignette illustrates the somatic basis of the orienting response. Maria was orienting to an internal stimulus which clearly felt vivid and present to her; she literally was keeping an eye on threat. This is an example of implicit somatic memory (Siegel 1999: 28), and it was not necessary to work with the 'story' behind it in order to create a shift. However, had I chosen to explore the figure of the door, I imagine that Maria would have remained dissociated and there would have been no therapeutic value. In orienting towards her experience of the door, Maria was physically and psychologically anticipating some aversive experience. By focusing her attention on a different experience, she was able to obtain new information about herself and her surroundings, permitting the emergence of a resource which interrupted her tendency to relive the trauma. In order to integrate this resource it was necessary over time to repeat the new orientation until Maria had learnt it for herself.

The neurobiology of fear

What follows is an overview of how neuroscience highlights the experience of trauma, specifically of fear. The writers and researchers I reference all repre-sent a western 'scientific' or medical model which seeks to explain definitively what is happening in the individual brain. As I have said, neuroscience is not the only way of making sense of some difficult experiences. I present these perspectives here for their potential contribution to understanding the experience of the people we work with, and of possible ways of supporting them.

Fear is both an innate and a conditioned response to threat. It is hardwired in us. Babies show fear in the presence of a loud noise or scary face, even if they haven't experienced these before. For trauma clients the response is learnt or conditioned in the Pavlovian sense. The effects of this conditioning may be long lasting. 'We have to learn what to be afraid of, not how to act afraid' (LeDoux 2002: 213). The brain is predisposed to associate fear with threatening stimuli, but completely neutral or meaningless stimuli can have this effect too (Panksepp 1998: 215). There appears to be a neural circuit in the brain which implicates the amygdala in fear processes (Panksepp 1998: 207; Damasio 2000: 61; Cozolino 2002: 242). The amygdala, sitting in the mid-brain, is assumed to trigger activation of the ANS and has branches to many areas of the body/ mind. It is this distribution of branches throughout the body that explains why the response to threat involves visceral, sensory and motor elements, making the experience a 'whole body phenomenon' (Cozolino 2002: 243).

The amygdala is believed to store fear memories in its circuits through association, and monitors the world for safety and threat. At the same time the hippocampus helps to evaluate and appraise the *context* of the danger, and contributes to the feeling that the traumatic event is ongoing (Rothschild 2000: 12). So, when you see a brawl on television or in a film you don't react in the same ways as you would if it were happening in real time in front of you. The response arises from a fear-laden ground without accurate appraisal of the threat. The site of these fear circuits in the subcortical area of the brain explains why we react to certain stimuli before we can think (Rothschild 2000: 239), the 'chatter' of the frontal cortex shutting down.

> As we move ... towards fear, then, we necessarily rely on lower and faster brain regions ... our responses are reflexive and under virtually no conscious control.
>
> (Perry and Szalawitz 2006: 49)

LeDoux (2002: 217) describes the relationship between the frontal cortex and the amygdala, suggesting that each inhibits the activity of the other. This is a closed, mutually reinforcing loop. When the amygdala is aroused it can modify the processing of sensory information in the cortex (LeDoux 2002: 227), and *increases emotional tone over cognitive function.* Meaning-making is compromised. There are clear implications for therapy with trauma clients who chronically avoid triggers or are hypervigilant, or both.

There are both neuronal and chemical reasons for the changes in the brain as a result of chronic stress, anxiety and fear. Recall Hebb's Axiom, that neurons that fire together wire together. Stress reactivates fear circuits which have previously been laid down (Cozolino 2002: 247). Stimulated repeatedly over time, the neural pathways involved in fear become 'hyperpotentiated'. This means that the resulting degree of fear is greater than the sum of the stimuli. Consequently, it takes a lesser stressor to reactivate the pathway (Cozolino 2002: 246).

Cortisol, which is a hormone released under stress from the adrenal glands, is a neurotransmitter which is key to information processing in the brain. Cortisol supports the organism in times of heightened stress, in particular increasing blood sugars to supply energy for the fight or flight response, and it slows down digestion which is not of primary survival value in the moment. It has a particular impact on the amygdala, increasing the intensity of fear reactions. Chronic release of cortisol has toxic effects on the body, and eventually the adrenal glands become exhausted and cease producing it. The result is that the protective function of cortisol is no longer available, and the individual is increasingly triggered by small stimuli.

Chronic exposure to stress is also thought to damage brain structures. This is particularly significant for people who have been subject to early abuse as well as those who live as adults in dangerous situations, such as war or domestic violence. There is a biological link between prolonged stress and reduced volume of the hippocampus, caused most likely by the presence of increased levels of certain neurochemicals. So, for chronically stressed individuals, it is easy to deduce that their ability to use contextual cues in the appraisal of threat is compromised, influencing 'the nature of emotional experience and emotion regulation' (Siegel 1999: 248). High levels of these chemicals in the bloodstream may also suppress the immune system and contribute to increased physical illness in some chronically fearful people (Cozolino 2002: 251–2).

Broadening the frame to a societal one, Taussig asks '[W]hat does it take to understand our reality as a chronic state of emergency, as a Nervous System?' (2004: 270). What happens, if a sense of safety is taken as a given, for people whose skin colour arouses suspicion on a daily basis? It is not uncommon for people of colour and Black people to be followed by store security because they fit a 'stereotype' of a shoplifter (Mackenzie-Mavinga 2009). How do you feel safe inside your own skin in such conditions? Or for those whose need of a social safety net proves to be more of a threat? There is evidence of victims of domestic abuse trying to access benefits to which they are entitled being 'subjected to further torment and placed at more risk by their mere interaction with the Welfare State' (McGarvey 2022: 176). A lack of safety is reflected throughout contemporary western societies. Could a chronic state of alarm in our collective nervous system account for the increased polarization of ideas and thinking, loss of flexibility, of the speed of 'cancel culture', the immersion in consumption and the operation of various forms of denial that we observe in contemporary western societies? Might we begin to value some of these for their defensive or regulatory functions?

Survival-based defences

The need to defend ourselves from threat is hardwired and inextricably linked with the need for survival. Defences are adaptive to circumstances so that, in ideal conditions, we have a degree of natural flexibility in response. In addition, we can see defences operating beyond the individual at the level of organizations and cultures: systemic fight, flight or freeze. Importantly, Cozolino (2002: 247) states that under stress we tend to regress to more primitive, subcortical defence mechanisms. Defensive systems are closely related to the orienting tendency in that the field of consciousness is narrowed (Ogden et al. 2006: 90). In trauma victims the problem is one of inflexibility of response (Ogden et al. 2006: 89). This is the result of defence mechanisms becoming conditioned over time: 'When a defensive behaviour is successful, it becomes recorded as effective; the chance of the same behaviour being used in a future threatening situation increases' (Rothschild 2000: 54).

However, repetition can be understood as an attempt to solve a problem for which there was no escape, no way of moving on until the situation can be completed. Janet, writing in the early twentieth century, said '[These clients] … have not been able to perform any of the actions characteristic of the stage of triumph' (Janet 1925: 669, cited in Ogden et al. 2006: 86). Along the same lines, Perls et al. ([1951] 1998: 77) write: 'It is a basic tendency of the organism to complete any situation or transaction for which it is unfinished.' So the defence continues to be a means of survival until the trauma can be 'completed' or processed.

The relationship between fear and danger suggests the possibility of escape, whereas shock relates to life threat, with no chance of escape. What determines whether someone develops a chronic trauma condition is not so much the degree of threat, but their inability to complete a defensive manoeuvre. If someone is overpowered or trapped, the instinct to mobilize towards escape is truncated, and fight and flight defences give way to more immobilized ways of dealing with the situation.

Fight and flight are active, mobilized defences, along with the instinct to reach or call out for others. The person being raped cries out for help; George Floyd called for his mother – the 'attachment cry'. In contrast to these mobilized defences are the immobilized defences of freezing and submission. Freezing involves alert immobility, rather like a rabbit in a car headlights. Submission is a state of collapse with profound inhibition of motor activity, more akin to the mouse in the cat's jaws feigning death. These patterns, or combinations of them, show up behaviourally, physiologically and posturally in many trauma clients. It is popular to summarize these defences as the 'Five F's': Fight, Flight, Freeze, Flop and Friend. 'When the mobilizing defences have failed entirely or produced only partial success in preventing trauma, the person may become traumatized' (Ogden et al. 2006: 92). A sequence of defensive responses has been proposed (Ogden et al. 2006: 98), as follows:

• Marked change in arousal
• Heightened orienting response
• Attachment and social engagement systems
• Mobilizing defensive strategies
• Immobilizing defensive strategies

This is a hierarchy of defences, and highlights the need to *reverse* the sequence in therapy where clients have become immobilized. Clients often experience flight impulses in their legs, but they can also be observed in 'twisting, turning or backing away' (Ogden et al. 2006: 91). Flight may be concerned with running towards safety or an attachment figure. Fight responses more typically involve the arms, hands and shoulders, narrowing of the eyes, jutting of the jaw or the impulse to kick or struggle (Ogden et al. 2006: 92). Clinically, it is helpful to be able to track and to work with these phenomena.

Clinical vignette

Maggie reported that she felt like running out of the therapy room. I encouraged her to stay with the sensations that she noticed in her legs and to make fast running movements while she was sitting. She found these rhythmic movements helpful and began to calm down. I then suggested that she made slow running movements, and then added a further stage to the experiment in which she slowly increased the speed and noticed the point at which she felt the impulse to escape emerge. Her comment was, 'I can do this, I can do it!' This sequence of movements helped Maggie follow her energetic charge while establishing some embodied control, and to fine-tune her awareness of her process.

Ogden et al. (2006: 101) observe that when hyperarousal accompanied by immobilization has been the habitual response to trauma, we often see arousal return to baseline through discharge and dissipation made possible by physical activity.

Risky behaviour

Let's take a look at the counter-intuitive *functional* value of risky and harmful behaviour. This is a complicated issue with no single explanation. Pain may be reduced as a result of secretion of opiates induced by *reactivation* of fear (van der Kolk and Greenberg 1987: 72). It is possible to experience analgesia as a function of immobility (Rothschild 2000: 49). Some trauma victims seek out dangerous situations, either deliberately or out of awareness. One young rape victim, for example, didn't think twice about accepting a lift from drunken strangers until later. Repetition compulsion can be understood as an attempt to complete the unfinished gestalt. It may be an attempt to relive and master the overwhelming feelings of the traumatic moment (Herman 1992: 42), or an act of bravado that preserves the integrity of the self – 'Nothing frightens me now' – and seeking stimulation can help organize sensation. The window of tolerance concept supports the notion that someone who is activated may feel more alive than in a dissociated or neutral state.

Bromberg suggests this:

Around each corner is potential trauma; peace is simply the calm before the storm, and if he goes too long without verification of the reality of his dread,

> he needs to find some event that provides evidence that justifies his felt
> need for vigilance in a world of traumatic reality.
>
> (Bromberg [1998] 2001: 260)

A client complained that life had become too calm and pleasant: 'I know I should like it, but I need danger', they said.

Risks are sometimes subtle because the behaviour links to passive defences. According to Kepner (1995: 61), 'We all tend to seek environments that match the self-functions we have.' So, if a client hasn't yet learnt to establish clear boundaries, for example, they may adopt a victim role in the pejorative sense and be repeatedly taken advantage of by others. Particular consideration needs to be given here to victims of domestic violence. It is a pervasive misconception that these individuals should 'just leave'. The issue is complicated by the nature of traumatic attachment (see below and Chapter 13). However, taking into account the theory of mobilized and immobilized defences, the riskiest time of all in domestic violence is the point at which the victim asserts their power and begins to act. Most victims know this implicitly, and fear justifiably keeps them trapped.

I think we need to be very careful about how we conceptualize risk and how we 'manage' it in clinical settings. It is easy to become moralistic about some behaviours (Fanen 2022: 148) without making sense of their function for the individual, and to fall uncritically into systems of control that exert power over (Taylor 2021: 121) and lack cultural sensitivity. Clinical experience shows that, as a sense of safety develops and fear is less figural in a client's life, so these risks diminish, but this can take a very long time. Clinicians and services need to manage their anxiety about this without imposing expectations of 'good behaviour'. Clients begin to be more attentive to their regulatory behaviour only when real alternatives are available. But for others, like the client needing danger, it is helpful to try to transform this tendency into healthy excitement.

A secure base

> Fear needs to be tamed in order for people to be able to think and be conscious of their needs. A person's bodily response of fear can be mitigated by safety of attachments ... and by a body whose reactions to environmental stress can be predicted and controlled.
>
> (van der Kolk [1996] 2007: 205)

Given that I position the experience of trauma as one of disconnection or dislocation, I think it is interesting to consider safety, the polarity of fear, as an attachment issue. By attachment in this sense, I mean relationships or structures that offer a sense of predictability at a minimum, and add depth and meaning to the sense of self in the world at best. Recall, if you will, Stolorow's comment about the destruction of the 'absolutisms' of everyday life (Chapter 1). These absolutisms include not only trusted personal relationships, but culture, community, routines, homes, places, schools and workplaces among others.

When I worked with young people, there was a terrifying attack at a local school, witnessed by a number of pupils. One young person came to see me after I was approached by their mother for help. We talked about everyday life, comfort and the things they enjoyed, keeping things quiet and familiar. A month later they were settling well. Another parent called in great distress, blaming the school, and pulled their child from it. I don't know how this young person fared over time, but I imagine less well. Their parent's reactivity, understandable in so many ways, would have been a factor in their recovery.

It is too easy for therapists, 'secure' in a neurobiological model, to assume that safety is an internal process, independent of external factors; an all-knowing position is powerful and misses the context. The experience of safety is not the same for any two people, nor across cultures. My assumptions were called into question when running a workshop series soon after the protests at the Belarussian election of 2020. One participant asked 'How can I feel safe when there are guns in the street outside?' I didn't know how to answer. Their fear was absolutely proportionate to the situation, and the theory unhelpful. Here, the predictability of the given order of political and social life was being rapidly undermined, regardless of political affiliation. We worked slowly over time to establish some trust in the group and could do little more than hold curiosity and compassion, which did make some difference.

The position of political, economic and climate refugees is another example where multiple absolutisms may be torn aside. Their journeys away from fear and towards safety have for so many added layer upon layer of trauma, perhaps through their contact with exploitative traffickers and dangerous means of travel. The ways in which they are received into their new country will either compound or serve to relieve the trauma of their dislocation. Having to recount their story to justify their entry into a host country may well be retraumatizing. Whose agenda does it serve to keep them in fear and enduring uncertainty as their applications for asylum are processed? Once in therapy, an interpreter speaking in their native language may become a more important attachment figure than the therapist.

Establishing safety

Safety as a concept is not accessible to all clients. Indeed, for some it can feel dangerous, implying that they must drop their hard-earned adjustments to a terrifying world. 'Safe' may be a word that has been used by an abuser and therefore its use may need to be avoided until it can be tolerated. Replace it with 'calm', 'peaceful', 'feeling quiet inside', so that you can develop a shared meaning.

- The establishment of safety is recognized as a primary function in recovery from trauma. Everyone needs to feel safe and it is a fundamental human right. We need to distinguish between environmental safety and an inner sense of safety. It is potentially harmful to work towards safety with someone who is living in a situation of grave threat, therefore the extent of safety possible is a function of the situation. It is more an inner sense of safety that is required, by which I mean the ability to recover a degree of equilibrium, to find the ground and to create boundaries. This relates to access to resources as implicit in the window of tolerance or ventral vagal states, not as ideals but as potentials. The premise of the ventral vagal state is individualistic, and to some extent one of privilege; Fanen (2022: 120) poses the critical question 'Whose oppression must exist in order for me to feel safe?' Personal safety may be predicated on access to resources, such as quiet and undisturbed time in nature. I suggest that a ventral vagal state is comparable to the Zen-like centre zone of the window of tolerance (Chapter 4) and does not necessarily give room for growth and healthy risk or exploration. Perhaps we have gone too far towards necessary safety and need to let the pendulum swing back a little. The premise of individual safety underlines the need for a body-based approach in therapy. Only if we feel safe internally can we engage actively with the environment and increase contact. Please try the experiment in the box here. It is crucial, as we shall see, that therapists have access to their own resources and sense of inner safety.

Dropping in

Here is a process that I have used or modified many times: one enquiry is to consider what kind of environment is needed to help you feel as settled as you know how, quiet and at ease. Can you begin to picture it or remember it if it is somewhere you know? It is helpful to make some simple conditions: it must be somewhere they can feel fully their self; no one can make any demands of them or have any expectation of them; nothing bad can happen there. Therapists may need to be quite insistent about this last point using a little bit of creative 'magic' to ensure that the tree-house can't fall down in high winds, for example. With an emphasis on slow integration, therapists should work with each of the client's senses in turn to build up a detailed experiential picture of the place; for example, using the sense of sight to attend to textures, colours, shapes, light, movement, and similarly for each of the other senses. Bring in also the client's sense of their body in this place, including posture, interoceptive awareness, movement and emotional responses. Really linger with each component of the whole experience, making it as vivid as possible. Find out what it means to your client to have this place, with these conditions, and how they could make use of this in future.

- This approach to developing a sense of safe place is not appropriate for all clients. It is a top-down method that leads to embodiment. A more bottom-up way is to suggest clients choose a colour, sound or other experience that represents calm, and to work to integrate it in a similar fashion. We need to encourage all the senses and cognitive modalities to build resources such as these because integration does not result from the activity of one system of the brain alone (Grigsby and Osuch 2007: 49). There is plenty of scope for creativity with this concept once you have grasped it. You are strongly recommended to try this for yourself before offering it to people you work with. An effective therapist understands safety or the absence of it from the inside.

- To a large extent, the figure of fear will only be mitigated when there is more focus on ground. There are far too many possibilities to name here, but relationship to gravity and the support of the earth is a fundamental consideration. Grounding, gravity and bonding take us closer to the earth. Grounding relates to 'our contact with the body, the earth, nature, other human beings, family, culture, country, God' (Anagnostopoulou 2015: 686). An important aspect of grounding lies in the body, providing a sense of continuity and ongoingness of self. Boadella (1987: 94) offers the opinion that we need to find our sense of inner ground, such as the stability of our spine, the regularity of heart beat, our inner rhythms. Coming home to the body is therefore necessary, by means primarily of a phenomenological approach. The bodily adjustments that accompany grounding may include a release of tension, a slowing of heart rate and of breathing, and greater perceptual acuity. There is a sense of greater safety and opening, while a sense of belonging and connection can also be expected. The feeling of being held, by the earth or by the chair, may be appreciated, while noticing how the individual may resist this by engaging their muscles. Implicit in resistance is lack of trust in support of anything external and overreliance on self. The process of grounding is therefore both physiological and psychological (Anagnostopoulou 2015: 686).

- An overarching principle of working phenomenologically to reduce fear is to limit the stimuli at any moment, by which I mean to identify the smallest aspect of experience possible and linger with it.

- The breakdown of the contact boundary that defines trauma points to working with boundaries. This not only reduces fear but begins to create a shape of the formlessness of undifferentiated trauma. A sense of where I end and you begin is absent for many traumatized people, and this is also culturally mediated, especially where working across cultures or ethnicities. The meaning of contact must be appraised on an individual basis. Awareness of boundaries is a valuable starting point and sensorimotor trauma therapy offers embodied approaches to this. You might, for example, suggest the person you are working with sit on the floor, placing a long loop of cord or rope around them to represent the boundary. Then slowly roll a ball towards them, coming to the edge of the loop or crossing it, and invite the person to notice their responses. You can try something similar by walking very slowly towards them, and stopping when you sense you have reached the boundary. Invite the person to use their hands to 'draw' out a boundary all around them, establishing a sense of how much space they need. Unpacking each of these is critical to integrating them and raising corrective experiences.

- Developing dual awareness supports a more accurate appraisal of current circumstances (see Chapter 5). The client needs to be able to recognize that they are remembering something that is over now, even where the memory is distressing; this is the difference between an actual event and a trigger. The important thing is to know that it is not happening now, and a reality check is helpful: 'Can you have a look around and see if anything bad is happening right here, right now?'

- Where fear tends to focus on particular figures of potential threat, it is helpful to be able to widen the aperture of perception. Simply enquiring about what else is happening in the environment or in the body at this moment can make a difference. The tendency to generalize fear diverts attention from neutral or positive experiences – a moment of ease or relief or pleasure may be ignored until you call attention to this. You might find words like: 'You feel tight and anxious in your belly and your breathing is shallow ... is there somewhere else in your body that feels easier than this, even a tiny place like the end of your nose or your little toe? ... Great, just stay with that...'. Well-timed, this line of enquiry will be welcomed by many.

- Learning to drop the story is another way of refocusing attention and down-regulating the process. This often requires the therapist's active intervention, by way of interrupting and supporting a shift in the work when the narrative strays away from the process. You may want to agree a limit to how much story comes in: 'What might be telling you that this is too much? How will I recognize that with you?' In this way, you work only with small slivers of memory which might be tolerated and integrated, returning to a more resourced state until the person lets you know they are ready to proceed.

- The notion of co-regulation is absolutely critical here. The therapist is working to help the individual learn their limits of tolerance and to drop into a resource when it gets too much. This may need to happen many, many times over before they can recognize and manage this for themselves.

Case study: Part 1

The background

Eve was in her mid-30s and working for a mental health charity when she came into therapy. She was a single mother with a 6-year-old daughter, Freya, from a brief relationship. The first story she told me was about her boss who was intrusive, bullying and sexually inappropriate. He was looking at her diary behind her back and cancelling meetings that she had planned. Eve felt undermined and humiliated by this, as though the remit of her job was being changed without discussion. It seemed to Eve that there was a hidden agenda which confused her. As we began to explore this current relationship, Eve was able to start telling me about a trauma that she had experienced in her twenties. She had been working for a medical charity in a refugee camp in Greece. One day she went to meet someone to arrange the delivery of some supplies when she was taken to a derelict building by two men, held hostage and raped. It became clear that Eve's current work situation was triggering old material. Interwoven with these themes was her strained relationship with her parents and her difficulty in communicating her need for support effectively.

Eve's feelings about not being taken seriously by her parents began to make sense when she spoke of a difficult time in her childhood years. Her paternal grandfather had come to live with the family when Eve was 13 because he was developing dementia and could no longer live independently. A symptom of his dementia was his sexually disinhibited behaviour and Eve had been the main target of his attentions. Eve's mother had responded by becoming depressed and taking to her bedroom, while her father coped by laughing the whole thing off.

Working with Eve

Eve's high level of anxiety when I first met her was an immediate concern. She sat tensely, seeming to have an unbalanced relationship to gravity as she tilted forwards and rested only her toes on the ground. She didn't stop moving her hands, eyes and head. Eve's voice was clear, unsupported by her shallow breath. I sensed a protectiveness in her crisp and efficient speech. She told me she felt abused and sorely lacking in protection. I didn't know why, but my felt response to her was a sorrowful but unspoken question, 'What on earth has happened to you?' I wanted to reach out gently, intuitively picking up that Eve was petrified.

As Eve told me about what brought her into therapy, feeling controlled by her symptoms, I registered viscerally that she felt unsafe in her work relationships, feeling fear for her myself. It puzzled me as my feeling seemed bigger than her story, but I trusted that this meant something that we did not yet understand. Because of this, and because it could do no harm, I chose to begin with talking about helping Eve to feel quiet inside. When we looked at the window of tolerance map together, it became clear that Eve related to both the phenomenology of hyper- and hypoarousal. Most of all, the map made sense to her and that gave us the opportunity to negotiate the way forward. It seemed a good way to meet Eve initially.

Eve's emerging trauma provided me with some relief as I made sense of my strong reactions to her. She began to be aware of the many ways in which she was being triggered, and that in turn made sense of feelings and sensations that accompanied situations in her current life. Eve was sleeping poorly and reported that she often woke with a start, which distressed her, though she had no recall of dreams. She was quite preoccupied with her relationship to her boss, feeling trapped and terrified of his presence, which she avoided often through taking sick leave when she was due to meet with him.

We worked consistently and carefully with safety, helping Eve to identify the feelings associated with her thought processes and finding ways of returning to a calmer state within her window of tolerance, by altering the focus of her attention, particularly using her safe place. While in Greece, Eve had dived off the coast and returned to the peace of that underwater environment in her imagination. I noted Eve's rapid glances at the door when she was hyperaroused, which I thought was her orienting response, imagining that she was being triggered in a closed space. I frequently worked to recover Eve's sense of where she was and her place in current time.

It was necessary to understand Eve's phobias, particularly of her pain and of body sensation. Eve had a recurring painful body memory which caused her to be fearful of approaching any charged topics. For her, learning to feel again might make the trauma real. Increasingly she was able to know for herself what she could and couldn't talk about and we discussed sometimes what might help her to feel more supported. In this way she was learning to recognize and manage her fears.

Eve invariably avoided busy situations like supermarkets, where standing in a queue brought her into too close proximity to others. She shopped at quiet times of the evening, even though this was not ideal for Freya. We worked on her sense of boundaries, and Eve had a great deal of difficulty in asking me to stop during an experiment in which I approached her slowly. She had no sense of her ability to say 'No' to me or identify what she needed from me. Over time, she developed the ability to ask me to have my chair at a certain distance from her; she became sensitive to any changes in my position; a more differentiated awareness. The concept of the boundaries of her own body, and of her skin as a container, was a complete mystery to her to begin with. 'Boundaries are out there', she told me. However, she began to get a sense of the difference that being wrapped in a blanket made to her, and she treated herself to a new fluffy throw to use at home.

I had to be quite clear with Eve that, given the lack of safety in her ongoing relationship with her boss, there were limits to the work we could do. Safety needs to be both internal and external, and Eve understood this. One focus of our work over time was therefore what she wanted to do to change this aspect of her life. As a single mother, there were of course financial considerations to keep her in her job. She worried that the amount of sickness absence she had taken would be used against her in finding a new job. The idea of speaking up about her boss caused her to have panic attacks, based on a fear of him becoming violent, without any evidence for this.

Summary

Fear is a symptom which may carry a story about past trauma and unfinished business. It is a major organizer of figure and ground in the experience of trauma victims. It carries with it elements of pervasive terror about both external and internal threat. The fear response in trauma clients is conditioned and may be state dependent. Because it has become generalized, as far as the client is concerned fear is related to current reality. It is a problem of perception in which past and present cannot be distinguished, leaving the client in a state of alarm. A state of heightened fear can be triggered by any object, situation, person or experience that is sufficiently reminiscent of the original trauma to have become associated with it. Clinically, fear presents as avoidance and hypervigilance as well as in postural, behavioural and physiological adjustments.

One consequence of fear is that clients tend to narrow their field of awareness, focusing on danger to the exclusion of other contextual cues. This tendency is referred to as the orienting response. The implication for therapy is that by widening or redirecting the focus of attention, new possibilities for orienting towards safety emerge. The orienting response is biologically driven, closely connected to survival instincts. Neural circuits concerned with fear and appraisal of threat operate in different areas of the brain, particularly in the amygdala and hippocampus, connecting to the ANS and the viscera. Coupled with these networks, chemicals related to stress play a significant role in the response to threat, and act very rapidly indeed. The hormone cortisol is particularly concerned with responses to threat and under prolonged stress can be damaging to structures of the anatomical brain. The felt experience of fear involves the whole sensory-motor body/mind. These responses are not within conscious control, the integrative capacity of the cortex having become uncoupled in the process.

Once the orienting response has initiated an emergency reaction, survival-based defence processes take over. These can be grouped into mobilized defences of help-seeking, fight and flight, or immobilized defences of freezing and submission. In cases of extreme danger there can be greater survival value in becoming immobilized, which can de-escalate threat. These defensive tendencies become deeply embodied and re-emerge in the clinical setting when the client is triggered. It is an important task of therapy to help the immobilized client to reverse the process towards **mobilization.**

A further situation where fear may present is in clients who take risks. There are a number of possible ways of understanding this kind of behaviour, and they may coexist in individual clients. There are important implications for risk management by therapists.

Learning skills related to safety is also survival-based and is essential for recovery from trauma. These skills may begin with an embodied sense of a safe place to which the client may 'return' in memory when needed. In order to support emotional regulation and tolerance of internal experience, the ability to feel grounded and contained is invaluable. To do so requires the development of a range of somatic resources, built slowly and carefully over time. For some, though, the development of safety cannot be approached directly, and caution and less direct routes to the same end must be found.

7 From helplessness towards agency

The sense of helplessness is a very pervasive and implicit experience for trauma victims. This chapter looks at helplessness as a feature of immobilized defences both for its psychological impact and its embodied effects. In contrast, Gestalt therapy principles of mobilization and fluid process are considered. The chapter continues by exploring changes in interpersonal dynamics and the locus of control shift which alters the client's sense of self and other. Autonomy and self-agency are discussed, setting up an enquiry into how trauma clients can be supported to regain control over their own bodies and feel more powerful. The role of anger as a differentiating emotion is explored.

The relationship between fear and helplessness is very close. Overwhelming fear paralyses us; we become 'scared stiff' (Levine 2010: 49). To be overpowered or trapped means to feel pervasive loss of ground in the continuity of self. Even finding the language to describe the experience creates helplessness. We literally do not know what to do with ourselves or which way to turn, or even that there might be something to be done. There can be a loss of sense of volition and intention in the body, and self-concept as someone with agency is usually radically altered. Trauma victims no longer have a sense of control over their life and immobilized defences of freezing and collapse are not appreciated for their survival value. In situations of societal oppression and injustice this loss of control is real and ongoing. More probably, clients will condemn themselves for not having taking action. So, the feeling of being helpless continues or repeats the original trauma. Bromberg ([1998] 2001: 302) recognizes helplessness as an inevitable though frequently hidden self-state of people who have experienced trauma. A sense of helplessness is therefore one of the most pernicious effects of trauma.

Helplessness and healthy process – a Gestalt perspective

In Gestalt therapy mobilization is privileged over immobilization because of its role in the healthy formation and completion of gestalts. Fluidity of process is a precondition for the creation of fresh, clear figures. An energetic charge supports the forming figure, building from sensate experience and pushing towards a peak at the contact point of the cycle of experience. The 'glow' of awareness (Perls et al. [1951] 1998: 75) translates into an impulse which may be thwarted, limited or develop at the point of mobilization. In the model used here it is the point of energetic change at which sympathetic arousal takes over from parasympathetic arousal. Mobilization is therefore rather like a fulcrum – an energetic balance point.

Mobilizing depends on sufficient support for action *from the environment* coupled with self-support. There is a point of differentiation in mobilization when an increased sense of 'I' is available. Mobilization therefore plays an important part in the process of 'selfing', moving the individual towards the contact boundary. Energetically, mobilization involves a gathering of self-support, the turning outwards of attention and a preparation to reach out. It is at the stage of mobilization that desires, needs and intentions begin to translate into expression; the possibility of aggressing – acting at the contact boundary – into the world becomes real. It is a point at which there is choice, potential and agency.

Through the lens of trauma theory, however, *im*mobilization is also adaptive because of its survival value in the face of inescapable threat. We have seen that when active defences under environmental threat are not possible the organism's instinctual response is to become immobile. Fogel (2009: 151) suggests that there is a relational and co-regulatory mechanism involved in immobilization. A predator may become more activated by fight or flight reactions and therefore the victim modulates the escalation of the threat by becoming still or feigning death.

The Gestalt therapy premise that in all situations we are doing the best we can is perhaps nowhere more pertinent than at times of literal fear for our lives. Viewed this way, there need be no cause for recrimination or self-blame for the failure of active defences, though as we shall see it is often extremely challenging for clients to accept this. Immobilization has a radical impact on the victim's view of themselves in the world. The victim often experiences severe conflict arising from the wish or impulse to act and the impossibility of doing so. Trauma clients are by definition highly attuned to the wider field, and may lose their sense of capacity to act in situations which are reminiscent of trauma. From a cognitive perspective, a limbically driven immobilized defence is not a function of conscious voluntary control. However, understanding the defensive function of immobilization is invaluable to the therapist, and for the client in developing compassion for the self.

When immobility is chronic, lack of fluid process presents as a fixed gestalt because it does not relate to the actual situation, regardless of how real it may feel. Immobilization is rarely total in the life of a trauma victim, but may rather involve changes in the energetic capacity to maintain the figure formation, and will likely vary under different conditions. Until the stage in therapy has been reached at which a client can restore mobilized responses, we have no alternative but to consider immobilization as a healthy and creative adjustment. Immobilization resulting from trauma needs to be distinguished from resistance, stuckness and impasse, though these may also exist as part of the whole clinical gestalt.

Two kinds of helplessness in the body

One way in which immobilization manifests in trauma clients that sets it apart from 'neurotic' resistance, stuckness or impasse, is that it is not only a psychological construct but is also physiologically and structurally embodied. *In addition* to the physiological responses to threat involving the autonomic nervous system, the muscular and skeletal systems of the body are major players in immobilized responses. Kepner defines what he calls 'adaptive body structure' which 'profoundly affects our physical being in the world' (Kepner [1987] 1999: 48). These structures are characterized as being:

- consistently and persistently used over time
- either frozen into the musculature so that the structure is continually visible, or preprogrammed muscular responses that channel energy and movement into a stylized movement pattern
- automatic and involuntary (under most circumstances)
- not easily or comfortably modified merely by trying to stand or move differently (i.e. behavioural change).

Such structures develop as subjective phenomena in the context of the total field, and have meaning. Kepner ([1987] 1999: 51) describes the inhibition of movement as a disowning of body self, the removal of 'I' from embodied experience. Tensions of the body might represent 'a person's frozen history' (Boadella 1987: 7). Similarly, Fogel (2009: 40) states: 'the memory of the situation becomes frozen in the flesh that has tightened in reaction to it', which can happen on a cellular level.

Dropping in

You can do this experiment standing or sitting.

1 Gather your energy around you, loosely, letting it occupy a space a little larger than your body. Notice how it feels to be with your gathered energy for a moment or two.

2 Now shake it out or pat yourself down.

3 Now gather your energy and allow it to drain out of your body, noticing how the rest of your body responds and in what ways this feels familiar or not. What quality of action might be possible in this state?

4 Shake it out or pat yourself down to return your energy to centre again.

5 With your energy gathered once more, draw it in, to the very core of your body, right in front of your spine. What happens in the rest of your body as you do this? What would it be like to follow through with an impulse in this state?

6 Shake it out or pat yourself down, returning to your state of gathered energy.

7 Make some notes about this experience.

Keleman's thinking about forms of somatic distress (Keleman 1985: 103ff) includes helpful descriptions of the rigid body and the collapsed body, which correspond roughly to the two patterns of helplessness deriving from trauma. Both structures may be observed in one individual, changing according to fluctuating levels of arousal. Keleman (1985: 104) describes rigidity as arising from loss of basic emotional support, which is a condition that many trauma victims experience, including the possibility that their fear may cause others to withdraw. This loss of support from the environment results in the individual becoming overly reliant on themselves, the skeletal bracing both holding and separating. Muscle tone increases in 'strength, thickness and endurance' and there is little sense of inner support (Keleman 1985: 108) or in relationship to the environment. One client told me that freezing was helpful because it allowed them to separate mind and body. Clinical practice shows that there is much effort involved in sustaining this kind of rigidity.

In Keleman's view, the collapsed structure, by contrast, is seen as an adaptation to lack of emotional nourishment and may convey a need to be rescued. Therapist, take note! Keleman (1985: 136) describes low levels of excitement in the collapsed form, with pools of excitement 'gathered ... deep inside in a private place'. The collapsed person has weakened muscle function, a sagging quality unable to resist the force of gravity. The inner core of the body lacks structure and collapses in on itself, and pulsation dies down. Rather poignantly Keleman (1985: 141) says, 'Nothing can move through the organism.' There is a kind of stagnation in which energy, impulse and memory become pooled in the body's systems. The collapsed state needs to be distinguished from the restful recovery of the parasympathetic state; it is more giving up than letting go, which has more conscious and voluntary potential.

Both muscle tone and energy are implicated in the structure of these somatic forms. Body therapists divide muscle tone into hypertonic and hypotonic, which can be tracked by observant therapists. The ability to respond is facilitated by the maximum adaptability of muscle tone, providing control over a maximum of possible responses (Bartenieff, interviewed in Johnson 1995: 277). In either state of immobilized defence there is a pattern of muscular contraction and release that is interrupted by extreme threat. In the frozen state there is heightened contraction, and in the collapsed state there is insufficient containment.

Laura Perls (1992: 126) calls this kind of paralysis a 'half-orientation' with a 'dim … awareness of the responsibility of motoric activity for whatever changes in the situation'. Contraction of a muscle or group of muscles is really only half a movement; an incomplete action. Any fully expressed movement requires both smooth contraction and expansion of muscle. Consider the action of preparing to throw a ball: the arm and shoulder draw back, gathering or mobilizing energy before releasing into the forward thrust. Muscular contraction and release occurs naturally also in breathing, here frozenness being associated with inhalation and collapse with exhalation. Breath is one of the bodily functions over which we have a degree of voluntary control, which has implications for therapy with immobilized trauma clients.

It is but a small step now to link muscle tonus to states of arousal. In hypertonicity, more energy is held in the system than is required for optimal functioning, while in hypotonicity it seems that excessive energy is required in order to complete actions. It is possible to 'map' the theory of muscle tonus onto the cycle of experience whereby hypertonicity relates to sympathetic arousal and mobilization, and hypotonicity relates to parasympathetic arousal and immobility. Muscle tension is one way of suppressing unpleasant feelings (Fogel 2009: 197), and changes in muscle tension are related to changes in emotional state (Fogel 2009: 192). Freezing is not just a lack of movement but 'an integrated, functional behavioural pattern' (Fanselow and Lester, cited in Ogden et al. 2006: 94).

The psychological impact of helplessness

To experience a state of helpless immobility is in itself terrifying because it resembles fear of annihilation or of death (Levine 2010: 16). Fear generates the helpless condition in the first place; fear hinders trauma victims from fully experiencing the helplessness and impulse that otherwise moves towards completion; and fear then prevents an exit from the helpless state. Thus a self-perpetuating feedback loop is established, in which the linkage between fear, immobility and trauma paints a 'complex and nuanced portrait' (Levine 2010: 62).

Devastating events radically alter our ways of being in the world cognitively, emotionally, somatically and relationally: 'Confrontations with violence challenge one's most basic assumptions about the self as invulnerable and intrinsically worthy, and about the world as orderly and just. After abuse [or trauma] the victim's view of self and world can never be the same again' (Reiker and Carmen, cited in van der Kolk and McFarlane [1996] 2007: 15).

I cannot exaggerate the damage to a victim's self-concept after traumatic events. Clients who have experienced a lifetime of trauma may never have had experience of relative safety and agency and therefore may not appreciate the loss initially. There is a myriad of possible manifestations of specific difficulties in relation to self-concept, in multiple combinations. Some broad themes, however, stand out.

The fact that a trauma victim has been unable to complete an active defensive movement and has of necessity resorted to an immobilized defence may lead them to feel betrayed by their own body. They do not have a way of understanding the significance of their adjustment. Add to this the numbing effect of opiate-like hormones released in situations of extreme danger, inherent difficulties in modulating arousal, and the loss of balanced postural support, trauma clients may come to profoundly shut off from any sense of relationship to embodiment. The body may be viewed as simply supporting a cognitive life by providing nutrients, air, locomotion and so on, which mirrors the objectifying of the body that often features in interpersonal trauma.

The ability to feel sensation and impulse may barely register for some people, and they therefore have difficulty organizing a clear figure around awareness of needs. In the absence of a clear sense of body it becomes more difficult to orient appropriately to the demands of the world and to a sense of the present. More positively, however, these clients may function well in education and the workplace where intellectual ability is important, and yet many underachieve.

Levine (1997: 100) links the bound energy of frozen or collapsed states with the high emotional charge of terror, rage and helplessness. For him, helplessness is an emotion. He suggests that it is this linkage with overwhelming emotion that makes it difficult for humans to move out of an immobilized state (Levine 1997: 101). I propose that the terror comes before loss of physical agency and the experience of oppression in the face of a dominant power.

Core beliefs of trauma clients centre around weakness, cowardice and being out of control: 'The helplessness … that follows inescapable shock is due to lack of control rather than to the shock itself' (van der Kolk and Greenberg 1987: 67). Victims may scorn what they perceive as weakness in themselves and others. This may present as a lack of tolerance of personal needs, a belief that it is 'selfish' to privilege one's own interests over another's, or the complete inability to make a decision. For trauma victims there can be strength in self-denial, and value is placed on masochism or self-sacrifice.

Interestingly, helplessness may be another generalized conditioned response to trauma, which affects multiple areas of the victim's life. Flannery (1987: 218) suggests that learnt helplessness is a 'condition in which patients lose their capacity to appreciate the connection between their actions and their ability to influence the course of their lives'. Conversely, some clients may assume an all-powerful position which, having an unstable ground, turns out to be brittle. In such a case there is a disowning of the vulnerability that is part and parcel of helplessness. Trauma clients can get stuck in the roles of victim, rescuer and persecutor which arise from their helplessness.

The shame of helplessness

It takes a tremendous amount of courage, determination and endurance to live with the lasting effects of helplessness. There is also much to grieve for as survivors connect with what wasn't possible. This may lead to a sense of existential despair that takes much resourcefulness to face. Trauma clients may blame themselves for not having protected themselves actively. While the subject of shame is the focus of Chapter 9, it is relevant to the discussion here too. Flannery (1987: 220) considers that people who hold themselves responsible for a situation are more likely to report feeling helpless.

However, blaming oneself in the face of environmental threat may also serve to mitigate the feeling of severe helplessness (Ogden et al. 2006: 263) by creating *an illusion* of having been in control. According to Herman (1992), the inability to act with autonomy sets up conflicts that lead to shame and doubt. She states that 'shame is a response to helplessness, the violation of bodily integrity and the indignity suffered in the eyes of another person' (Herman 1992: 53). It is easy to understand how this leads to confusion about self-as-agent and further withdrawal from the field. Previous experiences of mastery are erased from the self-concept of these clients, with a deep sense of loss of the 'self I once was' or of potential.

A last aspect to consider is that trauma clients tend to identify strongly with their trauma. This may be as a consequence of their loss of a sense of their previous selfhood, but equally it will be because of their excessive focus on the trauma. The all-consuming enterprise of hypervigilance, avoidance and warding off intrusive thoughts and images tends to define the victim's self-concept. 'I am not in control' is a recurring theme in the lives of these clients. Perls et al. ([1951] 1998) describe two processes of the self/other field at the contact boundary: identification and alienation. There is a reciprocal shaping of self and other according to what aspects are identified with and alienated from. In a healthy contact process, these aspects are dynamic, choiceful, flexible and engaged. From a trauma perspective, however, the client identifies with those aspects of the field that relate to traumatic events and their associated survival functions. To the extent that victims perceive the field as traumatic and identify with it, they alienate from aspects of self.

In trauma there is a radical denial of personal power. It is relinquished to those aspects of the field that are identified with, perceived as holding the power to determine the course of one's life. In the actual traumatic moment, 'almost by definition, the individual's point of view counts for nothing' (Herman 1992: 53). Equally, impulses and desires become embedded over time as unresolved and immobilized defences. The victim's life is often at the mercy of others, the situation becoming fixed and incorporated into their belief system. The locus of control in life therefore gives way to the perceived other; this is a shift in the boundary of responsibility. People and situations that have been hurtful continue to be a forceful presence in victims' lives long after they have moved on or ceased to exist. The field is not only dangerous, it is powerful.

Locus of control shift

Immobilization often results from the organization of power and oppression between the self and other/environment. The locus of control (Rotter 1954) in the victim's life is shifted away from the self, with consequences for their sense of self-as-agent. In essence, the concept of locus of control is about how people give away or hold their power. When people perceive the locus of control as outside themselves they feel as though their suffering is not of their own making, and therefore that they can do little to change the situation. Indeed, the social, cultural and material machinery of someone's life may make this all too true. A homeless person in the UK cannot receive benefits without an address, and cannot access accommodation without an income (McGarvey 2022: 159). Sometimes the thing that makes a difference lies in the power of language, but not so for those immigrants who don't have the luxury of being fluent. Rotter's theory suggests that high external locus of control is associated with higher levels of stress, while high internal locus of control is associated with lower levels of stress. I suggest that this is too binary a proposition, at risk of overemphasizing individual responsibility. What instead, if we were to think of external locus of control as being potentially adaptive, or internal locus of control as dissociative?

Sometimes clients' extreme passivity creates a relational position in which they are simply waiting for the next wave of events to overtake them, lurching from one crisis to another. It can be that clients only feel safe in a submissive state, echoing the defensive function of helplessness, which, for example, is protective in ongoing abusive relationships. Unreflective attachment patterns are often problematic, and the shift in power serves to prevent self-destabilization (Bromberg 2006: 7). By displacing attention from self onto the other, the integrity of the self is less under threat. Philippson (2001: 66) considers that fear of loss of control always implies a split between self-states, one part remaining 'in control' while the other is massively dysregulated. Passive clients may come into therapy in order to be 'treated' (Clemmens [1997] 2005: 32), current conditions in a medicalized mental health system reinforcing this position. While we emphasize the need to restore agency, this must not be at the expense of the interpersonal (Wheeler [1991] 1998: 99). Instead, we assume that increased relational skill brings with it some personal power.

Furthermore, not knowing one's positive impact on another reduces a sense of personal power, which shapes the relational field. Clients with complex trauma cannot have a clear sense of self when self-regulation has not been supported relationally. This further has an impact on their ability to be empathic, dialogic and to mentalize. When the outer field has betrayed them, they cannot turn to themselves reliably. Rather than relinquishing control to the other, some clients respond to helplessness by becoming overly controlling in different contexts, and may feel as though their autonomy is threatened by therapists' interventions (Loewenstein and Goodwin 1999: 80). In such ways, the locus of control becomes dichotomized and rigidified. Trauma theory requires a perspective that also includes *actual loss of control* at the moment of trauma and neurological function in its aftermath.

It is wise also to consider the impact of helplessness on the therapist. It is not uncommon to hear of a parallel loss of capacity or confidence in response to helplessness in the field. There is nothing, in my experience, quite like trauma to pull on a rescuer position in the therapist, which I have explored at length elsewhere (Taylor 2021). The depth of the suffering in the people we work with and our personal histories can converge to create a therapeutic field that is difficult to tolerate. Caught in the energetic collapse of helplessness and over-whelm, the therapist may be at a loss to know what to do, or doubt that they have the skill to intervene. This may overlap with a sense of dissociation (see Chapter 8). Recognizing this as familiar is a useful first step, in part because it adds perspective and normalizes the process. Because this can be an accurate reflection of the other person's current experience, admitting that 'I don't know what to say just now' may paradoxically be a potent response; the not knowing is named and shared between you.

Agency and choice

Having a sense of personal power supports the making of choices, which in Gestalt therapy is viewed as an indicator of healthy process: fluidity, 'response-ability' and individuation. A goal of effective trauma therapy can therefore be defined as expansion of the field of choice: 'To be empowered means to be able to choose between options, move towards the chosen object with grace and accept the consequences of one's actions' (Melnick and Nevis 1986: 43).

Intentionality and purposefulness of action are important features of agency:

> The ability to act ... in new ways with intention towards a goal is what we call *agency* or *being an agent* in one's own life. Agency compris[es] [the] capacity for deliberate action as well as the *sense* of agency, or the *feeling* that one is able to act as an autonomous agent.
>
> (Grigsby and Osuch 2007: 38, original italics)

An act of agency is a way in which the organism can alter its own state, and is dependent on its physiology. Getting your own needs met is regulating in a way that helplessness cannot be. Some trauma clients have learnt early in their lives that feelings, impulses and actions are dangerous, and so could not develop a sense of agency or initiate in relationship with others (Sapriel 2012: 107–8). Other functions of agency are to 'notice or empathize with the other and perception of the other as an independent agent' (Fogel 2009: 223). Naranjo (1993: 202) evocatively suggests that to be in action is to be oneself.

Jacobs states that 'The experience of autonomy and agency is *not a product of independence, but is an emergent phenomenon that is utterly dependent on smoothly functioning interdependency*' (Jacobs 2006: 14, my italics). Thus she places the development of agency within the context of the relational field, or, as we might now translate, as an emergent property of an interdependent locus of control. With limited sense of agency, one is not living one's own life.

Taking action

All of the ways of working described below challenge the client's traumatically generated procedural and implicit ways of being in the world; their potential agency increases as does their sense of themselves. Kepner (2002) associates a sense of personal capacity and strength deriving from muscular and movement capacity with the sense of being able to cope. Feelings of mastery and of competence can develop from this work: the sense of 'I can' which has not been available before. This in turn provides a basis for increased resilience in the face of demands and challenges in everyday life.

In the real world outside the therapy room, precise gains in sense of agency may be severely restricted in practice. Returning to a core theme in this volume, agency can only ever be understood in its context. How power operates in the wider field is a determining factor, which includes the availability of resources and opportunity (see Taylor 2021).

A first consideration in resolving helplessness may be to put words to experience. Feeling immobilized and speechless increases the sense of terror that most traumatized people live with. Reclaiming language begins to reconstruct a narrative and the possibility of dialogue that may have been lacking, especially where silencing has been a part of the relational field. A caution is that words need to be held provisionally – the best fit for now. A simple and effective entry point may be to ask, 'Does this feel better or worse? More or less comfortable?' I have found it helpful to offer a 'menu' of possible words such as: 'Does this tension feel bracing, stretching, constricting, pulling … or something else? What's the most accurate word you can find for this?' In this we are not only assisting in dialogue; we offer choice, and in the sense that this is provisional there can be no right or wrong answer.

Offering a framework in which choices are available without judgement or fear of retribution is therapeutic. Many everyday choices do not have consequences – a preference for either marmalade or peanut butter on toast only serves the individual – and some people need to learn this over time. Other choices may have consequences – perhaps going out for the evening because you can't say 'No' to a friend, while leaving your child without a sitter. Moving from the everyday to the therapeutic setting, choices can be woven into the work. 'Last week we agreed that it might be time to look at your relationship with your mother. What do you feel as I remind you? Is it possible to go there today or do we need to do something else first?' This kind of enquiry can be viewed as attentiveness to the ever-shifting parameters of the window of tolerance. 'Tell me when you've had enough' or 'Take your time to check if you are willing to try this' are other approaches; this kind of slowing down may create space for them to take in your support and increase their tolerance for the new experience. Increasing relational capacity might support exploration along the lines of 'How much would you like me to know about this?' or 'How can I support you as we look at this together?'

Someone who is in a helpless state is not actually doing nothing. In essence, they are implicitly working to regulate their environment in the service of survival. There is a great deal of energy tied up in a frozen response, while a collapsed response conserves energy. The question for therapists working with such people is how to reverse the defensive sequence, from immobilized passivity to mobilized action. 'The core of self-agency must lie in the body' (Fonagy et al. 2004: 58). Herman (1992: 160) was probably the first of many trauma therapists to make the link between the experience of safety and control of the body. This brings an increased sense of safety, volition, directionality and energetic flow. Working with and expanding the range of movement holds a lot of possibility. Where movement does not seem possible, you can trust that the eyes are most likely to be able to move. 'Find three shiny things in the room' became a regular invitation for one such person, leading naturally to a turn of the head to find them. Later, they reported how valuable this had been. Try bringing awareness to any impulse to move, and invite the person to follow it. Someone else often picked at the cuff of their jumper, and it became possible to capture this tiny movement and work to enlarge it into a deliberate rhythmic movement. Squeezing a stress ball can help, or pressing the feet into the ground, all the while inviting awareness of *how* they do it and the muscles involved. You may like to support this movement by doing it yourself alongside your client – 'Let's try this together.' It is surprising how transformative such minimal actions can be, orienting the client to the safety of the present. Movements involving the trunk or the limbs may also be quite small but nevertheless have a considerable impact in reorienting the client and mobilizing their energetic shift towards a more regulated and adaptive state.

The use of purposeful or rhythmic movement is helpful for some people. With one young person I offered a large physio ball that they could bounce on. The suggestions were to bounce slowly, to bounce fast, and to accelerate and decelerate between the two as smoothly as possible. This was not only fun, but provided a sense of the body that they felt they had no control over.

Breath is one aspect of bodily experience over which we have some control. Many popular breathing methods are accessible and can be introduced to the therapy. Particular attention may need to be given to the outbreath, which is associated with a parasympathetic phase of the ANS, through deliberately lengthening it, or perhaps blowing a feather away from the hand. With practice over time, people can learn to 'breathe into' different parts of the body. Attention to breath is exquisitely experience-near and gives rise to a sense of 'self-as-breather'. It can bring about a sense of expansion and flow in the body and a release of muscular contraction. 'We must recognize and sense the connection between breathing and bodily movement and bring about their correlation' (interview with Gindler in Johnson 1995: 10). Does an inbreath or an outbreath better support you in standing up from your chair, for example?

A further sense of agency can be developed through the experience of resistance. Pressing the feet into the floor or lengthening the spine a fraction are the beginnings of resistance. Other options include leaning with the hands on a wall and noticing where in the body the support comes from, or pressing into a cushion that you hold up for them. Finding such resistance, something or someone to come up against, is a precursor to finding a sense of 'No' in the body, which relates to the boundary exercises in Chapter 6. This is a crucial function in recovery – knowing and acting on one's limits – which has probably not been possible before. Where in the body can you find the support for your 'No' – from the feet, pelvis, spine or somewhere else?

There is a link here to anger, which can literally be the backbone of recovery after mistreatment by others. Of course, for many trauma clients anger evokes either terrifying memories or an intolerable intensity of emotion, or both. Anger and rage need to be handled in a sensitive and nuanced way. In terms of Oaklander's (2000: 267) statement that 'anger actually is the essence of taking care of oneself, getting one's needs met, making one's statement, establishing one's position in the world', anger is an entirely appropriate and necessary response to the incapacitating experience of trauma, and its emergence in therapy can indicate a turn towards greater mobilization and response-ability. Therapists who have difficulty working with anger need good training, personal therapy and supervision to be supported to bear the intensity of the feelings that trauma can engender.

Case study: Part 2

Eve's experience of hypoarousal soon became clear to me when she went into a tired, dizzy and floppy state, telling me she needed to lie down. The first few times this happened in sessions I felt pleased that she could tell me what was happening and ask for what she wanted. I thought this was a parasympathetic response, and duly provided blankets and cushions so that she could 'recover'. I needed to change gear quite rapidly when I learnt that this didn't have the desired effect, Eve having gone from a potentially balancing parasympathetic state into collapse too fast, without any control over this process. Eve took a very long time to recover from these episodes, which became more frequent.

In relational terms, she agreed that she now felt safe enough to let me know how her body was remembering the terror and inescapability of the rape. Increasingly able to observe and put words to her experience, Eve told me that she felt enormous heaviness in her chest at the start of these episodes, as though she had woken during an operation unable to move. The challenge of gathering her energy and taking action was considerable. For a long time we had no way of helping Eve find her way out of this state, other than by slowly introducing deliberate movement, especially in her legs.

As she entered a collapse, I noticed that Eve would move her left leg outwards, and although I didn't know the meaning of this I imagined it might be based on a memory of a truncated defensive action. There was little energy in this small movement, but I wanted to capture it and see what potential there was in it. The sensations associated with rising energy triggered Eve because she feared losing control, until she learnt ways of managing and containing the charge in her body. Setting up experiments in which she could begin to turn this movement into a small push felt strong and enlivening to Eve, and we paid close attention to her integration of this somatic resource.

The downside for Eve of finding this movement was that she contacted her anger, an emotion that held a sense of danger for her. She recalled trying to talk to her father about her grandfather's behaviour, and his dismissal of her feelings. More than her grandfather's behaviour, Eve was angry with her parents' reactions, even as she relied on them. It took a lot of painstaking work to unpack her feelings about anger and herself as an angry person, needing to calibrate carefully and slowly what she could tolerate. Because Eve imagined anger as being out of control, she made sense of her helplessness as a way of retaining some degree of control. Any feelings of anger towards her attackers were outside of her awareness for a long time. Interestingly, it was an expression of frustration on my part towards Eve that opened up the space for her to grow into her own anger. She began by quietly telling me that she was upset with what I had said, and later found the capacity to stand up for herself more with her father.

Initially Eve was triggered by attention to her breath, because it reminded her of how her breathing changed during her rape. Over time she became more confident in working with breath because she could observe for herself how it settled her and deepened whenever she entered a more resourced and present state. Now she became more choiceful, using her breath consciously to manage dysregulated states, both in and out of sessions. Using techniques and resources for herself helped her regain the power that had been taken away from her, and slowly dissolved the helplessness she had developed.

Eve told me: 'I feel buffeted, badgered by the situation at work. It takes me to a dark place, where I need to defend myself and get it right for other people, and I don't know how to do that. I don't know what's right for him any more. But it's not about them, it's about me. When I push with my legs I feel anger, and it's scary and it's good too. Anger, it's energy isn't it? It's unjust when my boss shows me up like that, and when I say those words I feel more alive.'

Summary

The ability to make choices based on well-formed figures of contact is valued in Gestalt thinking. This supports a sense of existential freedom, response-ability and differentiation in self-functions at the boundary between self and other. The role of mobilization is key to the formation of such figures, which arise from sensation and awareness. Mobilization is the point on the cycle of experience at which energy is gathered and parasympathetic arousal turns to sympathetic. Under conditions of extreme threat, however, active mobilized defences may come to be aborted where survival is more likely by entering a submissive, helpless state. Immobility is therefore a creative adjustment which is physiologically structured and it can become generalized to many situations in a trauma victim's life. Furthermore, helplessness can be understood as definitional of trauma, because its link with terror produces trauma reactions.

An embodied sense of self can be profoundly affected by immobilized defences. The helpless states felt by trauma victims involve frozenness and collapse. A frozen state may include agitation or paralysis, or both. Either state may be present in different forms in a single client or in a single moment, varying by degree according to current perceptions of safety or danger. Helplessness is embodied through breathing and muscle, where the energetic charge needed to support an action or movement through the cycle is not available or organized. Rigid and collapsed body structures organize energy in recognizable ways and reveal much about the client's habitual ways of being in the world.

Because of the overwhelming impact of events in the field of experience, trauma clients' sense of self is greatly impaired – the world is something that they are unable to influence, and they may feel less able to determine the course of their lives. Shame, weakness and cowardice may become aspects of the client's experience of self in relation to the world. These clients can have difficulty incorporating the trauma into their former or idealized self-concept. In feeling that they can never be the same after a traumatic event, they tend to allow the trauma to define them. Thus the locus of control over their lives shifts towards the environment, and they become acutely field-sensitive. It is difficult for clients to understand their immobility as the creative adjustment that it is, and they carry blame for what happened to them.

In order to restore a sense of self-as-agent it is necessary to reverse the immobilized patterns held in the body. Many experiments are possible to support the reorganization of somatic experience to include a bodily sense of power, which can be linked to restoration of safety. Such experiments can be built around increasing sensation and developing a sense of directed and purposeful movement. Resources can be established which recall moments of mastery in the past or imagining mastery in the future.

8   From dissociation towards contact

Dissociation is a feature of trauma reactions that is both biologically and psychologically driven. This chapter explores this phenomenon, arguing that as necessary for survival, it can be seen as creative. The effects of dissociation on the body are discussed, placing them in the context of neurobiology. Further, the effects of dissociation on the self, causing fragmentation, are developed, and the Structural Dissociation Model is presented. The implications of fragmentation for relationship are explored, before the chapter moves on to describe some thinking about how contact can be increased for these clients. Eve's story is continued.

Traumatic events call into question basic human relationships. They breach the attachments of family, friendship, love and community. They shatter the construction of the self that is formed and sustained in relation to others ... Traumatized people feel utterly abandoned, utterly alone.

(Herman 1992: 51–2)

In the aftermath of trauma the ground on which one's existence rests is shattered. Such deep disconnection inevitably raises questions about the self in relation to the world. This profound existential crisis is deepened by a sense of alienation from the vital, experiencing self. Traumatic experiences often lead to dissociation, which is particularly challenging for clients and therapists alike. Trauma-based dissociation is a kind of living death, like perpetually 'going through the motions'. People who experience dissociation following trauma can feel as though they barely exist in any meaningful, authentic way, and may describe themselves as being in a fog for much of the time, not knowing. This is the quality of unformulated trauma.

Theoretical perspectives on dissociation

The capacity to dissociate is normal and something we all do at times. Take daydreaming for example, getting lost in a book or film, 'highway hypnosis' when driving and 'missing' a chunk of the journey, or other ways of coping with boredom or overstimulation. Dissociation has other important functions in day-to-day life, such as helping us deal with tiredness and pain. Dissociation 'organizes the mind's responsiveness to novelty' (Bromberg 2006: 4) whereby we adapt our self-state to the demands of the present moment. These dissociative responses are fluid and adaptive.

Dissociation resulting from trauma is quite different: it can feel like trying to catch smoke in a net. It may help to define dissociation by means of what it is not: it is an *absence* of association, integration, assimilation, coherence and engagement, the difference between ethical presence and dissociated absence (Chapter 1). Dissociative experiences can over time lead to a more fragmented and structural aspect of the personality. It is important to remember that degrees of dissociation vary depending on circumstance; dissociation is field-sensitive, and may range from mild and temporary to severe and chronic – the so-called dissociative 'disorders'. In addition, I consider that collective dissociation is a prevailing phenomenon in contemporary western social systems.

The window of tolerance is concerned with contact boundaries, and I see dissociation as a radical boundary function. At the boundary, the ways in which we make **modifications to contact** are the subject of debate about what can be observed and what may be interpreted.

One experience-near modification to contact is **desensitization**. This is a tuning out to certain physical stimuli, though the process by which this is achieved is only vaguely described. If we understand this as an energetic shift, desensitization can however be placed on a continuum with dissociation. We might for example become habituated to some discomfort such as a daily commute, a noisy, smelly or dirty environment, or to a degree of cold if we can't afford heating. Individual sensitivities will vary, particularly for people who are neurodivergent. Indeed, difficulties in regulating stimuli for such individuals may suggest variations in the ability to desensitize. Or we might defensively 'live in our heads', rush our food, overwork or pay scant heed to bodily sensations as a **contact style**. These forms we can call desensitization, and we can see their function in regulating contact; but neither is traumatically induced.

Trauma-related dissociation is at the other end of the continuum, and involves dealing with stimuli that are not obviously connected with the present situation. Dissociation has clinical features that are recognizable as problematic by both client and others around them, even on an unconscious level. Philippson (2001: 64) uses the term 'splitting' (into different self-states) as an interruption to contact; it is certainly a feature of dissociation. Typically, dissociation involves a change in awareness, withdrawal of one or more contact functions, and a disengagement with current reality which may take different forms. Kepner (2002) describes dissociation as withdrawal of the energy of awareness, a fleeing from embodied life. Dissociation may create distortions in memory, perception, identity or consciousness.

Dissociative episodes last from a few moments to many days in the extreme. The idea of the long slow flashback is helpful for making sense of longer dissociative experiences. Phenomenological observation indicates a slowing down of response and deadening of contact, a sense that the client has left the conversation or gone somewhere else. If you are tracking energetic shifts both in yourself and the person you are sitting with, you are likely to spot that something has changed. Some trauma victims are capable of operating on several different levels at once, with partial attention to different figures; a question then is to what degree someone is able to remain present.

Dissociation is thought to develop as a result of overwhelming experience that cannot be contained, processed or reflected on. If an individual dissociates at the time of the original trauma, or experiences threat to their bodily integrity, dissociation will probably become a greater problem in later life, which can be predictive of future 'PTS' (Nijenhuis 2004: 89).

In normal life, conflicts between the competing needs of self-states can be resolved by internal dialogue, a self-function that is damaged by trauma. Here, conflicts centre at their most basic level around the disjuncture between the need for a safe and predictable world in which one can continue to function, and a reality that threatens, destabilizes and is unbearably painful. The process of selfing moment by moment is not fluid or organic, and the capacity to reflect on experience is limited. Bromberg calls this 'a thought without a thinker' (Bromberg 2006: 65), neither rooted in nor arising from embodied experience. Dissociation creates a terrible cost to authentic life.

Depersonalization and derealization

There is a wide range of possible dissociative experiences or symptoms. Nijenhuis (2004: 108) considers that there are far-reaching alterations in behaviour, affect, sensation, perception and knowledge which result from dissociation. Broad categories of these include depersonalization and derealization. Depersonalization is the feeling that something is happening but not *to you*, or that you are 'outside' of the body observing the event from a distance. For example it is common for clients to report that during childhood abuse they 'floated up to the ceiling' and watched from there. Many dissociative trauma victims have a degree of difficulty sustaining a reasonably coherent sense of themselves, and may feel as though there is more than one 'self' which takes control at different times. Thus identity confusion is common.

Derealization involves feeling that events or people are unreal, or that common things are unfamiliar; derealization may include distortions in the perception of distance or time (Boon et al. 2011: 17). One person commented, for example, that my therapy room had 'got bigger' between sessions. Blanks in the continuity of time are common, and more highly dissociated clients sometimes 'lose' periods of time – but this is different from substance-induced blackouts (Ross 1997: 138–9). Total amnesia for traumatic events in particular, and often for significant parts of childhood, suggests a dissociative process. Where there is some memory of traumatic events it may be experienced as fragmentary, sensory and discontinuous; victims report that their trauma memories have a different quality from memories of day-to-day events or other significant occasions. Other somatic experiences may include pain without medical explanation, temporary loss of speech or use of part of the body. A hallmark of these dissociative symptoms is that they are involuntary (Boon et al. 2011: 14).

Making sense of dissociation

As a normal function which becomes overused in response to trauma, dissociation should not be treated as pathological. Dissociation is a necessary, biologically driven means of coping with fundamental threats to the integrity of the individual, which allows ongoing functioning and basic attachment systems to survive 'given that from their point of view the trauma is not occurring' (Ross 1997: 65). Dissociation is the means by which trauma victims *maintain* a sense of personal continuity, coherence and integrity of self. One person declared 'They can't hurt me now because I'm not there' – a great defence! The mind plays tricks with reality: 'The dissociative patient in his or her normal state may insist "I was not abused", or there may be intransigent beliefs such as "I am weak, helpless and unworthy" or "I am strong and aggressive"' (van der Kolk et al. [1996] 2007b: 317), neither of which contains the whole picture. This fragmentation is an extraordinarily creative adjustment to events that cannot be contained in an integrated self-state. It involves an active disowning of the traumatic experience at major cost to the self, effectively conveying that 'I want out from that whatever the cost.' Notice the operation of agency in this process. Dissociation is both an active boundary process and a resource.

Victims may have been subject to threats from their perpetrators to deny, to remain silent or to 'forget' what has happened. Sometimes threats have a psychotic quality, for example 'that didn't happen', which can lead victims to doubt themselves and to feel crazy for remembering. The family may cast the victim as the crazy one in order to protect the perpetrator and the family system. Dissociated people can occupy the margins of social relations, living in a liminal space between belonging and alienation. A vicious reinforcing cycle of denial is set up at multiple layers within the 'laminated' field (Parlett 2005: 51), creating the ground for further dissociation.

Dissociation and the body

Where there has been some sort of assault or abuse, the victim will have been treated by another person as being less than human – their dignity and humanity subsumed to the desires and control of the other, their body treated as an object, their sensibility discounted. The physical body is a dwelling place, the centre and ground of our being and humanity. On it are imprinted the desires, beliefs and denial of our ancestral inheritance and of the collective. This is gifted to us through changes in the expression of genes, a process called epigenetics, which 'deliver[s] and translat[es] messages from the environment that "tell" the genes what to do' (Maté 2022: loc 1520). In every sense, in every cell of our body, the environment finds expression. The human body has the unique ability to ground awareness of self and environment and to integrate experience. The loss of connection with an embodied self is therefore disastrous. The trauma victim may no longer be able to inhabit the truth of their story (Goodwin and Attias 1999a: 5). A dissociated person may tell their story in a disconnected way, but the truth of it cannot be known and integrated until it can be deeply and fully felt.

There is no sense of an 'I' in the disconnected body. The bodily betrayal makes reclaiming of an embodied sense of traumatic events essential to recovery. We might say that dissociation has to do with knowing: 'knowing about one's body and knowing about one's self, one's past, and one's relations to others'.

Sometimes dis-identification with bodily experience is in conflict with self-states that need attention for pain (Goodwin and Attias 1999b: 172), perhaps where medical help is sought too late, like delaying to seek advice for a breast lump. Although apparently contradictory, however, to withstand pain may represent a last hold on personal identity (Scarry 1985: 347). But '"out of mind" does not mean "out of body" ... bodily symptoms allow the person to express mental distress without having to acknowledge [it]' (Bakal 1999: 52). I believe that self-harm sometimes fulfils this function of making distress manifest. The body holds many memories of trauma, including those of actual pain which can be relived intensely. Somatoform dissociation is a term that refers to a wide variety of bodily based phenomena, which may involve almost any of the bodily systems, each with its own meaning and function; I will give an example shortly. Other bodily disturbances, sometimes seemingly bizarre, may be symbolic representations of hurts or somatic reactions caused in traumatic circumstances. Either involuntary or deliberate dampening of emotional reactions may generate physical distress (D'Andrea et al. 2011: 383).

It is not uncommon for clients to experience physical pain during a therapy session as memories and feelings come to the surface. People may be very alert to pain and sometimes misinterpret it, as they do with other sensations. To witness an identity formed around the experience of pain affects me, as therapist, to the core. Pain is a distortion both of somatic experience and of the self. It is common for victims to self-medicate in various ways: by distressed eating, substance abuse, overuse of opiate-based painkillers, or self-harm for its analgesic effects. The ambiguous relationship many trauma victims have with pain can be seen in their avoidance of medical care on the one hand, and recurrent seeking of medical attention on the other (Loewenstein and Goodwin 1999: 77). This reflects the confusing twin states of 'feeling too much' and 'feeling too little' which coexist even in the shut-down state of dissociation. The story told by the body is not necessarily what the 'self' tells (Goodwin and Attias 1999a: 3). For example, one person was keen to understand their condition but dissociated whenever we approached the reality of their felt experience.

The neuroscience of dissociation

There are indications of neurobiological processes at work in dissociation alongside the psychological ones. Dissociation seems to go hand in hand with profound hypoarousal of the ANS, and an apparent disconnection between thoughts, sensations, behaviours and emotions (Cozolino 2002: 24). How this separation is involved in the fragmentation of felt experience cannot be explained by current knowledge. Possible breaks in the integrated organization of neural networks affect emotional regulation, attachment and executive functioning (Cozolino 2002: 267). It is thought that the release of endogenous endorphins serves as an analgesic (Cozolino 2002: 74), helping victims to deal with the pain of trauma. Damasio makes an interesting suggestion that there exist in the frontal cortex 'multiple master control sites' (Damasio 2000: 354–5), and switching between them involves the thalamus. Parallels with the switching between self-states are interesting and unknowable at present. Dissociation appears to inhibit the insula (part of the cortex) and the hippocampus from binding the traumatic memories into coherent packages, so trauma memories become free-floating, bound instead to sensory or motor functions, which allows the memories to 'lurch into awareness' (Fogel 2009: 258). The primary executive role of the left hemisphere of the brain might explain the neutral emotional tone dissociative clients often present, suggesting an interruption between right and left hemispheres (Siegel 1999: 320). We can postulate that alteration to the corpus callosum, the 'bridge' between the hemispheres which is rich in neural connections, is involved.

The fragmented self

Separate self-states are probably shifting combinations of psychological and physiological factors, which we all have to some degree. One way of understanding the fragmented self is to consider each changing figure of interest, in Gestalt terms, or somatic phenomenon as an expression of a part or self-state. Equally, separate self-states may contain different fragments of story or memory. Dissociated parts are not usually seen in dramatic switches but present as more subtle changes in energy and the quality of contact. The discontinuity of contact is not always obvious, but may be picked up by the therapist as confusion about how 'we got from there to here'. Dissociation often has a quality of something not quite making sense; not quite fitting. When someone resists something helpful with an excuse or a 'yes but', you might guess that the conflict between competing needs indicates another self-state has switched in. Bromberg ([1998] 2001: 193) helpfully suggests that state switches are most commonly felt by the therapist rather than observed.

Gestalt therapists are familiar with 'top dog' and 'underdog' representations of part selves. Polster (1993) wrote extensively about 'selves' with diverse roles and qualities. To return to Philippson: 'Inherent in the concept of self as relational is the possibility that, in the interaction of a person with the environment, she can form more than one self, each one emergent from a different way of relating to the environment' (Philippson 2001: 64), and aligns this thinking with self-as-process or function of the field. Philippson is not necessarily talking about dissociation, because this splitting is created in response to circumstances rather than to life threat, though the process is similar. Some degree of splitting in this sense is common to all of us; according to different roles, moods, and other factors, I may come across differently even to people who know me well. But, importantly, in each self-state I have a sense of a common thread of 'me-ness', which is absent in dissociated states. Stern suggests that self-synchrony is an essential feature of self-coherence (Stern 1998: 84), and it is this synchrony that seems to be disrupted in dissociative responses to trauma.

Bromberg (2006: 113) states: 'If all goes relatively well in one's early life, one's own self-state shifts are normally as unobservable as the beating of one's heart, and self-state coherence goes on without disruption.' According to Yontef (1993: 269), fragmentation of the self 'is not only a loss of wholeness, it reduces the person to an it, a structural entity. "It" gets cohesive or "it" gets fragmented. And that is a disowning of responsibility, a loss of agency.' Arguably, coming close to the idea of personality, Polster (1993: 42) refers to 'essential' selves which can become fixed.

What happens in the fragmented traumatized person is not reducing, but rather becomes a complex layering of self-states. Ogden et al. point out something perhaps obvious but nevertheless crucially important: that 'parts' are simply metaphors which help us to understand processes rather than *actual* divisions (Ogden et al. 2006: 137). Bearing in mind the Gestalt maxim that the whole is more than the sum of the parts, we turn to a model of the dissociated self, based on functions, which helps make sense of the process in terms of creative adjustment to trauma rather than of pathology.

The Structural Dissociation Model

The Structural Dissociation Model (van der Hart et al. 2006; see Figure 8.1) takes the premise that with increasing exposure to trauma a person becomes more fragmented. In order to deal with inner conflict and continue some semblance of 'normal' life, trauma victims tend to reorganize their 'self' into different functions, one which holds the trauma and one which fulfils the tasks of everyday life, sometimes apparently functioning very well.

This is called 'primary structural dissociation', perhaps following a single trauma event. If the trauma is ongoing or repeated, the *traumatized* part may split further in ways that relate to truncated defensive functions, called 'secondary structural dissociation', while the ongoing functional self continues as before. Secondary structural dissociation will be the main focus of this discussion. This level of dissociation really defines complex trauma, and is likely to be present in *most* traumatized people in regular clinical practice. A further level of fragmentation, 'tertiary structural dissociation', relates more closely to the dissociative 'disorders' and specialist therapy.

Figure 8.1 The structural dissociation model

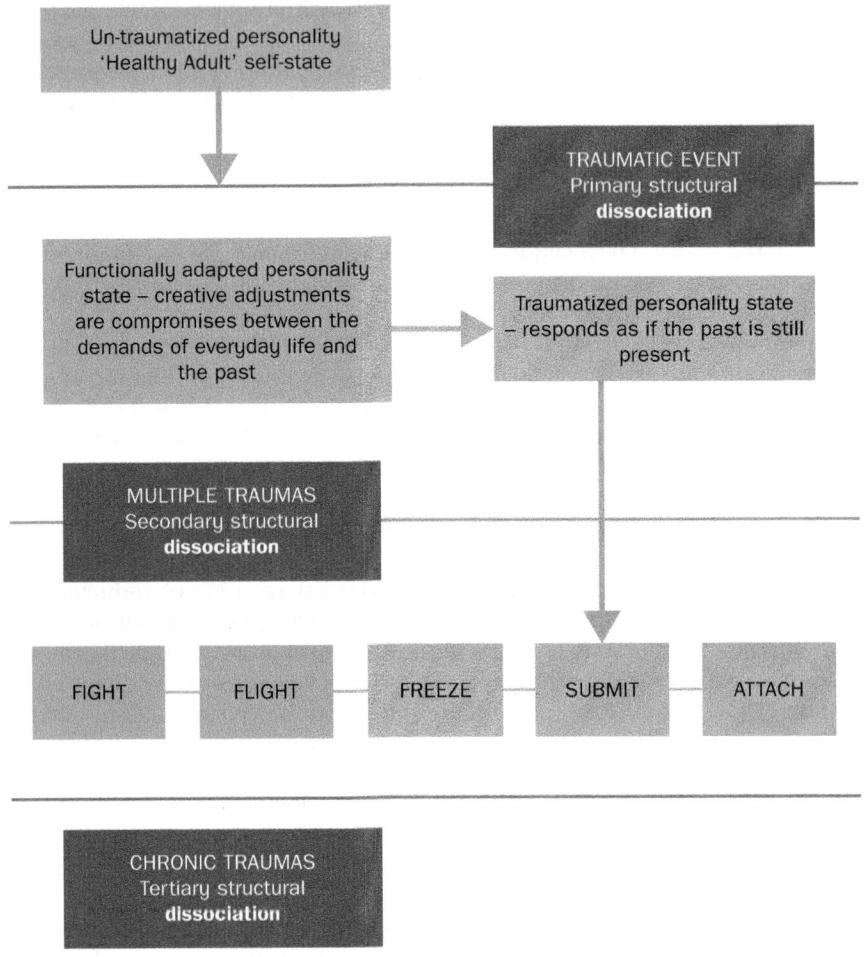

Source: Adapted from O. van der Hart, E. Nijenhuis and K. Steele (2006) *The Haunted Self*. New York: Norton

In Chapter 6 the three mobilized and two immobilized survival defences were described: fight, flight, freeze, submit and attach. Trauma victims have difficulty resolving the conflicts inherent in these five survival functions, which because they are not completed become fixed as structural but dis-synchronous aspects of the personality. The individual is, outside of awareness, perpetually concerned with a search to engage with and to complete any one – or all – of these defences in order to get some respite. What seems to happen is that one of these self-functions might take over 'executive control' at any time, including the part that gets on with daily life.

When triggered beyond their window of tolerance, the client is effectively hijacked by a distressed part.

It would be a mistake to think that these parts are as discrete as the model implies; the matter is not quite that simple. Sometimes parts come disguised as positive traits, such as a submit part having an easy-going approach to life when field conditions support this, while at other times their contributions to survival functions may be puzzling. A suicidal flight part may believe that they are protective, for example. The model implies that all the defensive functions are represented in the internal system, even where a client may perhaps disown their fight part or need for attachment.

This is not to suggest, however, that all parts are aware of one another; 'co-consciousness' is the technical term for awareness between self-states. As with amnesia, some parts or functions may be effectively hidden behind a dissociative barrier, as though they were shut in another room. In some states many clients are able to acknowledge their other self-states, while in others they are not. There can be an 'insularity and concreteness of each self-state as a black-white-island of "truth" about who one is at a given moment' (Bromberg 2006: 65), which paradoxically keeps changing. Just as in the top dog/underdog concept, even when there is awareness between the dissociative parts, they may be antagonistic towards one another. Trauma clients can feel murderous towards or frightened or rejecting of one or more of their parts. I have seen this in someone who wanted to get rid of a sulky adolescent part that was preventing them from making a life choice, and in someone else who became phobic of a frozen child part and the 'stories' they held. Inner conflict characterizes the process of dissociative fragmentation.

Disconnection between self-states is key in understanding the difficulties that trauma clients have in resolving conflicts, mobilizing or making decisions. A lack of balance between part selves is considered problematic in Aboriginal thought (Yunkaporta 2020: loc 1092). However, it only takes a little imagination to recognize parts as resources. What is essential to understand is the *creative and defensive role that each and every part represents and the positive contribution they make to the life of the victim*. The implication of this for therapy is that by understanding the parts and the relationships between them you arrive at a new appreciation of the whole.

One thing missing from the Structural Dissociation Model is the concept of a healthy adult self. It is, after all, a model of dissociation and not of healthy functioning. The implication is that however the self was organized before the trauma took place, it has been disrupted. This is an unnecessarily pessimistic view of the situation. There is no recognition that there may continue to exist a part of the individual that has not been affected by the trauma, a part to which they can return, or which they can use as a guide or a resource in the process of their recovery. The optimistic idea that not all of them have been damaged by the trauma is comforting.

A view more consistent with Gestalt values of health is offered in Schwartz's Internal Family Systems Model, whereby a leadership role can be taken up by one part. Using the metaphor of an orchestra, he suggests that 'the individual musicians are analogous to the parts and the conductor is the self' (Schwartz 1995: 39). No matter how tiny that potential may seem, people can often access the notion of an adult 'conductor' self in themselves, establishing the dual awareness perspectives of 'present and past', 'adult and child'.

Broadening this discussion, which rests on a western notion of self, we might consider also how the experience of part selves may be perceived in other cultures. I think here of how some First nations people of North America treat non-binary people as 'two-spirit people', sometimes known as berdache. They are shape-shifters, which ties in with the Trickster archetype that I use as a metaphor for trauma (see Taylor 2021). Dissociative Trickster qualities include changing identities and distorting perceptions. The notion of spirit 'possession' is included as a recent perspective on Internal Family Systems (Falconer 2023). Possession-like phenomena occur all over the world and throughout history, and are a psychological capacity available in all societies. Furthermore, these possession states are either desirable or scorned according to the meaning that the society places on them (Falconer 2023: loc 4341). Falconer calls these spirits or entities 'Unattached Burdens', which may not necessarily be identified as self-states, explaining why they are 'unattached'. In some cases these are seen as 'legacy burdens' carrying dark and malevolent energy across generations or cultures. For all their apparent power, Falconer proposes that these are frightened and suffering 'beings which need to be expelled to the light in which they can be healed'.

Falconer recognizes that to the western mind all this may sound fairly 'woo', but there is a history of thought in psychoanalysis that marries the tradition of making the unconscious visible with this notion of 'haunting'. Freud considered that 'haunting' might be the mechanism for repetition (in Alleyne 2022: 62). 'Something' moves across space from person to person, even at a distance, the collective becoming the experience of the individual (Alleyne 2022: 62). The Structural Dissociation Model discussed here is drawn from the work titled *The Haunted Self*. 'This has its professional vocabulary attached to it ('transference'), but in truth it is close to occult ideas about thought-transmission or telepathy' (Frosh 2012: 243). Frosh refers largely to the Holocaust and Judaism in his paper, but Alleyne introduces the term 'racial haunting' to focus on the experience of Black people. I have had the experience of working with people who I sensed were carrying something, particularly shame, that did not belong to them, and on occasion the sense of facing something evil. I am curious about the similarities between unattached burdens and the Trickster. However we frame this experience, it seems that a marked shift in energy is common to both dissociated self-states and possession states.

Dropping in

Just becoming aware of different parts can be very helpful. When you are with someone who has experienced trauma, try to simply track their shifting self-states as they report what they have done, felt or thought. Do this by telling yourself as each new figure emerges: 'That's a part, that's another part, that's another part' and so on. You don't need to do anything or to say anything about what you notice, just allow it to register in your awareness. I suggest that you maintain a steady eye on this shifting of self-states for a few minutes of a session, gradually getting used to this process over longer periods. Later, reflect on what you noticed, how the experiment helped and what patterns emerged, maybe making a few notes about them.

Collective dissociation

Trauma is a field phenomenon, and reactions to it are functions of that field. Cultural splits about the body and about trauma are acutely reflected as dissociative phenomena. Dissociation is a natural response to trauma at personal, familial, societal and political levels, and in individual cases there may be deeply held collective attitudes and beliefs that reach beyond generalizations. The individual is a barometer of the field and vice versa. As an illustration, I offer the following example.

In 2023 I taught a trauma workshop in Warsaw, which happened to take place in the area of the ghetto. Over three days, it felt as though the energy of the group kept draining out of the room, like collective freeze and collapse responses. Some people voiced the feeling that they might not return the next day. The vague, undifferentiated and confused process was familiar enough to me. I named this as unformulated trauma – something shapeless that had no form or meaning – referring to the black hole of trauma. I needed to take some particular steps to ground myself, walking the streets and confronting the area's history myself. I was struck by the need for everyday life to continue, and by the fragmented identity of the redevelopment in the area, as though that obliterated the history under my feet. I responded to requests for help in managing the here-and-now experience in the group, which helped build a ground for connection and the safety to tolerate some risk. Experimenting with the contact boundary, the group were eventually able to position themselves in relation to the black hole, represented by a loop of string on the floor, and they named it, chillingly and touchingly, the Star of David, giving it form and meaning. We had broken through many layers of dissociation seeping into the room from the ground, without recourse to personal narrative. A postscript to this workshop presented in the form of physical sensations, perhaps best understood as somatoform dissociation. While we were together, several people in the group happened to complain of problems with their eyes – soreness, dryness, weeping. I came back to the UK with Covid-19, the worst symptom of which was eye pain. It was just too painful for us to see.

Similar levels of mass dissociation seem to exist in relation to the damage of colonialism, slavery, pandemics, racial segregation, genocide and climate change.

Dissociation and relationship

The greater the trauma, the greater the boundary difficulty. And the levels of structural dissociation are boundary issues. The person who dissociates is actively redefining a boundary, removing their self from a seemingly intolerable situation; these people can be experienced as being hard to reach in therapy. For someone who is deeply traumatized, a catastrophic sense of alienation underlies *all* interactions, *all* self-concepts, *all* hopes, *all* longings for connection. And for the therapist working with this, there can be a parallel sense of loss and loneliness.

When abuse or trauma stems from childhood, the victim may never have felt a true sense of belonging: 'Trauma ... individualizes us, but in a manner that manifests in an excruciating sense of singularity and solitude' (Stolorow 2007: 41). Delisle (2011: 83) comments poignantly that 'Often these subjects have not been held closely enough to sense that they are in the world.' The need for contact is simultaneously imperative and terrifying. 'Profound isolation, longing and loneliness are hallmarks of traumatized people' (Hillman 1996: 54). As a victim, you are cast outside.

The Gestalt view of relationship is that we are hardwired for contact, which is confirmed time and again by neuroscience. Crucially, Bromberg ([1998] 2001: 277) considers dissociation to be *an interpersonal process*, an idea developed by DeYoung, whereby dissociation is more likely to be an accommodation to another than self-sufficiency (DeYoung 2015: 7). Abandonment by betrayal is an attachment dynamic in the interpersonal field which becomes mirrored in the internal world of the victim. Sacrifice of the authentic self in the service of attachment compounds the unbearable experience of actual abandonment in the wider or historical field.

There are several possible boundaries that involve the organism and environment. At different stages of therapy other boundaries (e.g. skin) may become relevant, but for the most part our concern is with establishing a safe enough interpersonal space in which the client can be as present as possible. Our therapeutic presence can be either a trigger or a support, and we may find ourselves navigating an extraordinarily delicate line between the two.

Trauma clients are often exquisitely sensitive to distance and closeness, and may have intense reactions to signs of intrusion, however subtle they may be. Someone might manage the therapeutic space by asking the therapist to position their chair 'just so', in order to begin to feel safe. An opportunity presents itself here to experiment with finding just the right distance. Therapists can learn to sense the edges of a kind of energetic bubble around the people they are working with, an embodied sense that they do not have permission to come closer, or an awareness that they have already invaded that space (Cook, n.d., 3.1). Carefully calibrated, it is possible to ensure that distance is 'not too much' and 'not too little'.

This dissociative bubble is, I suggest, crucial to take account of, for as therapists we can easily become enveloped in it. On the one hand this may be understood as accurate embodied attunement (Hoppenwasser 2008), giving us an insight into the experiential world of the person we are with. On the other hand, we are going to be lost in this space if we cannot recognize it and find a way out. *Closeness is not necessarily the most therapeutic position*, and *we may do better maintaining a greater emotional distance*, keeping outside of that bubble, than we are used to.

Far too often trauma victims are disbelieved, their stories denied or misunderstood. This may result from the 'not quite present' quality of the victim, which makes it harder for them to be taken seriously. The disembodied nature of their communication feels incongruous. A tendency towards immobilized defences lays the victim wide open to misunderstanding, and sadly sometimes to being further taken advantage of. The more functional part of the personality too often 'goes it alone', sometimes disavowing all need for contact which is dissociated from awareness. There is much deep mistrust in traumatized people, which corresponds to their fundamental lack of safety in the world. Dissociation also protects attachment relationships, keeping 'bad' aspects of the relationship out of awareness; this is characteristic of traumatic attachments whereby the abused person feels inextricably bound up or identified with their abuser. Disclosure and the search for connection involve the loss of hard-earned survival-based adjustments.

Typically, these individuals are fiercely independent, highly defended against exposing their vulnerability and distress. Unaware of their limits of tolerance, they may endure extraordinary adversity without asking for help. They haven't had the chance to experience support, that in healthy relationships people reach out to one another. Others are acutely vigilant for signs of abandonment or rejection, and may pick up the therapist's changing presence or availability for contact. Traumatized people need to learn to tolerate aloneness and solitude, which can regulate arousal, uncoupled from associations with abandonment.

A further consideration with fascinating implications comes from neuroscience. Research highlights a qualifier to the relational perspective, presenting a challenge to integrate into established thinking about self, other and contact boundaries. We now know that empathy, a relational skill, can be developed through the *individual* practice of mindful awareness. Siegel states that 'We can ... imagine that the social nature of our brains may have something to do with our minds in solitude' (Siegel 2007: 170, my italics). What this seems to suggest is that a process of *neural reconnection takes place in solitude which helps create the conditions for social connection.* This underlines the need for the middle zone of the window of tolerance, as discussed in Chapter 4. The need, in technical terms, is to restore the wiring for contact. But if dissociation is an interpersonal process in its genesis, maintenance and in recovery, then we can postulate that this neuronal repair in solitude is also a function of the relational field. It is in neither the realm of the individualistic paradigm, nor that of the other, but both. 'Movement of the flow of states of mind can involve activity both within the mind itself and in interactions with other minds' (Siegel 1999: 320).

Supporting contact

The overall principle in working with dissociative people is to support developing integrative capacity and a reclaiming of self in the world. 'Rehabilitation is to restore someone to his/her rightful place in the community after some kind of disjuncture or relational rupture' (Levin and Levine 2012: 8). At the same time, the creative defensive role of dissociation needs to be seen and appreciated. Here lies a paradox, the paramount need being to 'preserve the dissociative structure while surrendering it' (Bromberg [1998] 2001: 199). The first task is to learn the skill of staying present in the body, and the second is to work with fragmented self-states. These are examined in turn below.

- Begin with yourself – manage your breathing, orient to the present, make small movements like wriggling your toes, take a sip of water. Gather your energy gently, and pace your interventions. Your energetic presence may need to be a little greater than that of the person you are with – not so much as to be jarring, but not so little that you get caught in the absence that is in the room (see Taylor 2021). A healthy degree of hypervigilance is valuable to enable you to observe the flow and catch changes as they happen. Noticing your own somatic responses is important, such as tiredness, confusion, unexpected pain, or tension.
- Keep interventions simple and concrete; saying too much can confuse and disorient the person you are with. Tell them if you are about to do something and ask if it is okay with them.
- One concrete strategy is to ask clients what percentage of them is present in the room right now, and enquiring about what would increase this, even a little. It is helpful to 'rediscover a middle ground between complete dissociation and unbearable suffering inside the hurt body' (Goodwin and Attias 1999b: 172). It can be supportive to offer a narrative for what is happening: 'It looks as though you need a little time out just now. I wonder if you can take that time for yourself while staying present in the room with me?'
- To counter derealization, gently bring the person into the present by asking them to name some things in the room: 'What can you see (or hear) that lets you know that you are here now?' Let that be an anchor to the present. If you have done a safe place exercise together, you might ask them to remind you about the quality of the light there or some other feature. Asking about how they travelled to your consulting room, or their journey home, can also help to orient them.
- The out-of-body feeling associated with depersonalization points to using the senses and interoceptive awareness in order to come back to the body. Keep any invitations neutral or pleasant, perhaps offering some drops of essential oil on a tissue, a small object to hold and investigate, or a weighted blanket or lap pad to ground and heighten a sense of where their edges are. Inviting curiosity, using your own as a model, will help to re-engage the thinking brain.

- Contrary to what might be assumed, it is important to address directly the issue of part selves in therapy. Clients need to have their process confirmed and normalized, and their resources acknowledged. We also need to be clear about what we mean by integration between parts. The goal of this work is to 'repair the short circuits, not to remove or replace parts' (Ross 1997: 304), enabling a fluid movement between self-states. Integration is *not a final blending* of all the parts into a 'single' unified whole, which would not fit comfortably with a view of self as a complex and emergent process. Once clients are comfortable and familiar with parts, they tend to be reluctant to give them up. You will also need to be comfortable with the functions of your own part selves.

- Develop awareness of parts. You might begin by referring to younger or child parts that have been wounded, and to older parts that are more able to function day to day. You may need to support this by tracking the parts as they emerge and recede in the session, noticing shifts in energy, tone of voice, patterns of speech, movement or eye focus. Trust that you will know, and perhaps comment: 'I got the impression that something changed just then – did you notice that too?'

- Honour the splits as necessary for survival, relating them to defensive functions. Therapists need to elicit awareness of parts, together with a compassionate understanding of their functions and how they came to be this person, in order to achieve a greater degree of co-consciousness. Access to this can be supported by means of enquiry into the fears and needs of particular parts by 'befriending' them (Fisher 2017: 74). We cannot work with parts in isolation, but have to take into account the relationships between them as well as their functions and contributions to the whole. The client needs to learn to tolerate the underpinning internal conflict between parts to support integration (Bromberg 2006: 69).

- Establish whether or not there is co-consciousness, and work towards it. The image of a house, with parts occupying different rooms, is helpful – some doors locked shut, some partly open. I have used the idea of 'knocking on the door' and waiting to see if an exiled part is willing to make contact. Suggesting that the distressed parts 'drop into their feet' sounds odd but makes sense to some, or asking a perpetually vigilant insomniac part to let the 'others' go to sleep. The idea is to become increasingly conscious of disowned or exiled parts, so that they don't hijack the person to the same degree. This is co-consciousness, and when well developed it is possible to imagine the parts meeting around the kitchen table. This increases inner collaboration and reduces conflict.

- While the person you are working with needs to increase communication between parts, it is wise for you to avoid engaging directly with part selves. Where this cannot be avoided, specialist training and supervision are called for. You might say, 'I know that you have important things to say, but it would be helpful if you could ask (client's name) to tell me what they are.' That way you keep the relationship with the adult who is sitting in front of you, and don't get drawn into 'group therapy'. Working actively to support the development of a healthy adult self is best strengthened by encouraging this part to narrate *on behalf of the others*.

- Introduce the idea of protector or compassionate wise parts, perhaps enquiring what they would say or do in response to what is going on. Protection has been sorely missing for many people with complex trauma and it needs to be developed along with a sense of boundaries and agency.

Case study: Part 3

There was something remote about Eve, a combination of her low energy, the protectiveness carried in her voice, her functional use of language and her guardedness with me. I wanted to reach out for more contact with Eve but felt subtly pushed aside, and learnt that she had few expectations of having her needs met relationally. Eve said that she felt abandoned by other potential sources of support. She had no close friends and excused herself from social events at work and through Freya's school. Away from the safety of her home she felt, to use her words, 'as though I'm watching a film, and I'm not in it' – the experience of derealization.

This was something we worked with in the immediacy of the therapy setting and Eve became more able to sustain her growing presence, which we could monitor together. We worked directly on many things that could help her engage, in the therapy room, in her external world, and importantly in terms of her inner experience. There were moments, particularly when she went into a state of collapse, that Eve reported my voice becoming very faint to her, and said that she was floating away from her body. Therefore we worked in a sustained fashion to support safe body awareness and feelings of strength and fluidity, and to reconnect Eve with a sense of bodily competence. Eve used the additional support of a massage therapist and yoga classes, and returned to her former interest in swimming as the closest she could come to the safe experience of diving.

Eve's struggles with anger were very much at odds with her tendency to give in to others. Along with psychoeducation about trauma and dissociation, which Eve found helpful, I introduced the language of parts to help shed light on Eve's conflict. We recognized that there was a dimension of attachment in her behaviour towards her boss, that she needed him for the security that came with the job, regardless of his treatment of her and the stress she often felt. It was important to honour the purpose of her attachment, while seeing it as an attempt to keep herself safe that wasn't working well. Eve understood how submissive she had needed to become in the face of terrible threat and we worked with different parts to establish inner dialogue. Eve noticed that some of her confusion cleared when she could appreciate that aspects of her personality were both courageous and vulnerable.

As therapy progressed, Eve began to feel less isolated and more engaged with the outside world. She said that she could see more clearly and commit herself better. 'I no longer felt mad or that I was a square peg in a round hole', she told me later. Still, she remained extremely anxious about mixing with other people, and was able to notice the inner arguments which held her back. Crucially, Eve was learning to pay attention to somatic signals and could interpret their meaning with some accuracy and act appropriately.

Summary

Dissociation is a natural, biologically driven function, which we all use in order to switch off from boring or stressful situations, to daydream or to lose ourselves in a book or film. However, this is quite different from the dissociation that results from trauma, which may involve either depersonalization or derealization, or both. In this kind of dissociation there is a marked loss of contact functions, and a sense of the energy of contact being withdrawn. Dissociation is a major modifier of contact, redefining the boundaries and sometimes putting the client out of reach. A level of dissociation is likely to be found in the majority of trauma clients. For the client this can result in feeling as though they are deeply disconnected and just going through the motions of life. The role of therapy is to help create a way back, to reclaim the body and establish a more cohesive sense of self.

Dissociation is a creative adjustment par excellence, enabling the trauma victim to continue with some semblance of normality, though at enormous cost. Trauma victims sacrifice a cohesive and integrated sense of self and flee embodied life in order to survive threatening levels of inner conflict and intensity of feelings. The Structural Dissociation Model explains the process of fragmentation of the personality. Primary and secondary structural dissociation are the two types most commonly seen in clinical practice. These involve the splitting of the self into traumatized and functional 'parts'; in complex trauma or secondary structural dissociation, the traumatized roles are reflections of the five defensive functions under threat: fight, flight, freeze, submit and attach.

The sense of alienation in dissociative processes can be quite profound; alienation from self, body and from other. The inherent distancing in dissociation is a self-imposed boundary which isolates rather than includes. Restoration of connection involves work on different levels, harnessing the potential integrative capacity of the fragmented self-parts and of the body in order to increase connectivity with the wider field. Establishing compassionate understanding of the contribution of each part and of relationships between them, called co-consciousness, together with increased capacity for inner dialogue, is essential. In working to reclaim the sense of the body as a safe dwelling place and container, work on the core of the body is needed.

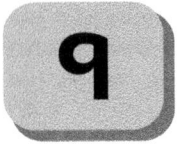

From shame towards acceptance

This chapter explores the experience of shame as a particular response to trauma. It looks at how shame can be understood as an attack on the self, often mirroring the attack of interpersonal trauma. Perspectives on shame, blame and responsibility in the context of trauma are discussed. The chapter moves on to issues of self-harm and suicidality, and the somatic response to shame. The experience of shame is placed in a trauma field context and there is an exploration of the dynamics that operate to keep shame in place. Acceptance is offered as a polarity of shame, and ways of increasing this are explored, including the role of compassion and pyschoeducation.

Shame is a universal experience that pervades traumatic experience, and indeed goes hand in hand with it. Bromberg (2011: 23) considers the emergence of sudden shame to be a 'threat equal to that of fear'. The seeds of shame may lie dormant from before or at the time of birth in the case of an unwanted pregnancy, or a baby not being welcomed lovingly. More classically, though, shame is an emotion that develops alongside an emerging sense of 'I' from about 18 months to 5 years of age, an aspect of omnipotence and developmentally healthy narcissism. It is this budding 'I' that becomes vulnerable to shame, when one or more aspects of the 'self that I am' is not seen, acknowledged or prized by others. Thus we can construct shame as a relational dynamic. Indeed, consistent with our growing understanding of regulation, 'Shame is the experience of one's felt sense of self disintegrating in relation to a dysregulating other' (DeYoung 2015: 18). Gestalt therapists understand shame as a creative adjustment – a reorganizing of the contact boundary because of a rupture or threat of rupture between self and some aspect of the wider field. Shame is also linked in Gestalt to the theory and process of self: the self that is formed in contact at this acutely sensitive boundary (Lee and Wheeler 1996). The boundary, as reorganized, is fragile because of the fixed gestalts that constitute it.

Shame-prone people are highly attuned to relational cues about the receptivity of the field, where attention may be turned to the needs of the dysregulating other as a substitute for getting their own needs met. Poignantly, such attunement on the part of the trauma victim is the inverse of their experience of misattunement by others, and leads them to draw damaging conclusions about their intrinsic worthiness. 'She is thereafter in doubt both as to her own legitimacy as a person and the reality of her internal experience' (Bromberg 2011: 43). The forcefulness of the emotion is such that a range of defences against it come into play, including hiding, denial of desires, attack against self and other, perfectionism and defensive justifying.

The major themes of fear, helplessness and disconnection in the lives of trauma victims become constellated around shame, each living at a different depth within the individual, shame arguably running deepest. That is not to say that these people come into therapy with awareness of shame processes; they may tend to avoid recognition of this intense emotion, which must be hidden and which in turn masks authentic contact. They may give other names to their experience which belie their sense of unworthiness, self-disgust and humiliation, and need to come to this language in their own time. There are mutually reinforcing shame loops at play; shame upon shame builds a laminated experience of the world, personally, relationally, socially and culturally. Personal history, current situations and internal and external fields all clash here, and no one can control how we are seen in the eyes of another (Schultz-Venrath 2022: 91). In particular, relational styles informed by the 'there and then' field (Yontef 1993: 260–1) are internalized; perceived expectations become the template for contact. Shame processes are embedded in fear through hypervigilance, in helplessness via the locus of control shift, and in disconnection through a deep sense of not belonging. Because of psychophysiological similarities between them, 'there is an *intrinsic* association of shame and trauma … [shame is] an almost structural component of trauma' (Levine 2010: 60, original italics). In trauma, shame is therefore a given.

Shame through the lens of trauma

The experience of shame is searingly visceral, complex and multifaceted, 'usually continuous with moments of more intense pain' (Orange 1995: 97). It is closely related to physiological systems concerned with threat and fear: a 'threat that we are about to be violated' (Bromberg 2006: 190). There is a high potential for reactivating trauma responses when an environment is perceived as shame inducing. First, traumatized people orient defensively towards potentially shame-inducing situations, becoming hypervigilant for signs of receptiveness or dismissiveness of the field. They are exquisitely attentive to signals of rejection, more even than to signals of acceptance, which may often be misconstrued or mistrusted. The expectation of being shamed escalates, which tends to preconfigure the field. Bringing to the encounter, as trauma victims do, the experience of being overpowered by some external force shapes their physiological, psychological and emotional ability to make contact.

The sense of shame is itself overpowering and as difficult to regulate as other trauma responses. Layered into this is shame for the inability to regulate, for not having 'got over it'. Shame relates to the states of high arousal and intrusion so characteristic of trauma, and naturally comes to be avoided. Trauma victims can experience shame for any of their trauma-based responses.

Furthermore, they can have vivid flashbacks to previous shameful experiences (Boon et al. 2011: 289), including the traumatic event itself. For some victims there are such intolerable levels of shame and disgust at what was actually done to them, most particularly – but not only – in respect of sexual trauma, that avoidance may be their best defence (Turner et al. [1996] 2007: 543).

The correlation between shame and helplessness has already been mentioned in Chapter 7. The relationship between the experience of helplessness and physiologically based immobilized survival defences was explored through the lens of creative adjustments. Immobilization is experienced as a *failure* to defend, which becomes inextricably bound up with shame. Sadly, trauma victims are vulnerable to feeling shame for so much that they have done in the service of survival. Any healthy sense of potency is destroyed, any memory of having been capable erased, the sense of having belonged in 'another life' or having been a different person 'back then'; then, but not now, no longer. The wounds of shame feel so permanent that there is no hope and they feel unworthy of healing contact. In their own eyes, and often in the eyes of others, these shame-prone clients believe themselves to be weak, unable to stand their own ground.

Drowning at times in an ocean of shame, with an eye constantly on the next incoming wave, trauma clients habitually refer to others by means of comparison: others who keep things in perspective, who manage their emotions, who don't seem out of control. The paralysis of helplessness is reflected in chronic indecision, for fear of making the 'wrong' decision. When the validity of one's existence is threatened, the abilities and rights of others assume a greater significance – the locus of control shift. It may start like this: 'The other holds the power to destabilize the child's mental state by rupturing a relational connection that organizes the child's sense of self-continuity' (Bromberg 2011: 43). The conclusion that 'Something bad has happened to me, therefore I must be bad' is common. Kepner (1995: 38), however, helpfully recontextualizes this as: 'I feel bad about what was done to me.' In recent years this has become more mainstream through the Power Threat Meaning Framework (see Taylor 2021) or *What Happened to You?* (Perry and Winfrey 2021). The experience of helplessness can be seen in the strong sense of injustice that many trauma victims experience. Indeed, viewed compassionately, shame is an indicator of sensitivity towards basic unfairness in the world.

Traumatic experiences evoke existential crises for many victims: shame-laden cries of 'Why?' and 'Why me?' may go unvoiced, unheard or unanswered, but are nevertheless central and intrinsic concerns. People need to gain a sense of order in a world that seems unordered, and explanations may be a search for a sense of control and safety. I think about adding a sixth defensive 'F' of 'find out'. For those whose spirituality or faith system is threatened by trauma there may be a sense of abandonment by their God: 'How could He let this happen to me?' The pull to make sense, to explain to the self and to others how their world has changed so dramatically, to find words for the experience, to be understood and therefore to be received and to reconnect, is strong.

The rupture of the boundary between self and other is experienced as both deeply alienating and deeply shaming. The conclusion drawn may be that one is so disgusting as to be unworthy of belonging in the world. There may be dissociative parts of the personality which are persecutory and shaming. In any victim of abuse or trauma there may exist a part that seeks vengeance on those who have caused their suffering, and it can be challenging for clients to accept and integrate these powerful forces. Shame is so intolerable that it may itself become dissociated, reorganizing the sense of a coherent whole (Bromberg [1998] 2001, 2006, 2011).

There are some further considerations of shame that are particular to trauma. Shame is a rather different experience for people whose trauma is a result of accident or natural disaster and those who have suffered deliberate interpersonal attacks, in which betrayal of trust is often central. In the case of the former, it is now recognized that the availability of support in the immediate aftermath promotes recovery; in other words, acceptance and receptivity in the relational field are crucial. If attachment bonds are not destabilized by misattunement or misunderstanding, the individual may fare well in the long run. However, adult traumas of this kind may reactivate earlier attachment difficulties, and feelings of shame may be rekindled. Additional shame may be caused when a perpetrator is known to the victim, which buys into cultural myths that in some way the victim asked for the attack or could have prevented it. Further, for some the issue of survivor guilt may greatly impinge on recovery:

> Feelings of guilt are especially severe when the survivor has been a witness to the suffering or death of other people. To be spared oneself in the knowledge that others have met a worse fate, creates a severe burden of conscience.
>
> (Herman 1992: 54)

Attachment shame

Because shaming experiences are fundamentally relational, they become the template for our attachment patterns. Contemporary theorists understand the link between this achingly painful feeling and the absence of interpersonal regulation or repair following ruptures:

> Feeling intense affect and with no regulation from another person, this [person] will dissociate in order not to feel the pain of a self disintegrating with no hope of repair. Her acute, core shame will be strongly laced with fear, panic and disorientation.
>
> (DeYoung 2015: 49)

The dilemma for this person is to resolve the contradictions between the need for dependency as a developmental stage, with the presence of the abandoning or 'scaregiving' other:

> To need you means to be both afraid of you and confused by you. It hurts, but since feeling anything is shaming, I'll have to dissociate these frightening experiences from my consciousness and instead learn to control my environment.
>
> (Badouk Epstein 2022: 51)

Figure 9.1 The relationship between fear and shame

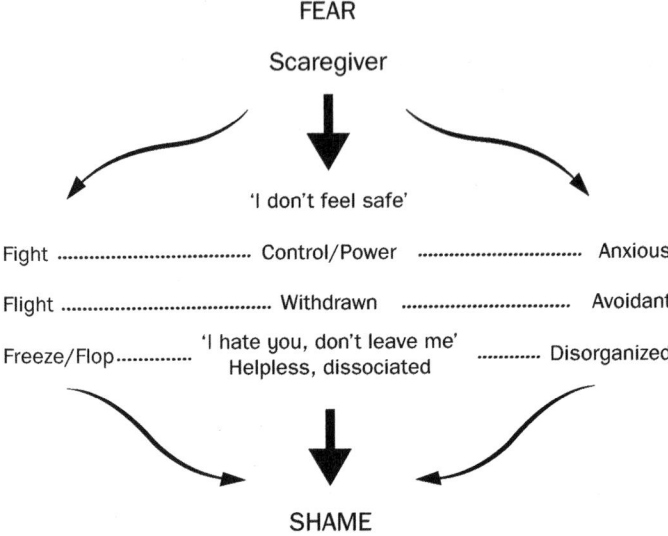

This makes it possible to pull together some ideas about the relationship between shame and fear. The need to adapt to the fear-inducing other requires a defensive manoeuvre, which can be associated with attachment styles, as illustrated in Figure 9.1.

The correspondence shown here between defensive systems and attachment styles is intended to be indicative rather than definitive. We see here the approach/withdrawal relational styles as well as the unsolvable dilemma of approach *and* withdrawal. A feature of a yearning for control may be what Chefetz (2022: 61) describes as 'attackments', 'the quality of relating that simultaneously feels desperate for connection while remaining intolerant of being met or known and urgently needing to keep others at a distance'. We can imagine these contradictions being distributed between disparate parts of an individual's personality structure.

Traumatic events are commonly seen as threats to bodily survival, and the physiological response serves to optimize survival. Shame, on the other hand, is primarily associated with an attack on the self – a threat to the integrity of personhood and identity which 'typically calls forth dissociative processes to preserve self-hood' (Bromberg [1998] 2001: 295). It begins in relation to the dysregulating other and becomes an internalized attack.

We can also look at shame through the lens of boundaries, in particular the breakdown between self and other. Lee shines light on how *'the need that is not received by the other is disowned and made "not me"'* (Lee 1996: 9, original italics). Difficulties in determining boundaries between self and other may involve a shame-bound disowning of any personal right to determine their own boundaries. There is not only a disorganization of the self/other boundary: other experiences of self are threatened by shame processes. Connected with the sense of being 'defective' and unworthy is a denial of the basic right to a place of safety, or to be treated with dignity.

Where it may be painful to be seen by an attuned other, it can also be painful to 'see' oneself. Bromberg (2011: 43, my italics) considers that 'the struggle to *self-reflect* is mentally disorganizing'. The question of identity is at the heart of the issue in some specific minority groups: 'Identity shame is perhaps the single most important variable that overarches so much of what is seen in the psyches of wounded people' (Alleyne 2022: 115). Who I am is felt to be irredeemably wrong, and there is nothing to be done about it. 'Identity shame is observable in black clients where, even when successes are achieved on full merit, there seem to be deep and troubling doubts about personal entitlement to such accomplishments' (Alleyne 2022: 116). As a hallmark of intergenerational trauma, this is neither a state of victimhood nor numbness: 'rather this should be recognized as a *perpetual* state of feeling held back and being held back' (Alleyne 2022: 25, my italics).

Loss of dignity, of value and sense of welcome in the world becomes the foundation for how shame-prone people treat themselves. As a solution to a relational deficit, it makes sense, for it is better to be bad than banished (Howell 2022: xvi). The conclusion that 'I am no good' is painfully compounded by this sense of loss, the perception of self being skewed. Yontef (1996: 354) describes shame as 'a learned sense of not identifying with self as is'. By disowning or hiding important aspects of the self, the shamed person cannot comfortably grow into their fullest humanity.

Shame, blame and responsibility

Clients who are prone to shame tend to take a disproportionate degree of responsibility for the difficulties in their lives. Self-blaming becomes more pronounced. By locating power in key people in the wider field, the locus of control shift tends to locate blame in the victim. Responsibility becomes polarized, especially given the characteristic of perpetrators to deny responsibility. Present-day cultural narratives about victim blaming reinforce this propensity. 'They shouldn't have been drinking/dressed like that/walked in the streets at night, 'They should have fought back/told someone/left the relationship' are all myths that organize power into the hands of the perpetrator and blame to the victim. Therapy often involves a reorganization of the complex responsibility boundary, accompanied by a reorganization of power and control. To realign boundaries of responsibility can mean relinquishing a small degree of control that might have been a resource previously. It may therefore be more regulating to assume responsibility for the traumatic event.

It is through the lens of the co-created relationship that the fixed gestalts which maintain the dance between victim and perpetrator are best understood.

Perls et al. ([1951] 1998: 216) frame it like this: 'you are creative in your environment and are responsible for your reality – not to blame, but responsible in the sense that it is you who lets it stand or changes it'. Here is the theory of co-creation, which points to an uncomfortable realization: trauma victims had a part in their trauma. This does not in *any way* apportion blame to them nor suggest *equal* responsibility; the participatory part may be a very tiny percentage of the whole. This is simply a condition of being in any relationship. Responsibility is shared, and only the victim can take ownership of their helpless response, for example; the key is to come to understand how it made sense to be helpless in that moment. For some people, acceptance of their part in the relationship can bring relief; it is far easier to forgive oneself for something small, reasonable and proportionate than for the whole catastrophe, and more true to their subjective experience. It is a more active position to take than that of being unable to do anything about a situation.

An even more sensitive issue exists for some victims of sexual violence who may have become aroused during the attack. The belief that goes with this is along the lines of 'If I enjoyed it, then I was to blame; I consented', without recognizing that the body will respond to certain kinds of contact by becoming aroused, *regardless* of context, relationship or consent. They may be more angry and ashamed of their own bodily nature and less of their attacker's. Later, victims of sexual trauma may become ashamed and avoidant of their sexual desires, with an impact on later relationships.

Not only do trauma victims identify with their trauma and a sense of victimhood, they may also identify with the person who has caused their hurt, be it the perpetrator of an assault or 'the driver of the other car' involved in an accident. For someone who has been raped, for example, there may be a complicated attachment to their rapist, a greatly feared but ever-present intruder who comes into their life by means of flashbacks and other trauma-generated experiences. Traumatic attachment patterns are common, of which so-called Stockholm Syndrome is an extreme, and we will return to this in Part 3. Identifying with victimhood is part of the narrative: 'I'm worthless' is one side of the coin, and the perpetrator voice 'You'll never be anything without me' is the other. The abuser's treatment of the victim can become the critical lens through which the victim sees him or herself. Their words, threats and displacement of responsibility become a kind of 'truth' for their victims, who make them right and give away their power. I remarked to one person that the way they treated themselves was reminiscent of the way their abuser treated them. 'Yes', they replied, 'and it's me who chooses it.' Shame is not only an experience of how we see ourselves, but a perception of or preoccupation with how others see us. No wonder that the need to hide, to not be seen or 'found out' (for being human), is a clinical feature of shame. So often it is other's' views of us that define us, making us smaller than we really might be, or in the case of grandiosity, larger. Van der Kolk (2014: 11) writes of the lies which make us suffer most; I think this is also true of the lies we have been told about ourselves by others.

Shame brings with it the harshest judgements of self, sometimes in the form of vitriolic and vicious self-attacks, an extreme form of the top dog/underdog dynamic. Self-judgement can make a new shape of chaos, making it more containable. The victim may interpret the trauma and its consequent suffering as a punishment for not actively defending themselves or for putting themselves in a vulnerable position. It can be hard to accept that they were simply in the wrong place at the wrong time, for to do so demonstrates that the world is unpredictable and sometimes random, over which they have no control. Self-blame permits 'an illusion of potential control. Ironically, there is evidence that rape victims who blame themselves fare better in the long run than those who do not assume this false responsibility' (van der Kolk and McFarlane [1996] 2007: 15).

Shame-full bodies

To have experienced overwhelming trauma means for many victims that they must bear the scars of that trauma, whether visible or invisible. For some, these scars are so unbearable that they must be hidden and disavowed: 'I hurt too much to bear to let you see.' Pennebaker (2000: 309) reports that trauma victims who do not talk about their experiences tend to have more physical illness; I wonder about the cost of shame in holding this silence. Victims may be so acutely conscious of the burden of shame that they come to see their physical selves as sick, defiled, toxic or violated, and it may feel better to pretend that the body and its needs don't exist. There can be such a rawness in the pain of trauma. 'Because of complex boundary problems, there is severe confusion, and patients may experience their own wounded self as fatally toxic if seen ... and the reality of the abuse as a fatal image that must be concealed' (Attias and Goodwin 1999: 161).

Body shame is a key factor in reducing self-care and body awareness, caught between the need to feel invisible and feel seen. Schore (2003a: 154) says that shame, 'perhaps more than any other emotion is so intimately tied to the physiological expression of a stress response'. Shame triggers defensive responses of blushing, postural change, reduced eye contact and withdrawal which are different from the instinctive survival responses of fight, flight, freeze, submit and attach. In shame there is a loss of footing, one cannot stand one's own ground because one is standing partly on the ground of the other.

Unable to find a way to fit in, the shame of being in a minority group or holding a perceived divergent identity is profound, and brings with it unremitting stress (see Taylor 2021: 47). Living in your own skin is a whole different paradigm for BIPOC (Black, indigenous or people of colour) people, who suffer the indignities of micro-aggressions at first sight and on a daily basis, and for whom 'white passing' or white skin is seen as the 'ideal'. It is sobering to learn that skin-lightening products form a multibillion-pound industry in sub-Saharan Africa.

Dropping in

If you are able, with your shoes off, stand upright, feet hip width apart, with your shoulders relaxed and knees unlocked. Attending to your breathing, allow a softening in your body on your exhale, allowing a sense of your whole body breathing. Bringing your attention to your feet, and to the contact between the soles of your feet and the ground, notice the areas of your soles where the contact is most vivid and the areas where there is less contact. Compare left and right foot, noticing the differences; it is rare for both sides of the body to be the same. Following your exhale, begin to allow your weight to drop through your body into your soles and the ground underneath, a sense of yielding into the ground.

Now, increasing your attention to the soles of your feet, add a small push from your soles as you inhale, clarifying your sense of contact with the ground. Widen your focus of awareness to include your whole feet, your ankles, calves, knees, thighs, hips, spine and whole body, alternating pushing and yielding as you continue to breathe in and out. Stay with this experience for a few moments, resting in it, enjoying this natural state perhaps. Now take a step forwards with one foot only. Notice the differences, paying close attention to how your focus changes and how you now orient and reorganize yourself.

Begin to make a list of some of the things you appreciate about your body – your eyes that can see, your legs that can move, your heart that has beaten since you were a few weeks old in your mother's womb. Does anything feel better, worse or no different?

Shame and self-harm

There is a close relationship between shame and self-harm. The experience of early trauma increases the likelihood that the victim will self-harm in adulthood (van der Kolk et al. 1995). To feel endlessly terrible about oneself erodes the sense of self, and becomes externalized in self-inflicted acts of violence against the body. This may include pursuing injurious relationships such as engaging in reckless sex. Self-harm is a reflection of the degree of pain trauma victims feel. 'This state of shame ... may ultimately be followed by self-destructive impulses ... to do away with the self in order to wipe out the offending, disappointing reality of failure' (Kohut 1971: 181, cited in Orange 1995: 100). This is not to say that incidents of self-harm are necessarily triggered by states of shame, at least not overtly.

However, the desire to attack the body speaks clearly of disconnection from embodied life. Fisher makes clear the link between self-harm and the need to relieve tension in those who have been abused and have not learnt to seek soothing from others (Fisher n.d.). For some, self-harm is related to the reversal of more immediate relational concerns, by providing an alternative to dealing with conflict, the setting of boundaries and the risk of relational rupture. Shame gives rise to physiological reactions. Its emotional and physiological dysregulation mean that episodes of self-harm occasion the release of endogenous endorphins which substitute for the attuned other who is unavailable (Cozolino 2002: 278–9). Self-harm can 'paradoxically act to shield the individual from overstimulation or attack (by putting the self in control of the infliction of pain)' (Attias and Goodwin 1999: 161).

The physiology of shame

The experience of shame is agonizingly physical, a more visceral experience than guilt, a 'powerful, preverbal, and physiologically based organizing principle' (Cozolino 2002: 195). Schore (2003b: 154) describes some of the acute physiological and phenomenological features of shame: heightened body awareness, intensified perceptual functions, uncoordinated motor movements, cognitive impairment, blushing, cardiac deceleration, thus implying there is a 'more primitive, biological base'. It is a state of heightened sympathetic arousal, accompanied by self-consciousness and hypervigilance. Blushing is caused by the dilation of small capillaries of the face, triggered by sympathetic arousal of the ANS (Cozolino 2006: 160), and may serve to reduce self-exposure and self-exploration (Schore 2003b: 154).

The relationship between shame and fear is clear. Panksepp (1998: 27) considers more specifically that shame may emerge from 'separation distress' systems in the brain, the relational and attachment function. Cozolino (2002: 119) proposes that shame is a feature of a bias in the brain towards right-hemisphere and more 'negative' emotions. 'Prolonged and repeated shame states result in physiological dysregulation and negatively impact the development of networks of affect regulation and affect' (Cozolino 2002: 194). Shame is not only associated with regulation; there may be a physiological correlate to the feeling of being toxic or dirty that so often accompanies this feeling. In the muscular contraction that accompanies shame states and heightened arousal, toxins can be trapped in the muscles – the literal presence of something bad in the body. However, on a positive note, Attias and Goodwin (1999: 172) observe that 'the bodily suffering is not as endless or as shameful as the patient's traumatic cognitions have constructed it', or at least it need not be.

In an unreceptive world

Kepner writes that shame is not simply an emotion, it is an experience of the field (Kepner 1995: 39). Shame is therefore a conclusion you come to about yourself and your needs in an unaccepting world, associated with the need to make relational bonds, defensive attachment systems, and the breach of those attachment bonds. Shame calls out to be received by the other, to be made wholesome and tolerable. When the other is unable to bear the pain of trauma alongside the victim, the shame is so much greater.

The way society deals with the unbearableness of trauma creates a precondition for shame. A number of factors come into play in this respect. First there is a palpable sense of shock when traumas are publicized, whether natural disasters, man-made or individual. Shock is a defining characteristic of trauma and this is held collectively. Shame shapes commonly held denials about atrocities against other people, because these are far removed from our agreed standards of acceptable behaviour. A victim of domestic violence may feel ashamed for loving their partner when everyone around them is saying they should leave and move on. 'The shame of abuse is compounded by the ultimate shame of denial: nothing happened, you imagined it, your very reality and experience are not wanted or received in the field; relationally speaking, you don't exist at all' (Wheeler 1996: 225). These days we would speak of gaslighting.

Collective shame and cultural norms

Such denial is organized at multiple levels: family, social groups, institutionally and in the legal process. Terr describes a situation in which doctors failed to examine for evidence of abuse in a group of nursery school children, and considers that this was a group-held response to shame: 'the physicians, in other words, may unconsciously have preferred not to look' (Terr 1990: 121). Wheeler also comments on societal shame related to trauma. He says: 'In a Gestalt field model, [the factors contributing to PTS are part of] a field characterized and organized by deep internalized shame' (Wheeler 1996: 225), and this results in a tendency to pathologize the victim. Protection is often afforded more readily to perpetrators than to victims, in families and more widely; whistleblowers are vilified and scapegoated.

High-profile cases of recent years, for example Jimmy Savile, Harvey Weinstein and Jeffrey Epstein, illustrate some of the powerful dynamics around abuse. Their actions were writ large for all to see, yet the magicians waved their wands and entire nations fell asleep for decades. On waking up, the collective sense of shame for the failure to protect becomes tangible. Such dynamics are repeated in families and communities on a daily basis, across the world. In the face of collective shame, the offer of protection to victims is defensive rather than authentic.

Anonymity provided in law to victims of sexual violence, while providing necessary protection, also speaks to the shame of trauma and suggests that there is something to hide; this is reflected socially, in medicine and the media. People are, however, beginning to emerge from behind the veil of anonymity, though the position of the 'whistleblower' is still a vulnerable one; defence against reputational damage is a powerful force. Within the wider field there remains a split between 'undeserving' victims, the clean-living virgin who needs protection, and those who were 'asking for it' by virtue of their chosen lifestyle. Further, we live in a culture that endorses active humiliation as a means of control and oppression; 'naming and shaming' of those who stray from given standards of behaviour, even in our own psychotherapy profession, is in vogue. In this climate, silence moderates how we act.

Working with shame

Much has been written in the Gestalt literature and elsewhere about how to work with shame; the general principles of a dialogic attitude apply no less to working with shame in trauma clients than to shame-prone clients in general. In Gestalt theory there is no one polarity to shame. Wheeler (1996: 49) suggests luck, Yontef (1993: 493) suggests pride and Lee (1996: 10) proposes support as polarities of shame. The two latter concepts are more relational than the first. It is helpful to consider acceptance as another polarity in relation to trauma victims; so much of their experience has been disavowed. What is most needed in therapy for trauma clients is a restoration of their sense of humanity, by which I mean acceptance of their fallibility, vulnerability and dignity. This term has some subtlety in this context. It implies both relational and self-acceptance, a coming to terms with who one really is, and repair of the alienation of dissociation. Acceptance requires integration of body awareness and honouring of instinctive survival defences. It also includes acceptance of the past, a stage of grief equivalent to the third stage of Kepner's Healing Tasks Model – undoing, redoing and mourning. Finally, it is consistent with the Paradoxical Theory of Change (Beisser 1970).

Traumatized people struggle to be authentic and suffer greatly to be accepted by others. I suggested earlier that the threat to survival of the sense of self is a major concern for people experiencing relational trauma. Rejection, being ignored or unseen are experiences equivalent to annihilation. Shame then becomes an organizing factor in everyday life – how to avoid it, how to live with it, how to mask it. Impossible standards are imposed from others and also on ourselves. Perfectionism and a myriad of 'shoulds' and 'oughts' become a tyranny that defines the parameters of being in the world. So many survival adaptations involve disowning aspects of self, that acceptance of the whole messy human self is also critical.

Inhumanity is one of the factors that govern the behaviour of perpetrators and oppressive systems alike, and comes to be understood as being personal. 'I am pond life in my organization' said one person. Restoration of dignity becomes a central developmental relational need. The tenderness and unconditional respect we offer to those we work with can be transformative. Not that this is easy, as so many traumatized people will regard this with mistrust or fear of your 'agenda', or expect that they must give too much of themselves in return, or feel that they are deeply and irrevocably undeserving of your care and attention. And this does not obviate the space for therapeutic challenge and holding other perspectives on the person and their situation. One person held an intransigent belief that their abduction was their fault, and I resolutely offered a different perspective. When eventually they were able to tell more of their behaviour in that situation, I commented: 'It was terrible, for you to have no alternative but to stop resisting. Had I been in your shoes I might well have done the same.'

The thorny subject of forgiveness often comes up in therapy with trauma victims. Forgiveness has many meanings for different people. Harris (2007: 114) defines three possibilities: seeking forgiveness for wrongdoing, forgiveness of those who have caused hurt, and forgiveness of self. A focus on the last two is most pertinent to trauma work. Harris (2007: 107) considers that forgiveness is 'a choice about how one deals with the present experience of past betrayals'. It is a way of completing unfinished business, but it is unlikely to be a choice that can be made without first fully understanding one's pain, in the spirit of the Paradoxical Theory of Change. Forgiveness is in one's own self-interest, by virtue of 'letting go of one's hurt, bitterness, and anger, which prevents the hurtful act from controlling one's life' (Harris 2007: 109). He cites a number of research studies which demonstrate improvements in health and well-being resulting from forgiveness. Forgiveness in these terms does not mean denial or apportioning of blame; it means acceptance. My own position is that *forgiveness is not a requirement of recovery and should not be asked of or expected from anyone*. What I do believe, though, is that forgiveness of self, as evidence of acceptance, is necessary. To be able to forgive yourself for having been small, vulnerable, helpless, for doing the best you could in impossible circumstances, for having made unwise choices – ultimately for having been human – is a powerful reclaiming of selfhood and reality.

We need to accept that shame will accompany the relationship we form with traumatized people; it is part of their experience and how they have learnt to relate. We might attend to shame potential, perhaps signalled by a withdrawal of energy or an unexpected attack. By bringing attention to something happening between you, and being curious rather than defensive, the possibility of repair opens up. I shall say more about rupture and repair in Chapter 13.

Shame inevitably arises in the therapeutic relationship, and needs to, in order to be borne relationally. 'For individuals experiencing intense shame, no words can capture the assaultive intensity of the experience. It is only through *reliving* the trauma through enactment with the analyst that its magnitude can be known by an "other"' (Bromberg [1998] 2001: 296, original italics).

Work towards acceptance that suffering is part of life and that experience of pain is part of being human, and what happened is not personal. We cannot control everything. Consider also 'the acceptance that comes from being oneself … in relation to significant others or others in one's expanded context' (Davies 2022: 8).

Therapists must be alert to the risks associated with self-harm, first and foremost by demonstrating the care, compassion and acceptance that are needed. It is important to develop a shared understanding of the phenomenology of self-harm and what precedes harming episodes, so as to recognize and accept the likely regulatory function it serves. There can then be agreement that the aim of therapy is not to stop self-harming, but to develop alternative ways of finding soothing.

There is a place for psychoeducation about trauma in order to reduce the impact of shame. Explanations and knowledge normalize experiences which feel marginalizing or incomprehensible and therefore shameful. Finding commonalities with other victims limits the sense of being unacceptably different, and comments like 'Some people find that ...' are helpful. Appropriate interventions may range from making clear and simple statements like 'What he did to you was a crime', 'That was a disgusting thing to do to you', to explaining the role of immobilized defences and demonstrating respect for creative adjustments.

Developing resources representing previous competence, mastery, pride and confidence can be pivotal in therapy, bringing a realization that shame does not define you. It is also helpful to attend to the qualities that the client feels they need to overcome their trauma, and if they cannot find them in their own history, they can be encouraged to think of someone they know, or know of, who holds these qualities – a role model as a resource. If they can find other ways in which they identify with their role model, so much the better.

Ultimately, developing some self-compassion is healing, because it helps create dis-identification with the victim position and allows perspective on the extent to which one has been wronged. This opens the space for rightful rage and anger to come into the frame; relational safety in the therapy is required for this to be possible.

Case study: Part 4

The more Eve struggled with feeling and expressing her anger, the more she continued to treat herself as an object of contempt. She felt a great deal of disgust for her body, especially since 'it' had done nothing to get her out of the terrifying situation of captivity in which she was raped. Eve saw herself as weak and useless, and felt that the trauma and this belief about herself defined her. She felt permanently damaged. Eve's shame was greatly compounded on those occasions when she deliberately injured her genitals to regulate her pain. A momentary relief was quickly followed by guilt, greater self-loathing and a fear of discovery. It was a very long time into therapy before she could stay in a conversation about self-harm with me. She expected me to react with horror and disgust, rather than compassion when she disclosed this self-harm to me.

It helped a great deal when I explored instances of Eve's self-harm phenomenologically. Together we made sense of the distress that she was in and the relief she felt, however fleeting. It was important too that we could understand that even though she was in some ways inflicting the same violence on herself as her abusers did, she now had a degree of control. This provided us with another opportunity to work with making choices that felt better, even where Eve found choices that challenged her shame in sometimes uncomfortable ways.

The position I took in respect of some of the hardest aspects of Eve's current and historical field was consistent and gave her a bridge to a less terrifying world. I genuinely felt warm and compassionate towards Eve. I repeatedly asked her for the kindest things she could tell herself, and looked for ways of encouraging her to increase her self-care. My biggest concern, though, was the lack of care she took of herself in relation to others. Out of compensatory guilt, Eve was letting Freya run rings around her, and Eve was afraid that if she said 'No' Freya would be harmed. Eve had protected herself during her attack by not protesting. Her work with the mentally unwell echoed how she had pacified her deranged attackers in Greece. Eve was overextending herself in an attempt to make things better.

As we looked at the processes and beliefs that kept Eve in this difficult position and she learnt more about trauma, she came to recognize for herself the part that she played in her current relationships. Eve developed an awareness of the choices available to her, even where it was difficult to act on them. Her relationship to her trauma changed when she could begin to be sad for the pain she felt, rather than attacking it in the belief that she should be different. She understood more about the defensive role she had taken during her ordeal and this helped her to feel better about herself.

Summary

Shame is an emotion that everyone is familiar with, regulating our interactions with the environment to keep personal identity, dignity and integrity intact. Somewhat different from other responses to trauma, shame is experienced as an attack on the self of the victim, and therefore deeply personal, rather than an attack on the physical body. The experience of pervasive shame profoundly affects the way clients perceive themselves and others, and their capacity for full engagement at the contact boundary. These are clients who have difficulty accepting themselves for who they are, and, as for trauma responses, do not update information about the current field easily. Shame tends to loop back on itself, clients feeling shame for being ashamed, shame upon shame. It therefore has a role in maintaining the cyclical reliving of trauma which defines PTS. Although shame is a broader problem than that of trauma, the two are inextricably linked.

Shame is present in the primary features of fear, helplessness and disconnection. Coupled with states of high autonomic arousal, avoidance and intrusion is shame, which can be triggered by any of these trauma-related experiences. When shame or humiliation has been an explicit feature of the original trauma, shame is also a trigger in itself. Helplessness is a precursor to shame, because it places power in the wider field and relates specifically to immobilized survival defences. Shame feels so interminable as to give rise to hopelessness and resignation. It is a profoundly alienating experience, disconnecting the individual from a world in which they feel shunned or unwelcome. The intense bodily involvement in shame is such that it may be denied or dissociated, and in addition dissociative parts may hold shame or be felt as shaming.

Shame-laden attacks on the self often indicate a shift in the locus of control – victims taking more blame for the situation than is reasonable or necessary. This is related to ruptures in attachment bonds, and applies specifically to the configuration of the victim's relationship to the perpetrators in the case of personal attack or abuse. In this process, blame becomes polarized in the dynamic between the victim and the perpetrator. Gestalt therapy treats relationships as co-created, neither party taking full responsibility, but correspondingly neither party necessarily taking an equal share. By this token, we come to understand that trauma victims have a small degree of responsibility for the events which have overtaken their lives, if only in so far as their reactions are theirs and theirs alone. It is phenomenologically consistent to allow victims to accept this minor role in the evolution of their story, which is more proportionate to the event and allows some sense of control.

When terrible things happen to people's bodies, they may feel themselves to be disgusting, dirty or contaminated. Embodied life and its vital needs become shameful and may be disowned or denied. Body shame often leads to an inability to take appropriate care of oneself, and victims may ultimately resort to self-harm. This is often a response to terrible pain, regulating the arousal that cannot be contained. Acts of self-harm or mutilation make visible, and therefore manageable, that which cannot otherwise be tolerated. Risks of self-harm of one sort or another increase after therapy sessions when there is inadequate containment and regulation within the session. Shame is understood as a state of dysregulated arousal associated with prevention of relational rupture. Different physiological defences come into play in shame processes, linked biologically to the networks and systems that deal with fundamental emotions of fear and threat.

The way society or the wider field deals with traumatic events is not dissimilar to the way individuals respond to them. Shock, disgust and fear arise along with denial, disbelief and dissociation. The reality of some victims' experience is so intolerable that it cannot be borne by others in their immediate world. Such reactions only serve to compound the shame and secrecy that surrounds much trauma, and the stigma of being treated for a medicalized 'disorder' makes matters worse. It has been suggested that such factors reflect a shame-laden society.

Acceptance is proposed as a polarity for shame in work with trauma victims. While much of therapeutic work with shame is the same for trauma clients as for anyone else, there are a few specific considerations for this client group. Developing compassion over time for one's considerable wounds is seen as key to healing. Forgiveness is a way of letting go of the emotional ties to the past that are caught up in resentment and pain. The development of resources related to confidence and achievement is to be encouraged, along with a growing sense of gratitude and appreciation for survival and aliveness.

Part **3**

A relational home for trauma

10 The role of the therapist

The way the therapist approaches the work plays an enormous part in the healing process, providing a different embodied relational ground from which someone might safely move on from their trauma. How the therapist creates the conditions for change is the focus of this chapter, keeping safety at the heart of the work. The therapist's power and transference issues are explored in the light of relational trauma. Some exploratory questions and reflections support the reader in deepening their understanding of the relational impact of the work, and the self of the therapist.

The four dimensions of trauma described in Part 2 form a closed loop, reinforcing one another and maintaining the system, until circumstances arise that allow the loop to be opened. What, then, are the relational conditions that support change? Each moment in which a therapist facilitates a state shift away from a traumatic activation and towards regulation builds the ground for change; they are not the change in themselves, but create the possibility of replacing the closed loop with a more open system.

The therapist and change

In Chapter 3 I proposed that in an integrated model, change only happens under optimal conditions. What the therapist does to support the new conditions provides a relational perspective on change. In the Integrated Model of Change the therapist is positioned more actively than Beisser proposed in his Paradoxical Theory of Change. I think we need now to have a look at that. Philippson (2005) suggests that Beisser's position is idealized and somewhat naive. While I agree that as psychotherapists we do not impose our own ideas about change or work towards defined outcomes, the therapist's very presence creates a change in the environment at all times; it cannot not be so. Philippson goes on to claim that there are situations in which the therapist needs to be a change agent (Philippson 2009: 136), more active than simply being present, as interpersonal neurobiology confirms. A corollary of the Paradoxical Theory is that the therapist relinquishes the expert position in the interests of equalization of power.

How to achieve the fine balance between 'being a change agent' and horizontalization of power requires skill and consideration.

What trauma work points towards is something subtle: that the therapist temporarily takes responsibility to the degree that the client is unable to do so. The Paradoxical Theory of Change rests on the assumption that the client can take responsibility for their own process and has the relational skills to support this. But this is not realistic in traumatized clients because of their neurobiology, relational history and creative adjustments. Neither is this a fixed position but one that will vary moment by moment, and be adjusted according to the ongoing phenomenological process of the client. Therapists therefore need a degree of flexibility to track moment by moment, and their own supports, both internal and external, for this. The goal, for we must have one, is to establish the more horizontal position over time, in line with the Integrated Model of Change.

Beisser's caution against the expert therapist is principally against taking an objectifying position. It is obvious that this might replicate the dynamics of relational trauma. However, Hycner (1993: 7) observes that an objectifying position is necessary *at times* in order to accomplish certain goals. I have found the knowledge I have, held lightly, is immensely grounding when I feel lost or unsure; it helps me to stand back and observe what is happening and make sense of it. The meta position, provided by good supervision and reflection, supports us in separating from the hyperfocus of the black hole we can be drawn into. In order to establish reasonably reliable stability within the window of tolerance, the therapist must consistently call on the specialized knowledge supplied by neuroscience *and* the skill to apply it in a relational manner. It is these qualities of knowledge and skill that are the hallmark of the true expert. Having said all this, the ability to meet each client with the freshness of a beginner's mind stands as an abiding principle of Gestalt therapy. The phenomenological approach requires that we have the humility to unlearn what we already know and relearn what is unknown, afresh in each successive moment. This place of uncertainty, while uncomfortable, has much potential for emerging spontaneity (see also Taylor 2021).

The therapist and emotional regulation

By far the most important contribution the therapist can offer the traumatized people they work with is to be a 'steward of arousal'. The term is drawn from a comment made by Hycner and Jacobs (1995: 13) about the therapist as steward of dialogue. One client found the process of 'shepherding' (their word) them away from their story helpful, because they didn't have to grapple with it in a way that made them anxious. There is an ethical issue here, I think, concerning the potential risks of leaving people unsupported, dysregulated and out of contact. This suggests a different mode of therapy, requiring flexibility on the part of the therapist and a wide range of skills. However, this is more than simply a moment-by-moment management issue; the therapeutic value over time is in helping clients to distance themselves from emotionally uncontainable experiences without dissociating (Fisher 2001).

The therapist's attunement to and interest in another individual's state of arousal is a relational dynamic that the person may never have encountered before. Together you learn to collaborate around arousal, as your client becomes increasingly interested in and trusting in the process. There are times in trauma work when the therapist needs to build successful exchanges around less charged material, or you will both lose your footing and be lost. When the material is too hot for the person to tolerate, it is the therapist's responsibility to de-escalate the situation as quickly as possible. As discussed in Chapter 4, if someone moves outside of their window of tolerance they need help to return to it, because they are beyond the threshold of *self*-regulation. For example, when someone becomes triggered into a state that removes them from present contact, the switch can happen extremely fast and it is not helpful to try to explore what happened; it may even be extremely unhelpful to do so. The therapist needs to switch equally rapidly into a mode of taking more charge, knowing what to do or at least what might help. Cozolino (2002: 252) tells us that biological processes need to be reversed as soon as possible after being triggered to allow the body to do the job of recovery.

The Window of Tolerance Model can be considered usefully from the perspective of the therapist. A therapist is neither creatively indifferent nor taking on the mantle of change agent all the time, but shuttling backwards and forwards between the two as the energetic arousal between you changes. You and the person you are working with both need to learn early on in the therapy what specific changes in arousal look and feel like. You will often pick this up on an embodied level, aware perhaps of a shift in energy in the room, or of a change in muscle tone or orientation in the other person. Similarly, you both need to understand how to intervene for different degrees of dysregulation, for both hyper- and hypoaroused states (see Figure 10.1). This information is important in order to enable the ability to spot these changes almost before they happen, returning the client to the safe emergency within the window of tolerance.

The expansion of the window of tolerance happens in incremental stages, learning together the dance steps to re-establish the safety needed. Confidence in the process and in your reliability as a regulating presence is thereby increased.

The therapist holds the reins only for as long as is needed, staying present as much as possible. For example, they might sense that the client is in touch with a memory, and ask them to put it to one side for now and focus on their breathing, or something safe in the room. Choices can be offered within the dialogue, such as: 'Is it more helpful or less to be doing this?', and later: 'Would you like to tell me what happened or do you need to let things settle

Figure 10.1 The therapist's role in regulation

	CLIENT	THERAPIST
HYPERAROUSAL	• Past focus, creative adjustment • Unavailable • Unsafe • Chaotic • Choiceless • Overfocused • Implicit memory • Confusion	• Aims for safety, 'glue' • Drop content, new frame • Establishing ground • Moderate to high risk • Narrow attention • Focus on sensation • Leading • Directive • Grounded • Present • Embodied • Slow, soothing
WINDOW OF TOLERANCE	• Focused • Narrative • Processing • Choiceful • Response-able • Flexible • Available for contact • Present focus • Explicit memory • Meaning-making	• Aim – exploration, loosening fixed gestalts, 'solvent' • Open attention • Low to moderate risk – the 'safe emergency' • Process focus • Sharpening figure • Creatively indifferent • Following • Phenomenological tracking • Receptive • Curiosity • Experimental
HYPOAROUSAL	• Unfocused • Choiceless • Rigid • Disconnected • Unavailable • Past focus, creative adjustment • Implicit memory • Confusion	• Aim – presence, small drops of 'solvent' • Narrow attention • Moderate to high risk • Focus on mobilization • Establishing ground • Leading • Directive • Still, encouragement, adding some energy • Drop content, new frame

some more?' These enquiries help bring into the verbal and explicit domain the previously unverbalized implicit material, allowing reorganization and integration. The BCPSG (2010: 149) consider that 'The intentions of most interest to the psychoanalytic endeavour are those intentions to make and adjust the state of the relationship.'

Clinical vignette

Amy had been traumatized through her long history of medical treatment for a congenital bladder deformity. She had had unsuccessful surgery which left her in pain, and over time she began to require sedation to enable doctors to perform tests. To make matters worse, on the last occasion the sedation she was given for the procedure failed to work and she was left with conscious memory of the entire process; her shock and distress were misunderstood by the doctors. When Amy's difficulties increased, she did not attend her routine hospital appointment, delaying for several months. And when she became clearly unwell, Amy began to work more actively on her terror in therapy. Her initial impulse was to get herself out of the situation once again – a defensive flight response – and she entered a highly dysregulated state which endured over several weeks. Her terror of repeating this investigation was extreme, and she settled a little when I commented that she could not make a real choice at the moment because she was driven entirely by fear.

I negotiated with Amy to increase her choices by regulating her severe trauma reactions, to re-establish her window of tolerance and to develop some new resources specific to this situation. This was the territory we inhabited time and again in the coming weeks. Because Amy seemed to have been hijacked emotionally by a traumatized self-state, I actively supported her stronger, less traumatized self to emerge as a resource. Throughout this time I remained creatively indifferent about what decision she would eventually make, while at the same time working within a trauma-focused perspective in order to support the making of those choices.

Privately, though, I was concerned about Amy's illness, and hoped that she could reach a position in which she could access the help she needed without being retraumatized by it. With more ability to stay in touch with a host of new resources, Amy went ahead with the investigation; this time the sedation was effective and the hospital staff kind and supportive. What astonished me was the fact that several weeks later Amy told me in a quite matter of fact way that she had been for a routine smear test. This was something else she had avoided for many years because of its similarly triggering intrusive nature. This time she was able to handle the procedure with a degree of equanimity, and without my support.

Power and horizontalism

Adopting a beginner's mind opens up the possibility that the therapist will be changed by the client, as Beisser suggested. We might consider the space between us to be the salient factor in bringing about change. In trauma therapy this means allowing ourselves to be changed as human beings by highly dysregulated and disorganized people whose impact we might more intuitively resist. In this delicate situation, the potential for a more horizontal relationship still exists. The notion of creative indifference (Friedlander 1918) underpins the concept of the horizontal therapeutic relationship: 'By remaining alert in the center, we can acquire a creative ability of seeing both sides of an occurrence and [of] completing an incomplete half. By avoiding a one-sided outlook, we gain a much deeper insight to the structure and function of the organism' (Perls 1969: 14–15).

When the shift in the locus of control (Chapter 7) has reorganized the boundaries around power, trauma victims do not expect to find anything resembling a horizontal relationship. They may assume a position of relational helplessness, power dynamics becoming severely and habitually skewed. Those who have become controlling and manipulative are not exerting real power in relationship but employ a more coercive and sometimes bullying style of relating, because it is the polar opposite of their powerlessness. After all, while 'power' is a hot issue for many trauma clients, it is something that can be used for good or for ill: power may oppress, abuse and destroy on the one hand, and on the other it can facilitate and heal (see Taylor 2021). We need to recognize the quality of the power we hold and are perceived to hold by virtue of our role, and how to let go of it over time.

The imbalance in the consulting room is a manifestation of how the therapist holds the tension between horizontalization and power. The extent to which therapists can help to liberate the people they work with from the bonds of their past puts them in a very powerful position indeed; it is helpful to think in terms of the therapist's potency rather than dominance in this regard. Alongside this is a comment by Loewenstein and Goodwin (1999: 80): 'It is important to point out to the patient that the clinician, far from being in full control, is far more likely to be reactive to the patient's style of communication and statement of problems.' The degree of control exercised by the therapist may be reassuring or it may be threatening; either is grist for the mill.

The therapist does not decide how the client should live their life or who they are, but seeks to restore self-functions through the relationship. Therapists can be in too much of a hurry to try and hand over power to their clients, sometimes as a co-transferential resonance with their clients' lack of personal power. A therapeutic stance is one in which we act in the service of the other's recovery, while maintaining an attitude of creative indifference. Crucially, *the power we can creatively hold does not include coercion or pressure to change*. The experimental attitude of Gestalt therapy is a great asset in shifting power dynamics from the therapist-directed to the self-initiated: 'try this and see what happens' (Grigsby and Osuch 2007: 71). I value how Levin and Levine (2012: 6) highlight the difference between change as by expert practitioner and learning how to cure yourself with help or direction from a therapist.

Establishing the relationship

Harman (1982: 46) suggests that 'The Gestalt therapist must be willing to ask, tease, cajole, provoke or demand contact from patients.' Such a proposition is far too provocative for most clients who have a fragile process, but the spirit of this statement does encapsulate an important principle. Traumatized people are among those who find any kind of contact – with themselves, with others and with current reality – the hardest. The trauma therapist in the more evocative and dialogic manner of contemporary relational Gestalt must nevertheless insist again and again, 'Don't go there, find your feet in this room now, come back to me.' The paradoxical tension inherent in this invitation is part of the therapeutic rigour the work demands.

The therapist's orientation towards safety is likely to be at odds with the client's embodied orientation towards danger and threat. This influences the ways in which we are able to meet our clients. Often the most genuine and humane meeting available is to invest fully and intentionally in bringing about a moment of relief in which a more regulated state and relational contact become possible. While we can rightly question the therapeutic value of meeting the needs of the other, we do so to this extent only, for the individual concerned needs first and foremost to be shown the way back.

It is bound to be difficult to make any relationship with someone who is beset by phobias of therapy and of the therapist, who has difficulty staying in the present or whose relational history includes betrayal, criticism or misattunement. For these individuals a working alliance needs to be built around safety issues, emotional regulation, the relief of symptoms and the building of self-functions or resources, in keeping with the first two stages of Kepner's model. The support built into Kepner's model is primarily relational support. Some find that the possibility of relationship with a therapist is so fraught that it is more helpful to be given clear instructions about how to develop the skills they need. Handled as dialogically as possible, the person will come to recognize that it was you, the therapist, who offered these helpful tools, and thus the seeds of a relationship are planted.

Bromberg ([1998] 2001: 137) asks a pertinent question: how is the work of therapy to be negotiated with patients for whom negotiation is an art that has never been learnt? There is a particular implicit negotiated process with the person's state of arousal – of which you are the steward – and capacity to be present, which is at the heart of good trauma therapy. A simple and effective negotiation tool from sensorimotor therapy is to enquire over and again, 'Do you feel better or worse or no different when you try this [experiment]?' By considering this question, the person learns to begin to reflect on and discriminate their experience, to make choices and to ask for more of what they need. This question also has the effect of overriding habitual cognitive responses by going straight to the felt sense. Supplementary questions may include phenomenological exploration of *how* the client can tell if it's better or worse, and the specific physical components of their reported moment-by-moment experience, the awareness continuum. It is a task of trauma therapy for the therapist to provide the optimal conditions for change, most often a case of 'grappling', together with where to go and how to get there (BCPSG 2010: 101).

Transference issues

Among other things, the shift in contemporary relational psychotherapies places more emphasis on the relationship between two parties than on transference. Gestalt therapy, with its focus on how we meet, eschews the notion of 'counter-transference' in favour of the concept of co-transference, emphasizing the parts we both play in the encounter. Issues of co-transference in trauma work are often compelling and call for attention. For *both sides* of the therapeutic dyad, the other has the potential to evoke uncontainable reactions. The person who comes to us brings their fear, helplessness, disconnection and shame to the heart of the relationship; our co-transference, formed in response to the present moment and from our own histories and biases, may mirror these dynamics directly (see Taylor 2021). Clients' orientation towards these dynamics is a gravitational pull that the therapist must find a way to counter. Tracking shifts in the other's experience is demanding when at one moment the therapist represents safety, validation and even rescue – the resolution of deep yearnings for connection – and in the next moment may be seen as a controlling abuser. We enquire into the client's process and are perceived as intrusive; we hold back and are seen as neglectful. Shifts in arousal may represent dissociated parts which may be malevolent towards the therapist. In such instances '[i]t is not generally useful to encourage a transference reaction to reach full affective force' (Perlman and Saakvitne 1995: 20). The client is not yet able to tolerate such feelings, and the therapist may need to be active in shepherding the person away from them for the time being.

Therapists can very easily get caught in these splits as they emerge – it happens in the blink of an eye. Trauma can feel contagious: it is inevitable that the therapist will feel disturbed in some way as they enter the painful and fragmented world of their client. The ideas the other person has about the therapist can have a paranoid feel to them. 'We are asked to feel threatened, devalued, objectified, ignored, and hated – on the other hand we may be idealized and revered, and required to maintain a standard of perfection that splits off any disconfirming aspect of ourselves' (Davis and Frawley, cited in Perlman and Saakvitne 1995: 24). What, then, of the self of the therapist, which is brought into this heated and complicated mix of relational factors?

Dropping in: Part 1

The following exercise, comprising a series of questions for self-reflection, is presented in three parts in this chapter, each representing the three elements of the SOS model (Chapter 1). The questions provide a structure for you to reflect on the impact of working with traumatized clients and how you may respond to them. They also touch on aspects of your personal history which may shape your ability to be present to your client's trauma. If they feel powerful that is intentional; they are offered to increase awareness of your need for resilience and the role of personal therapy and supervision, among other things, that will support you in this work. These reflections lay the ground for the material in the next chapter. **If your answers to any of the questions in this chapter cause you unexpected distress or disturb you greatly, please take care of yourself and find immediate help. In addition, you may find**

Chapter 11 helpful. You are encouraged to take your time writing your responses to these questions. Be as honest with yourself as you are able; you do not have to share this writing with anyone unless you choose to do so.

- What is your response to difficult intense emotions? What is your experience of working with them or of resolving them?
- What response do you have to hearing stories of appalling abuse, torture and suffering? Shock, denial, shame, anger, blame or dissociation may be among them.
- What of your own need to be comforted or regulated by your client, or for contact when someone is dissociated?
- How do you support yourself, both in the moment and in life generally?
- What is your personal experience of and relationship to power?
- What is it like for you to recognize the influence you hold as a therapist?
- What do you think is your capacity for facing suffering? Are there ways in which you protect yourself from the suffering of others?

The co-regulatory approach to trauma therapy that is being proposed here does much to mitigate against the effects of vicarious traumatization. Extraordinary as it may seem, the work can be enjoyable, and this will be considered further in Chapter 11. There is inevitably a major impact on transference by working in this way. Our aim is to provide a regulating environment within which the therapist maintains a degree of neutrality, that may nevertheless be perceived otherwise. When we actively resist dysregulating material, when we take a respectful and compassionate position for the immediate relief of suffering and emphasize positive resources, we are more likely to evoke a positive transference, even though it is not our intention to do so. Philippson (2005: 16) cautions: 'If the relationship is an attempt to create change by mimicking some idealized parental relationship, it is less effective than if a real intimacy develops organically (and with great difficulty at first) between therapist and client.'

The issue of the trauma therapist's intention is crucial to working with transference. It needs to be the therapist's active intention *not* to replicate relational dynamics that have been detrimental in the client's history. In my experience, the refusal to accept the expert position and my ongoing working through of my own trauma (see Taylor 2021) serves as some protection from the hubris associated with being idealized. On this point Turner et al. ([1996] 2007: 553) comment that:

It is important for therapists to accept the fact that this need for idealization is not founded on their real attributes (which in their anxiety to stay in control, patients barely perceive), and that patients idealize them in order to replace the sources of security that were destroyed by the trauma.

Each therapist, however, inevitably brings their own complex and intersecting trauma history into the relationship as part of the co-creation, and the two may rub up uncomfortably against one another. Replication of trauma dynamics, in the form of an enactment, is most likely to occur if we allow a negative transference to develop, though it must be stressed that we cannot always avoid this. This is a situation that can become unworkable and unresolvable, in which the client cannot engage fruitfully in the process, and may be revictimized. It is far less risky to run some distance with an engaged positive transference, which builds the ground for the emergence of negative transference safely.

Therapist as (re)organizer

In Part 2 we explored the various ways in which traumatized people reorganize their experience and their field, especially relational boundaries. Trauma is first and foremost a neurobiologically based regulator of boundaries within the entire field. Trauma therapy offers clients the opportunity to understand their creative adjustments and to reorganize their experiential ground, principally somatically. Earlier, Chapter 2 focused on the ways in which the ground of trauma becomes sedimented and the figures arising from it rigidify. The therapist offers new ways of structuring the ground both functionally, through experiments and resourcing, and relationally. The therapist's embodied presence is invaluable. Delisle (2011: 65) observes that 'the therapeutic relationship, before it can be a reparative space, must be a space for reconstruction'. There is an important relational component in directly engaging to loosen fixed gestalts, whereby 'The therapist is pulling both parties out of the pattern' (Philippson 2012: 89).

One of the principal tasks of stewarding arousal is to actively intervene when the client moves out of their window of tolerance. The clues that such intervention is necessary may be sensed via a shift in self-state, or through the therapist's awareness of their own embodied response, or both. In such an instance 'it becomes possible for patient and analyst alike to use the other person's momentary self-state as part of his own. This process of *mutual borrowing* entails a permeability of boundaries, both between self and other and between self-states within each party' (Bromberg 2011: 51, my italics). Sensorimotor trauma therapy (Ogden et al. 2006) asks clients to drop the story as soon as signs of dysregulated arousal emerge, to 'park it somewhere else', and to find a resource in the present moment that feels better. These may be resources that have been created together in the past and can be relied on, or they may be developed organically in the moment. All trauma therapists need to develop the confidence to check regularly on how the client is feeling as they recount some life experience; we must hone the skill of interrupting, even insisting – kindly, supportively – that the client direct their attention to something more regulating. This not only supports the client in their reorientation towards more resourced states: it opens up choices and reorganizes the relational field. The therapist's refusal to go to those places for which support is lacking models containment and clear boundaries.

Dropping in: Part 2

- What personal history do you share with your client? How do you regulate yourself around this?
- What enduring relational patterns, taboo subjects, gendered roles, expectations or addictions can you trace to your ancestors?: 'In my family, we never/always …'
- How have you recognized the familiarity of these patterns being repeated in your own life, relationships or behaviour?
- In what ways have you sought to heal the wounds of your family, either directly and consciously, or implicitly and indirectly?
- What kind of ancestor would you like to become?

By embodying missing polarities and self-functions, the therapist models something different. This is another key way in which the therapist contributes to reorganizing the ground. This requires that the self of the therapist has enough resources to contain strong emotions, to remain grounded and in touch with their embodied senses moment by moment, to reflect on experience, to have curiosity and to demonstrate clear boundaries. The therapist needs sometimes to process the traumatic material themselves, before handing it back to the other person. In my description of collective dissociation during the workshop in Warsaw (in Chapter 8), I gave an example of this. It is therefore imperative that the therapist do their own work on healing their own fear, helplessness, dissociation and shame. No one wants to sit with a therapist who is scared, for example. The therapist's body becomes a mirror and representation of something that needs to be owned.

Among important attitudes that the therapist can model is curiosity and the capacity to tolerate uncertainty. Offering a 'menu' of possibilities helps the person you are working with to be able to determine and own what fits for them. For example, one person used only the word 'nice' to describe anything that wasn't actually unpleasant. It helped reanimate them to expand their vocabulary when I asked if perhaps they meant 'pleasant, lovely, comforting, delightful, kind or something else? What is the most accurate word for you right now?' This kind of precision, which is a valuable feature of the phenomenological approach, invites the differentiation of experience that is compromised by trauma.

The therapist and the here and now

First and foremost, the trauma therapist serves as an anchor to the present. The concept of dual awareness (Rothschild 2000) implies that the past trauma cannot safely be revisited unless the client also has a foot in the present moment, orienting them to current reality. The presence of the therapist can be a powerful influence in ensuring that the client does not fully disappear into the overwhelming terror of the past. There is a therapeutic skill in staying anchored and connected in the face of disconnection. Bear in mind that the disconnection may not be an immediate function of the therapeutic relationship, but of something outside the door. The demands of the field are always present, and the therapist becomes a representative of that wider context. How they are perceived in terms of socio-economic status, education, religion, sexual orientation is part of what is implicitly in the room, as it is for the other person (Johnson 2018: 105). These intersecting domains will constellate in the therapeutic relationship and re-present themselves in the here and now.

Dropping in: Part 3

- In what ways can you see the shaping of your culture and social systems – through education, race, class, gender or being part of a perceived minority – reflected in the way you bring yourself into the world?
- Is there more than one way in which your life space is circumscribed by such systems – an intersectional perspective?
- In what ways have you benefited, as we all do, from systems that oppress others?
- Who, or what, in your culture might have paid the price of any privilege you might have?
- How have you reacted to some of the big themes of contemporary life – Black Lives Matter, reparations for colonialism, #MeToo, climate anxiety or denial, fundamentalism, for example?
- How can you sit with the knowledge that you are neither entirely innocent nor entirely guilty? (From Chidiac 2023: 19.)

The therapist has a key part to play in holding the continuity of experience for the client. This can be supported by making links that the client holds outside of awareness, recalling previous sessions and highlighting the fluidity of experience: now this, then that. Self-disclosure of embodied phenomenological process by the therapist is one way of bringing continuity of experience into the room and has a containing effect on clients. Bromberg cautions against using self-disclosure as a technique, but regards it nevertheless as a human act, particularly when the therapist is 'free of internal pressure (conscious or unconscious) to prove his honesty or trustworthiness' (Bromberg [1998] 2001: 261).

'On another level, the therapist serves as an external neural circuit to aid in the integration of networks left unintegrated during development' (Cozolino 2002: 283): assuming that the therapist is able to maintain a reasonably regulated state, they will act as a kind of joint temporary cortex for the client, a brain-to-brain communication of calm, curiosity, attentiveness and safety. Bromberg ([1998] 2001: 136) quotes Kahn: 'It is for the analyst operating as an auxiliary ego ... to register dissociations and help the patient to integrate them.' Here is a function of holding the other in mind, a property of object constancy and mentalization, which is so necessary for those who have never mattered to another human being. For the therapist, the client is held as someone who continues to exist outside of immediate experience.

It is often assumed that the therapist needs to act as a witness to the trauma and to the suffering of the client. It is true that people who have suffered much on their own need the connection with a safe companion on their journey. However, the Window of Tolerance Model implies that *it is less important for the therapist to be the witness than it is for the client to be enabled to witness their experience for themselves.* From a relational field perspective, in which the therapist is not neutral and shapes the work through their presence, it is more accurate to suggest that both therapist and client need to find a way of *being participants and observers together.*

> Ultimately the therapist is powerless to *change* the patient, and sometimes the pain of wanting to make the patient's life better but being powerless to do so is keenly felt. The therapist who is present brings this pain too to the meeting.
>
> (Woldt and Toman 2005: xix)

Vietnamese Buddhist monk Thich Nhat Hanh (2012) speaks of the gift of non-fear, which I believe is perhaps the greatest gift therapists can offer their trauma clients; it cannot be achieved alone.

Summary

In revisiting the Paradoxical Theory of Change from Chapter 3, the different role of the therapist in trauma work comes to the fore. Beisser's claim that the therapist should not be an agent of change is challenged by the neurological condition of the client, who is unable to take their share of responsibility for the progress of therapy. The therapist takes a more active and directive role in the Integrated Change Model, which is somewhat more complex and subtle, responding to the emerging stabilization of the client and accommodating to this, moment by moment. The key role for the therapist is to establish safety for the client, both in their external and internal worlds and in the between of the therapeutic relationship. Technical ways of managing this can help in the beginning to establish a relationship with people who may have few relational skills or tools.

There are inherent power issues in any therapy, but in working with clients for whom power dynamics have overwhelmed their natural sense of agency, the therapist is in a more powerful or potent position. Many trauma clients come into therapy with the expectation that trauma-related power dynamics will endure because they have become fixed in the locus of control shift.

Therefore it is helpful to think in terms of a gradual transition of power from therapist towards a more horizontal position, the place at which Beisser's injunction can come into play in the spirit of the Paradoxical Theory of Change. There is necessarily an impact on transference issues that emerges from this relational shift, one in which the likelihood of an idealized transference is increased. It is argued that this is preferable to the risk of the negative transference which can recreate the traumatic relationship.

By emphasizing the resources of the client, the therapist contributes actively to reorganizing the ground from which the figure of trauma emerges. The therapist needs to be able to teach and model resources and integrative capacities, thereby transforming the implicit procedural learning of fixed gestalts into mindfully held explicit choices. In order to regulate arousal, when the client moves out of their window of tolerance a different set of therapeutic skills comes into play. The therapist must become more active in dropping attention to the figure that has caused the distress and supporting the polarity of safety. The here-and-now focus of the therapist supports the client to have a hold to some extent on current reality, in the service of being able to enter the traumatic past and process it within a widened and more resourced window of tolerance. The therapist holds together the discontinuous and fragmented threads of the client's experience with the aim of integrating a more coherent self-experience.

11 The well-resourced therapist

This chapter entails a temporary change of key and a more personal voice: its subject is the selfhood of the therapist as one part of the therapeutic dyad. It begins with stories about the development and use of resources, particularly embodied ones from my own experience, and offers a range of experiments for you, my reader, to follow and develop for yourself. The examples that are presented are not to be taken as a template, but more as an illustration of one therapist's journey into more resourced embodiment; each therapist must venture on their own path.

The impact of trauma on the therapist is explored in the light of co-transference and vulnerability to vicarious traumatization, and the case is argued for an increase in the therapist's personal resources. The chapter goes on to consider the therapist as wounded healer and proposes that the work can be mutually healing. Exploration is also made of how embodied resources make a contribution to therapist presence and to the practice of **inclusion**. The neuroscience of mirror neurons supports the work and is given a twist in considering the impact the therapist can have on the client's mirror neuron system. Theoretically, the two strands of dialogue and embodiment are woven together to develop a theme of embodied intersubjectivity, akin to Kepner's (2003) concept of the embodied field.

Trauma therapy profoundly changes the therapist ... These changes are both inspiring and disturbing, involving gains and losses. Rarely do therapists enter the field of trauma therapy with full understanding of the implications of their choice.

(Perlman and Saakvitne 1995: 279)

Personal story 1: Gathering resources

It was during my sensorimotor trauma training in 2007 that the need for resources in trauma work caught my attention. Presented in an experiential style, congruent with the work in hand, the training offered participants the opportunity to try out a range of somatic resources for ourselves. The impact this was to have on my work and my personal life was not foreseen, I think, in the design of the training. The more I inhabited these resources, dropped into my body and made them my own, the more I found that the work I did in the therapy room was more grounded, open and connected. This revelation came to sow a seed for the thinking in this chapter, which I suggest is the most important one in the book. Certainly, the ideas have become to some extent my trademark in the following years, and I have taught workshops on the 'well-resourced therapist' to thousands of people on several continents. I have developed this thinking about the selfhood of the therapist further in my second book, *Deepening Trauma Practice* (2021), especially in Chapter 6 of that volume.

Receptive though I was to this more resourced way of working, the ground for the seed had already been prepared in a number of ways. I had the privilege of visiting Esalen at about the same time as my sensorimotor training, where not only was my interest in neuroscience developed personally and professionally, and new horizons opened, but I discovered a book there that changed my life. This was *Body and Earth* by Andrea Olsen (2002), a book that defies genres but offers an experiential way of connecting the systems of the body to the systems of the natural environment. Alongside extensive therapy and the knowledge I gained from my training, these were just the connections I needed in my own recovery from personal trauma.

Here is one of my favourite exercises from the book; whenever I do it I find it loosens the grip of my ego.

Dropping in

The witness

Seated or standing in a comfortable position, eyes open:

- Choose something, living or other-than-living, on which you can focus your attention for several minutes: a tree, a pond, a bird. Find a comfortable position and allow yourself to witness, non-judgementally, for five minutes. If your mind wanders, bring it back to the process of conscious witnessing, observing whatever occurs.
- Pause in open attention. Now allow yourself to be witnessed by the 'thing' that you chose. Imagine that you are being witnessed by your tree, pond, or chair, non-judgementally, in whatever you are doing. 5 min.
- Pause in open attention. Write about your experience; read it aloud to yourself or someone else. Witness as you listen. 10 min. (Olsen 2002: 60)

I have added an element to this experiment for psychotherapists: imagine that you are sitting in front of a client in silence for five minutes, witnessing non-judgementally, observing whatever occurs.

- What is your embodied response?
- Now imagine that the roles are reversed and the client observes you, witnessing non-judgementally, for five minutes.
- What do you notice in your body now?
- Write about this experience too; then read aloud to yourself.

Your responses to these observations may well have had something to do with mirror neurons, which function to connect us to others, human or beyond human, in particular ways.

Mirror neurons

The discovery of mirror neurons came, sadly, from animal research. The presence of similar responses in humans has caused much interest and excitement, and yet there remains much to be learnt about these mechanisms. There is therefore a great deal of speculation about the conclusions that can be drawn from the research. The discovery came about through studying the firing of brain cells of monkeys, and their responses to certain highly specific gestures and movements by other monkeys. Importantly, it was noted that when the subject monkey saw the movement, the same neurons fired as if it was doing that movement itself, and hence the term 'mirror neurons' evolved (Cozolino 2002: 184).

Much learning of sensorimotor and other skills is thought to take place via the network of mirror neurons (Damasio 2000: 298): you first show a child how to tie a shoelace, before they attempt over and again to do it themselves, just as trainers demonstrate particular skills to their students. Siegel (2007: 350) considers a specific property of mirror neurons to be their action potential, differentiating them from purely sensory neurons. The mirror neuron system is linked closely to perceptual and motor areas of the brain, forming a circuitry for 'resonance' (Siegel 2007: 350, 165).

Mirror neurons are thought to be responsible for enabling us to make representations of the intentions of others, to understand their state of mind. 'Mirror neurons demonstrate the profoundly social nature of our brains' (Siegel 2007: 166). Perception and intention, mediated through the outer layers of the cortex, become 'linked to … limbic/emotional processing and … alter … limbic and *bodily states* to match those we are seeing in the other person [or being]' (Siegel 2007: 167, my italics). We do not necessarily have to be in the presence of another person to match bodily and emotional states; we all know that we can respond with fear or sadness to a powerful film, for example. Empathy draws on these bodily and limbic shifts in the process of interoception (Siegel 2007: 168).

It is this embodied quality of mirror neuron activation that is of most interest in our work as trauma psychotherapists. Fogel (2009: 207) states that 'The concept of mirror neurons in the neural networks for embodied self-awareness is therapeutically very important because it suggests an embodied approach to working with people who show body schema and interoceptive deficits', among whom many are trauma clients. Wilkinson (2010: 56) quotes Harrison et al. (2006), who suggest that mirror neurons offer a 'common neural representation for the perception of actions and feelings in others and their experience in self [and a] *basis for a neuroscientific account of intersubjectivity*' (my italics; see also Staemmler 2012: 169). Thus we can consider mirror neurons to be both a property of and a function of the field.

While this theory provides a clue to how we 'read' our clients – without which we can't operate – we can also use the concept of mirror neurons to consider other people's perceptions of us. Cozolino (2006: 231) suggests that for those who have experienced trauma, mirror neurons are employed to defend rather than to cooperate. This means that traumatized people are more likely to read others for signs of threat than for approachability, bringing the issue to the heart of the therapeutic relationship. The mirror neuron system is intersubjective, part of the co-created field, and *must work in both directions*. Clinical experience suggests that the way people read our bodies is critical to the establishment of safety, trust and a regulated embodied field. 'Our own body process is an intrinsic part of the transaction with the client' (Kepner 2003: 11). What is being proposed here is that the deep embodiment of the therapist needs *continual attention*, and that this is not only part of our development as therapists but *part of our ongoing day-to-day work*.

In order to practise the dialogic stance of inclusion, in which we remain rooted in our own subjectivity while at the same time attending to that of the client, we must be exceptionally clear about our bodily resources. The more resources we have, the more the person we are with will pick up on and use, even on an implicit level, through their mirror neuron system. Siegel comments that findings about mirror neurons '*verified the importance for each of us to be attuned to our own internal states in order to attune to others*' (Siegel 2007: 168, my italics); in any co-created relationship this is bound to work both ways.

Therapist vulnerability

While mirror neurons can be of service in the relationship between therapist and client, they have their downside. We can hope that we learn about clients' experience through our own mirror neuron system, and we hope also that our clients can learn about our resourced state through theirs. However, this is also the mechanism by which we pick up on distressed emotions and dysregulated physiological states in our clients, and this can be problematic. There is something about being in the presence of a traumatized person that can make their pain and terror contagious. So often this energetic communication can set our own traumatized system into a state of arousal. We need to take especial care of ourselves in order for this not to dysregulate us too badly, and in order to stay as present, available, open and embodied as we are able. And we need to be able to do so without becoming defensive or distant. There are particular ways, besides our own trauma activation, in which therapists become vulnerable when working with trauma in particular, and these have implications for the quality of the therapeutic relationship. We will consider these separately, even though in reality they may be layered together in our experience.

Vicarious traumatization

Vicarious traumatization is inevitable for therapists who work regularly with trauma (Perlman and Saakvitne 1995: 281). It is certainly my experience that a handful of particularly graphic tales told to me by clients over the years have stayed with me as images that hold considerable emotional charge. Vicarious traumatization means experiencing the same signs and symptoms as the client, but at subclinical levels (Perlman and Saakvitne 1995: 282). Sinason comments that 'We have been drip-fed traumatic narratives; we are watched to see if we retaliate, get ill, give up. Only when we show that we are still standing is it possible for the next drip to be given' (Sinason 2008: 84–5). How do we stop ourselves reeling when working with trauma that 'means taking on cruelty and pain on a level we may never have experienced' (Sinason 2008: 86)?

Alongside emotional and somatic activation, the therapist's frame of reference may change, meaning that their view of inherent goodness in the world can be profoundly altered (Perlman and Saakvitne 1995: 282); a trauma perspective can preconfigure perceptions, attitudes and relationships. When I worked with young people, I thought it was normal for 14-year-old girls to cut themselves, which stopped me listening accurately to individual sufferers. A sense of moral injury as a consequence of our work is perhaps inevitable. Furthermore, the identity of the therapist is affected, raising existential questions: who am I, with my history, experience and circumstances, in the face of my client's story? Do I consider myself superior in some way, luckier, or do I seek to find the commonalities between us in order to stay connected? Does this evoke pity, compassion, disturbance, **confluence**, loss of self-worth or efficacy, detachment?

For example, working with clients with abusive partners tends to evoke gratitude in me for the kind and respectful relationships that have been healing for me. This can be a defensive position, contemptuous even, in which I disengage from my client's unremitting and immediate danger: 'Thank goodness I'm not like you.' Another protective but detrimental strategy is for therapists to lose touch with their body in order to 'manage the onslaught of emotions connected to trauma' (Perlman and Saakvitne 1995: 284). As Sinason, above, implies, the therapeutic relationship is imbued with the signals of traumatic energy. These sometimes subtle imprints need sensitive attention. While there are bound to be parts of ourselves that we hold back, it is important to recognize that it is not the therapist's theoretical orientation that is so crucial in the healing process, but the wholeness and availability of the self of the therapist (Hycner 1993: 15).

Personal story 2: Feeling wobbly

Alice came into therapy after a very traumatic bereavement and a period in psychiatric hospital. We worked together over many months to stabilize and regulate her symptoms, and she had been discharged from all mental health services. Therapy is never a linear process and we had already successfully negotiated a number of challenges. Just as we were moving from stabilization to the processing stage of the work, one of Alice's colleagues died suddenly, reactivating her original trauma which was still unprocessed. For two weeks I worked hard to provide enough glue and resources to contain Alice through this crisis.

On some level I disregarded my rising anxiety and held fast to my belief in the approach I was taking and the strength of our relationship. I thought we knew how to get through this together. I did not want to listen to the nagging doubts I had about the differences I now saw in Alice: her loss of contact functions and shaky grip on reality. However, by the third session it became clear that Alice was in a full-blown psychiatric emergency, extremely agitated and having not slept for a week, triggered by violent nightmares and flashbacks to the original trauma. Alice looked very unwell. She was living in a volatile situation, with family and friends becoming very reactive to her deteriorating condition. I took the necessary steps to ensure Alice's continuing psychiatric care. On one hand, I could at least tell myself that I had done all I could, that I had not given up on her, but on the other hand I knew that I had returned her to a system that can be oppressive, and was likely to medicate her heavily and ignore her trauma (see Taylor 2021).

Once Alice had been transferred to other hands, I found that this didn't reassure me. I was unsettled and alarmed by what had happened; it is always horrible to watch someone you care about fall apart. In the immediate aftermath it seemed as though things were happening in parallel layers of my experience. Although I was absolutely clear that my actions were ethical and proportionate, and that no alternative was available to me, other thoughts were chaotic and disorganized because *I* didn't know where to begin processing this. My breath was shallow and unsteady, I was feeling agitation and distress in my chest and solar plexus, and I felt restless in my legs. Furthermore, my faith in the good work we had done was shattered.

I feared for Alice and for the future of our relationship. In the following hours, my thoughts changed from the chaotic to the ruminative and repetitive. I experienced fleeting images and sensory reminders of what had happened – little flashbacks. I felt less in control. I started to blame myself for my helplessness; something bad had happened and it was my fault, a belief rooted in my own history. I felt that I wasn't a good enough therapist, that I had let my client down for allowing this to happen, and I struggled to accept my own limitations, all of which I recognized as quite irrational.

My rational mind could see that I had become vicariously traumatized, and I was able to bring some gentleness to bear towards myself for this. But no amount of kindliness and clear reality-checking could initially settle the level of somatic distress I felt. My access to a range of somatic resources proved to be grounding, which settled me. I could later sit in awareness of both the disturbance in my upper body and the solidity of my lower body, knowing that both were true for me in that moment and that the disturbance was not the whole of my experience.

The wounded healer

In our day-to-day work with trauma victims we are repeatedly exposed to impressive forces which inevitably have something to do with our own history as well as our clients'. A therapist's susceptibility to vicarious trauma is greater when their own story includes experience of personal or transgenerational trauma; if this describes your interest in working with trauma you will need to pay *extra* attention to what resources you. Whatever your story, this work demands that we confront those parts of ourselves that we loathe or fear or ignore, including young, damaged and traumatized parts. According to Orange (2010: 87), I have 'a responsibility to understand my own traumatic suffering as meaningful insofar as it enables me to respond to, and suffer for, my destitute neighbour'. What therapist does not already know resistance and impasse from the inside? We can be pulled uncomfortably out of shape by clients who do not yet understand boundaries, and undermined by their attempts to take control. What, too, of the therapist's own fear, powerlessness, dissociation and shame? These may arise 'not only in response to narrative, but also to the patient's non-verbal communications and in the bodily movements or facial expressions that accompany flashbacks' (Goodwin and Attias 1999b: 171).

It is easy, for example, to become wary of a client's unpredictability, especially when it manifests through dissociated aggressive or destructive parts and we become more alert. This can then trigger in us a cascade of helplessness, distancing and shame, whereby we lose understanding and compassion for ourselves and for those parts of our clients that so immediately signal their wounds. 'The way we respond to these [signals] will be pivotal in helping traumatized individuals deal with those difficult sensations and emotions. If we recoil because we cannot contain and accept them, then we abandon our clients … if we are overwhelmed, then we are both lost' (Levine 2010: 46). Therapists' embodied awareness and sensitivity to their own process is therefore critical: 'Each of us has a different set of behaviours and emotions which we find it difficult to support in ourselves, and others; and we need to know what these are' (Totton and Priestman 2012: 46–7). Above all, we must remember that vicarious traumatization is a response to the *client's trauma* and not to the client (Perlman and Saakvitne 1995: 300).

The embodied therapist

In order to practise inclusion 'the therapist has to understand the experience of the client, and yet concurrently be able to stay in touch with his own experience. It is an exceedingly difficult task to determine which to focus on and when' (Hycner 1993: 16). The emphasis of this chapter is on the embodied nature of the felt sense in order to support increasing presence to painful and shocking material. Fogel (2009: 225) considers that 'Practitioners must learn, through their own intensive ventures into the pleasures and pains of embodied self-awareness, to remain in the subjective emotional present and access their own resources while working with someone else.' Frank concurs:

> We must attend to our own bodies in order to be aware [of] the client's embodied experience … only [by shuttling back and forth] can we 'lend our

bodies' to the client, offer our embodied selves as support within the relational field.

(Frank 2008: 19)

This in-between process both allows you to become present and opens up a space for something new to emerge. The embodiment of the therapist is a major resource in the therapy, and is essential in the practice of inclusion.

'It takes a remarkable amount of generosity … to consider what resources and support a clinician needs, when the clinician is lucky enough to maintain themselves adequately enough to have a job and function in it' (Sinason 2008: 84). This perspicacious comment invites questions: How can I know when I have enough resources? What resources am I entitled to? A straightforward answer is that, just as for our clients, 'too many resources' suggests being totally self-absorbed. My experience has shown that the opposite is more likely to be the case; therapists tend to have difficulty in taking their own needs seriously (see Taylor 2021). I have known experienced therapists become thrown by their contact with some severely traumatized clients, needing more resources. An embodied therapist has ways of regulating themselves, to restore balance quickly and effectively (see Figure 11.1). In the words of Staemmler (2012: 37), 'we need not only a willingness to identify emotionally, but also a well-developed capacity to regulate our emotions'. The concern is for the therapist's capacity to respond and to process in the moment. 'When the therapist's needs are not balanced and when he is struggling and failing to meet these needs in mature ways, he is more vulnerable to vicarious traumatization' (Perlman and Saakvitne 1995: 309). The range and variety of resources needed by therapists is much the same as for clients, bearing in mind that it takes years to develop a deep embodiment

Figure 11.1 The therapist's expanded window of tolerance

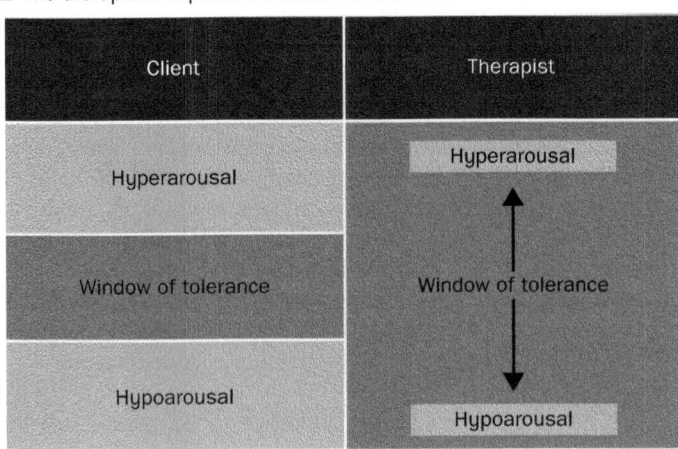

(Kepner 2003; Fogel 2009: 224). Carroll highlights the therapist's ability to regulate as critical to being non-defensive, which:

> [D]epends upon the therapist being anchored within their own body, able to bear and attend to sensation ... if this underlying regulation is there then the therapist can also allow herself to be knocked off balance, controlled or confused in the process with the client.
>
> (Carroll 2009: 102)

Dropping in

Bring to mind the range of resources you have – creative, spiritual, environmental, relational and so on. Which are most important to you? How often do you turn to them? How might you increase your involvement in these activities or ways of being? What do you need to let go of in order to be more resourced? Which support your presence most fully? Reflect on the physicality of these resources – which bring you most vividly into a sense of your body? Write about your resources.

Personal story 3: Developing capacity

I suggested in the last chapter that the therapist's capacity to bear the trauma they work with is a defining factor in the effectiveness of trauma therapy. 'The best yardstick for the enormity of the trauma lies in our own incapacity to bear witness to it; or in the level of dissociation that listening to it inflicts on the witness' (Sachs 2013: 25). The corollary of this is that the *best yardstick of healing trauma lies in our capacity to bear witness to it,* and the level of presence the witness can bring to it. I regard the ongoing development and maintenance of my resources as a *requisite* part of my clinical work, broadening my capacity, and the hours I routinely spend in doing so as valid work time. More than any other activity perhaps, this is what trauma clients pay me for, to keep myself available to practise as safely as possible. The ethic in this statement is, I trust, clear. I create healthy gaps between sessions, so that I am not left with the energetic residue of a previous session, clearing my body/mind of the content and the process, and regrounding myself. If I've been with a dissociated or hypoaroused client I generally do some stretches to raise my energy afterwards. I also attend to daily meditation, exercise, sleep and diet; I avoid consuming heavy food or potential toxins such as caffeine, alcohol or sugar before working. I nourish myself with art, music, film and nature. Considerable discipline is needed to sustain this lifestyle, for that is what my practice as a Gestalt therapist has called me to: a different way of life. It is a way of life that bridges the personal and the professional, and reduces intensity both from external demands and also from inner disturbance. Being human, I quite often veer away from this course!

My thinking and knowledge base is another invaluable resource – a meta-level that provides me with an anchor (Appel-Opper 2012: 90). Allied to this is my use of supervision. When working with one of my first very dissociated clients I was advised to seek specialist supervision, and it remains one of the best pieces of advice I have had. Severely traumatized clients need that implicit knowing of being held in mind by others, and their therapists are supported by greater holding for themselves.

These are the parameters, then, of supporting my practice, my functional external resources. I use internal resources when face to face with clients. From moment to moment when I am with clients I monitor the shifts in my presence and physical resonance. I check repeatedly on my breathing, on my seat in the chair, on any awareness that signals rising anxiety in me. The first thing I usually notice of becoming bent out of shape is a drawing inwards and upwards in my sacral spine, a micro-movement that initiates a whole body response in me. It changes my relationship to gravity and almost imperceptibly shortens my breathing: the crus muscles of the diaphragm are connected to the spine. The seat of my energy rises and contracts, and my thinking becomes more focused as I move into a state of higher alert. Because I rely on this keen relationship with this signal in my muscles, I can choose to change it and settle back into my grounded and soft spine, or not, as the situation requires. This is the skill of stilling the mind and the body to create a place from which I can listen, from which I can maintain my presence and hold my ground while attending to the other – in other words practise inclusion.

Dropping in

Take some minutes to scan your body and see if you can find a place that would be your first signal that your regulated state is changing. It can be very helpful to try to reverse the process in your mind: 'This I know, but what happens just before that … and just before that?'

Pay close attention to the minutiae of your experience. Feel your way into this awareness, experimenting with curiosity, settling your attention in this area. Ask yourself what the message from this part of your embodied self is, how it can support you, what it needs. Allow yourself to soften into your responses without judgement. Explore the quality and texture of your signal, its intensity and volume, its impulses and intentions. Deepening your exploration, shift from bringing your awareness to this place to letting this place be aware. From this awareness, establish a sense of connection with how the rest of your body responds to this signal. There is no need to hurry this important process of discovery; allow yourself to stay with it for as long as your curiosity remains alive.

You might like to combine this awareness with the subject of the earlier experiment, 'The witness', above, shuttling between your internal signal and the external other.

Somatic resources

Some general categories of embodied resources involve grounding, containment and breath. What follows are experiments for each of these.

1   Lying on your back on the floor, close your eyes, bend your knees; let your feet rest on the floor, slightly wider than your hips; let your knees drop together to release your thigh muscles; rest your arms comfortably on the floor, below shoulder height; allow yourself to be supported by the floor; allow your breath to move three-dimensionally through your torso; allow your eyes to rest in their sockets like pebbles dropping into a pool; allow your brain to rest in the skull; allow your shoulders to melt towards the earth; allow the weight of your legs to drain into your hip sockets and feet; allow your organs to release towards gravity; allow your mouth to gently fall open, your tongue to relax; feel the air move in and out through your lips and nose. In constructive rest, instead of controlling the body you allow it to be supported by the earth. As you release your body weight into gravity, your discs are less compressed and your spine begins to elongate. Constructive rest is an efficient position for body realignment. It releases tension and allows your skeleton and organs to rest, supported by the ground. (Adapted from Olsen 2002: 4.)

2   Building on the supports of the external environment – the ground or the chair beneath you – you might begin non-judgementally to notice the outline of your body, and the space you take up in the world. What is the volume and weight of your head, of your leg or your thumbs? How do you experience the contact of clothing, or any points of pressure on your skin and into your tissues? How deep does this sensation go? Notice the distance between your shoulders, and between your navel and your spine. Can you sense into your thigh bones and the flesh around them?

3   There are countless ways of focusing attention on breath, and you are encouraged to establish a regular practice involving breath awareness. This is just one method to help you. Lie in constructive rest, eyes closed. Notice air coming in through your mouth and nose: cool air coming in, warm air going out. Feel the air passing down through your throat to your trachea, the long tube ringed with cartilage supporting the front of your neck. Touch your neck lightly to feel this structure. Place your hands on your belly and allow it to expand on the inbreath and condense on the outbreath (without pushing). Imagine the shortening of your crus muscles at the back, pulling your diaphragm down towards your lower spine. Place your hands on your ribs. Notice them fanning out on your inbreath and softening on the outbreath. Allow all 24 ribs to move as you breathe. Notice your breathing pattern. Enjoy a few deep integrating breaths to finish your exploration. (Adapted from Olsen 2002: 117.)

Mindfulness as a resource

The experiments in this chapter, and indeed many of the experiments through-out this volume, involve mindful awareness, the process of attending moment by moment and without judgement to subjective felt and embodied experience: 'It is the subjective experience of the therapist that is often the key factor in the therapeutic relationship' (Hilton 2012: 28). Gestalt experiments in directed awareness are a form of mindfulness practice, and more structured forms of practice are possible, involving either focused or open attention (see also Chapter 5). Mindfulness is a primary tool for establishing greater body aware-ness and of stepping back from experience, both for ourselves and for our clients. For a fuller understanding of the role of mindfulness, I commend to you Dan Siegel's *The Mindful Therapist* (2010). Siegel illustrates the roles of integration, resonance, coherence and attunement that emerge from mindful states, and the impact of these on both therapist and client.

I suggest that *mindfulness increases practitioner resilience and relationality* – essential to trauma therapy. 'The ability to tolerate the truth of the traumatic experience involves a capacity to bear pain in the presence of another human being; this constitutes the core of mature intimacy' (Turner et al. [1996] 2007: 538). Furthermore:

> [A] therapists mindfulness contributes to critical relationship factors such as the formation and sustenance of the working alliance, countertransference management, and the provision of unconditional regard with difficult [*sic*] clients ... the more mindful therapists perceived themselves to be, the less aware they were of their countertransference.
>
> (Davis and Hayes 2011: 204)

Staemmler (2012: 226) argues similarly for the usefulness of meditation practices in prevention of practitioner burnout.

Mutual healing

This might seem far-fetched, but therapeutic work with trauma victims can be pleasurable. It must be so at times, for it is an indication that you are doing the work of regulation and interrupting the figures of trauma. Although this is not the whole of the therapy, the significant role of *reciprocal* resourced states brings benevolence and compassion to the work (Staemmler 2012), creating an energy field that is soft, deep, attentive and receptive. This must develop in a way that is genuine, because clients will be quick to spot when it is not; this is work that is not forced or artificial, but allowing of emergent relational phenomena. These are the I–Thou moments of therapy; they serve as markers in the ground, growth points, strengthening the alliance and opening up new possibilities. They 'can be considered pivotal relational influences that occur as a result of critical subjective colouring of experience on the part of both participants in the therapeutic encounter' (King 2012: 75).

More than this, '[w]hen the patient experiences true healing, it often serves to heal the wounded pole of the professional healer' (Miller and Baldwin 2000: 251). Hilton (2012: 33) deepens this argument:

> As the therapist accompanies the client on his journey back to the origins of his interactional failures, the therapist must know and understand her own relational failures and the solutions she sought for them. This dynamic interplay and all that is implied in it becomes the healing process for both therapist and client.

How we have each been failed by the others in our lives is echoed in how we bring ourselves to the therapeutic work. Therapists who bring their embodied selves, their whole selves, to the relational encounter risk so much and stand to gain so much; it is my hope that the gains outweigh the losses.

Summary

The selfhood of the therapist as one partner in the therapeutic dyad is an important consideration in all therapy, but there are particular reasons to pay attention to this in trauma work. Mirror neuron theory suggests neural mechanisms that enable resonance and empathy between individuals. It is suggested therefore that mirror neurons are the neurological component of relationship. Usually, mirror neurons can account for the therapist's attunement to the client, but it is possible to consider that the reverse may be operating, when the client's mirror neuron system is activated by the therapist's embodied and implicit resources. This is but one rationale for developing one's own accessible somatic resources.

The second reason is that the mirror neuron system is likely to be implicated in vicarious trauma, the subclinical residue of the client's traumatic material which can disrupt and reconfigure the therapy and the therapist's view of the world. This can also tap into the therapist's own history of trauma and relational wounds, creating a vulnerability to additional distress. The case is made for developing a wide range of resources, in order to enhance the therapist's resilience in trauma work. Particular attention is given to those somatic resources which reflect and support a deep embodiment, enhancing the dialogic dimensions of presence and inclusion. When the therapist is able to include both awareness of the client and simultaneously remain anchored in their own experience, the relationship is supported and strengthened. It is also possible for moments of healing in the client to include the healing of the therapist.

12 Embodied relationship

Being in a therapeutic relationship with a trauma victim is often enormously complex and challenging for both partners. Whether recent or historical, the trauma will have profoundly challenged and shaped their sense of self and other, their connection to the world and their capacity to connect. These issues speak to the very heart of the therapy relationship. Above all, trauma victims need to be able to tolerate being in relationship in order to heal. This chapter explores concepts of resonance and regulation from a relational viewpoint. The Window of Tolerance Model is repositioned as a relational framework. Examples are given of non-verbal ways of relating to trauma clients, attending to their embodied contact styles, strengthening the working alliance. So we explore some ways of establishing the embodied relationship, including the use of touch.

Relational dilemmas

One person keeps their coat on throughout the session; they have arrived, but not fully. Another keeps glancing anxiously at the door, as though checking for an escape route. A third learnt as a child to withdraw to 'a place where no one can find me' and dissociates repeatedly in sessions, in terror of being 'found'. The themes of trauma come into play in the therapeutic relationship. Chaos and rigidity become structurally embodied as contact styles, as mobilized and immobilized defences. As an example, someone who is unable to tolerate the immobilization of trauma *can* actively control and attack the therapist, which is a semblance of power. The fast-moving figures of a chaotic process can be extremely difficult to disentangle and reorganize; we seek coherence in order to make some meaning, but find ourselves trying to grasp smoke, the gestalts unformed and shape-shifting. Perceived cultural norms in the form of taboos, secrecy and verbal threats operate alongside bodily based beliefs about self in relationship and finding one's place.

How do you include the client as a participant when they are preoccupied with defending themselves against exclusion? How do you establish collaboration with someone whose experience is of being overcome by some outside force or individual? How do you make an impact on someone who is well armoured against intrusion, or who doesn't expect to make an impact on others? How can you feel into the world of a client whose speech and language are divorced from any emotion, the narrative delivered as though they are telling you what they had for lunch – where 'language holds the potential to trigger an affective reliving of dissociated traumatic experience' (Bromberg 2011: 17)? Many of these dilemmas arrive multilayered, and while connected can be tricky to unravel. The therapeutic stance is shaped by them. There is a relational message in each of these behaviours, which needs to be brought into awareness and made sense of together, and we will return to this below. This task is particularly figural for people with complex trauma, which usually involves considerable damage to their capacity to be in contact with others.

What we already know

If we understand that relationships are fundamentally embodied, the role of the implicit cannot be overstated. 'The more one knows about one's inner body/ self in conjunction to whatever emerges into figure, the more one can keep a healthy contact boundary' (Ruzany 2020: 178). The body is the ground of our relational self, the 'place' we inhabit: '[T]he body that is me ... my total self as I respond to the world which is with me in unending dialogue' (Kennedy 2005, original italics). The mechanism of this dialogue is an energetic communication. When I come into my body sense, I feel more grounded, present and responsive. We connect to one another at an energetic level, tapping into the vibrations that form a human energy field, as part of a far wider system of resonance in the whole universe. 'There is a fundamental assumption that all life is sustained by a universal, life energy' (Shields et al. 2016). In essence, all relationship can be seen as an exchange of energy (Siegel 2009: 166), involving sound and light waves. Many auditory vibrations occur at decibel levels that cannot be detected by the human ear, but we can assume that they have an affect beyond conscious or sensory awareness. Electrical currents within the body are captured in EEG and ECG tests; cells in a state of health luminate and pulsate (Boadella 1987: 181). In the natural world, homing pigeons detect the electromagnetic fields of the earth, responding to changes in gravity and barometric pressure, and sting-rays sense tiny electrical currents when a muscle contracts – even a beating heart – via electro-receptors which detect the presence of prey. Who is to say that we humans do not have such acute capacities as yet undiscovered?

There has until recently been little scientific evidence to support the notion of the human energy field (Shields et al. 2016), although in different traditions and times energetic shifts may be attributed to spirit or paranormal activity, chi or personal aura. The idea that the life force could be in either a state of health or imbalance is common to traditional philosophies, with the belief that it 'flows freely through and between living beings and their environment' (Shields et al. 2016). One argument proposes that both living beings and their environment *are* energetic fields, while quantum physics proposes that all matter is energy, an energetic field surrounding and within everything. The qualities of the flow are an indication of the state of well-being of the systems and the energetic exchange between them. We all know how to 'read' the atmosphere when we enter a room, when someone approaches us from behind, or we have taken an instant liking to someone; most people can also recall instances of having had a 'sixth' sense, or of surprising synchronicity or coincidence. In what ways, outside conscious awareness, is my response to another or to a situation – even of someone I have never met, perhaps meeting them as a supervisor, or in an online session – mediated and communicated?

The contact boundary, the connection between one person or being and another, may also be associated with some form of consciousness. Conscious awareness has energetic properties, imprinted in the pathways of the nervous system (Kepner 2002: 4). Energetic resonance speaks to something being implicitly *known* in the relationship (Lyons-Ruth et al. 1998). This is more than attunement, a unidirectional process by which we align ourselves to the wavelength of those we work with; it means allowing their energetic communications to reverberate within us.

Dropping in

1 Find some pieces of music that have different resonant qualities, perhaps drumming, melodic choral harmonies, ballads or heavy rock. Lying on your back, listen to them and allow the sounds to resonate in different parts of your body. How do they vibrate within the hollow spaces of your body – your skull, your mouth, your throat, your chest, the bowl of your pelvis? How do they reverberate on your skin, and where is this most clear to you? Notice the variations in pulses and your response to each of them.

2 Lie on your belly on the floor, with your forehead raised slightly. Create a closed bowl by cupping your mouth, one ear on the floor with your hands. Make the open sound 'ah' and sense the vibrations in your face. Continue and notice vibrations in your head, arms and torso. Make the closed sounds of 'ng', 'n', 'mm', and sense those vibrations. Play with other sounds. Where in your body can you move the vibrations to? What sounds vibrate the most? The least? Exaggerate the consonants. Exaggerate the vowels. Tell a story out loud, perhaps what happened this morning, continuing to sense vibrations. Pause. (Adapted from Olsen 2002: 82)

3 Lying on your back, take a few deep breaths. Slowly sense the contact you are making with the floor and settle into the sensation of contact. Take a few more deep breaths holding a wide field of receptive awareness of your whole body. Maintaining this wide field of perception, allow your attention to come to your physical heart. Simply orient to its pulsation. Place your hands over your heart if its pulsation is not clear. As the beating of your heart clarifies, again widen your orientation of listening to your whole body. See if you can, while not losing an awareness of your heart itself, sense its pulsation in different parts of your body. Can you sense it in your abdomen? In your belly, legs, chest cavity, arms, neck and elsewhere? Allow a more general sense of the pulsing of your lifeblood to arise while staying centred in your heart. (Adapted from Sills 2011: 77)

Schore explains that '*Resonance* phenomena are now thought to play one of the most important roles in brain organization and in central nervous system (CNS) regulatory processes' (Schore 2003b: 51, original italics). Resonance is not a merely passive process and probably involves mirror neurons. 'Mirror neurons and shared representations are not primarily the mediators of simulation but the enactment of direct intersubjective perception' (Lindblom 2007). By implication, the practice of inclusion is dependent on resonance within the energetic field. In order to support neural integration we need to create 'mindful fields', in which the client is held in mind by a coherent and mindful other. This involves a recursive generation of safety and internal attunement (Harris 2011: 27) – the internal and external sense of safety that comes to replace terror (see Chapter 6). Kornfield (1993/2002: 245) observes that 'the best of modern therapy is much like a process of shared meditation ... the therapist joins in the listening, sensing and feeling'.

What, then, is the clinical significance of resonance? Energetic patterns can be understood as changes in the ANS, signalling state shifts that represent either safety or threat. Primarily, the concept is relational, as suggested by Boadella (1987: xv): 'the most essential tool, in transforming blocked patterns [of energy] is the responsive life of another human being'. Staemmler quotes Stein: 'by his walk, posture, and his every movement, we also "see" "how he feels", his vigor, sluggishness, etc.' (Staemmler 2012: 38). The mechanism for resonance is thought to involve unconscious communication between one right brain and another, '*tuned to receive these communications*' (Schore 2003b: 49, original italics). Thus a degree of synchrony between the members of the dyad is formed, which is inherently embodied. We can imagine this to be mutually reinforcing in the therapeutic dance. It is captured neatly in the words of Sander (2000): 'I sense that you sense that I sense'. This is consistent with the Gestalt position of the formation of self at the contact boundary.

The self that has formed following a trauma is an adaptive and creative response to a novel set of conditions that cannot be assimilated. Each individual is a self-organizing system, creating its own states of consciousness which can be expanded into more coherent and complex states in collaboration with another (Tronick 1998). Resonance indicates the quality and match between the partners in the dyad: it is an interactive process of two closely attuned systems which allows them to amplify and co-regulate each other's activity (Siegel 1999: 336). The influence of this 'persists within the mind of each member after direct interaction no longer occurs' (Siegel 1999: 281).

I was seeing a fairly new client in the late afternoon throughout the autumn months. The season was changing and I realized one day that their session would start in daylight and end in pitch darkness. I 'knew' it was important to check with this particular person whether they wanted the curtains open or closed. Their solution was to have them half open. They referred to dark figures outside the window, which had never been mentioned before; it seemed to them that these figures might come into the room. Later in the session they allowed me into the story, for the very first time, of their mother's serious and crushing emotional neglect. The resonant intersubjective field is an energetic container in which the client and the trauma can be held. Any unsignalled withdrawal from that resonant field by either person will disrupt the other's state of mind (Bromberg [1998] 2001: 193), such as when a new figure emerges for either party.

Mutual regulation

Much research into the interactions between infants and their caretakers has become the territory of applied neuroscience, and these interactions are taken to be prototypes for adult psychotherapy (see Stern 1998; Tronick 1998; Beebe and Lachman 2002; Schore 2003a, 2003b). These writers take a dyadic or systems view of the regulatory behaviour between mother and infant or therapist and client: 'the dynamic engine of the therapy lies in the self-organizing properties of analyst and patient together as a dyad' (BCPSG 2010: 97). Intersubjectivity theory puts this thinking into practice, in what can be seen as a four-stage cyclical process: (i) I become fully present to myself (ii) so that I can become fully present to you (iii) so that you can become present to yourself and (iv) so that you can become present to me. This is a system of reciprocal mutual influence (Stolorow et al. 1987: 42).

We have already established the case for trauma clients to develop ways of rebalancing the dysregulated arousal that is so dominant in their experience. In Gestalt language, this is a process of organismic *self*-regulation (Perls et al. [1951] 1998). We have seen in Chapter 4 how this natural regulation is rendered inaccessible by traumatic experiences. Often trauma victims self-support by withdrawing energy from relationships – an overly self-reliant stance that allows little space for contact. Tronick suggests that too much focus on self-support sets the stage for psychopathology (cited in Beebe and Lachman 2002: 162), or in less pathologizing language, for disturbed relationships. For trauma clients, allowing anyone else to do something for them may feel like a betrayal of the self (Beebe and Lachman 2002: 193).

A relational perspective in Gestalt therapy puts increasing emphasis on the interconnectedness of self and other, understood as a co-created, intersubjective therapeutic space. For trauma work it is helpful to think of this as co-*regulated*:

> The two-person system is a dynamic balancing act, with the level of feeling often fluctuating as the interaction between client and therapist is managed both implicitly (through self-regulation and interactive regulation) and explicitly (as far as these processes are the subject of verbal exploration).
>
> (Carroll 2009: 103)

If self-regulation is 'a way of perceiving and knowing and understanding' (Carroll 2009: 103), a way of knowing through the body, then mutual regulation is a way of perceiving, knowing and understanding one another through our bodies.

Clinical vignette

Stewart comes to see me straight after work. He tells me: 'My boss was in a foul mood today.' Tightening in my lower back, I pull forward a little from the support of my chair; my breath is shorter, centred in my sternum; I notice my throat vibrate as though it is ready for something. Simultaneously, Stewart looks briefly at me and then down and slightly to the left. The energy between us feels loaded. He takes an effortful breath, and when he speaks his voice is strangled, measured. 'Yeah, made me feel uneasy ... tried to keep out of his way ... but he ... wanted to talk to me about something.' I maintain my gaze, and nod to convey my understanding that he is saying something important. Stewart glances at me again and then looks out of the window; he's a bit less present now.

In this moment I settle my breathing, drop my weight back into the chair; I feel more receptive. 'What was it like for you in this?' I ask; my voice is soft and steady.

'Scared ... I felt scared he was going to lose it', Stewart replies; his hands are tightening in his lap but he seems more connected. I feel this in my chest, a pressure, and some tension developing across my collar bone and upper arms; I take a deeper, more audible breath.

'Oh, I see ... are you willing to tell me more?', I respond. Stewart's energy rises.

'Yeah ... yeah ... I was afraid ... felt terrified, ... like I was smaller, and ... and ... like he was going to hurt me ... my dad ... .' Stewart shifts slightly in his chair, straightens his posture, gently rubs his thumb on his leg a few times, looks at me. The energy which had felt held now seems to open; we engage a soft eye contact, breathe steadily together for a few seconds before we move on. It was not necessary for me to verbally share my responses to Stewart in order for the mutual resonance to be felt.

Stewart came from Northern Ireland, brought up during the Troubles. His home was regularly searched by the British Army, and his neighbour was murdered at their front door while the children were playing in the street. Stewart's father, after being shot in the back, became a heavy drinker with a volatile temper.

As Fogel (2009: 223) remarks: 'Any kind of coregulated activity with another person is a way of establishing a felt connection', thereby linking regulation and contact. Each participant must 'come to know' the current state of the other if the regulation is to succeed (Tronick 1998). In this, both parties are implicitly reaching for integrated nervous system states that support the creation of coherent narrative over time (Wilkinson 2010: 134). As the example in the clinical vignette shows, regulatory processes are fast, often below levels of consciousness; they are intuitive, empathic responses to the other in the room (Wilkinson 2010: 33). Further, '[m]utual regulation implies no symmetry between the interactants, only that influence is bidirectional' (BCPSG 2010: 8). Fogel describes such shared emotional states as awareness expanded beyond the boundaries of the body (Fogel 2009: 224); this thinking critically redefines what we mean by 'owning' our bodies because they belong as functions of the field.

Non-verbal features of mutual regulation by either the therapist or client include contraction and expansion of energy, aversion of eye contact, turning of the head, small gestures of self-touch, prosody of speech, mood, the intensity of emotion, silence, breath, and changes in muscle tonus or skin colour or quality, among others. This list is an expanded phenomenological description of contact functions (Joyce and Sills 2010: 59), the pulsation of lived therapeutic engagement, usually representing habitual patterns in a form that is subtle yet recognizable by the other. These processes relate to what Siegel (2012: 19-7) calls the 'social brain', creating subcortical shifts that literally resonate with what is being perceived. Moment-by-moment adjustments to levels of arousal are an intrinsic part of contact. There needs to be a reasonable match between the regulatory range of each participant (Beebe and Lachman 2002: 220). Importantly, the trauma victim, by virtue of their impact on the therapist and the reciprocal response, becomes an agent in the therapy when the regulation is co-created.

Mutual regulation and the window of tolerance

The Window of Tolerance Model provides a conceptual framework for relational connection and safety. Far from being an individualist, reductive, biological model, it creates a way to restore the victim to relationship within a field which has been so painfully fractured by the traumatic event. We can think of mutual regulation as a way of bringing *both* parties into a shared state of optimal arousal. Optimal arousal thus becomes optimal support and connection. The implications of this are enormous when we recall that it is only within the window of tolerance that a traumatized individual is truly present and available for contact. Therapist and client collaborate on expanding this zone, using one another's support to explore the margins of the safe emergency within which processing of trauma becomes possible. The window of tolerance is not therefore simply a calm and confluent condition, but a state of being together in which things can happen.

Even where the window of tolerance seems initially to be inaccessible and beyond prior experience, it offers hope in the possibility of a different state of being. In presenting the model, the therapist can use language that indicates its relationality: 'I have some ways to explore this idea together'; 'I'll need you to teach me about your ways of coming in and out of this state'; 'We can find out what is helpful and what isn't.' Far more importantly, it is *you*, the therapist, who conveys the message, not just in words but in your being. Together, you negotiate the boundaries between the two of you and continually redefine the space.

Trauma clients are often consciously watching for what we can tolerate, waiting for us to be able to bear their trauma with them (Sinason 2008: 84). Sometimes they know our internal state before we know it ourselves. Their fear of not being received, believed or understood in the rawness and horror of their experience is immense. The risk is of rejection, alienation and disintegration. The fear of being too much – of you, their therapist, being unable to bear and support the fullness of the traumatic experience – is common. I might make this explicit by asking, 'Just check if there is something that you see in me that tells you that I can bear this with you right now.' The issue of therapeutic capacity is central, and this is why I have devoted much of my second book to this (Taylor 2021). You may well recognize that the more experienced you have become as a therapist, the more clients will share. Skilled at regulating others, their process of 'drip feeding' information is their way of keeping us both in the window of tolerance. This is a mutually regulating cycle: if I can bear something as a therapist, it makes it more bearable for my client, and the next figure can then come into the light. Incrementally, a sense of safety develops, a sense that we can together recover from the waves of trauma that can engulf us. This is therefore also a model for the foundation of trust.

An experience beyond words: making sense together

There are countless ways of making aspects of the client's embodied trauma relational, and their success depends on the therapist's ability to access their own integrated embodied resources (Chapter 11). To use the words of Totton and Priestman (2012: 37), we need to 'somatize the relationship'. The 'therapist must be able to hold a constant awareness and appreciation that the body is intrinsic to *all* human process' (Kepner 2003: 9, original italics). It is impossible to be prescriptive about processes that emerge in intersubjective phenomenology in the moment, fast and often subliminal as they are. What follows, therefore, are some thoughts about relating to the client's body/mind, and descriptions of clinical work.

It is very common for otherwise articulate trauma clients to be unable to express their felt experience verbally. Their emotional life is undifferentiated and vague (Orange 1995: 91). The technical word for this is alexithymia, which involves impaired ability to identify the somatic components of an emotion, to know what they mean, or to use them as a guide to appropriate actions (van der Kolk [1996] 2007: 193). Alexithymia is a manifestation of the deep disconnection with embodied life which is characteristic of trauma. It implies disconnection in relationship: 'The ability to link feelings and words ... relies on relationships to build connections between separate neural networks dedicated to affect and language' (Cozolino 2006: 231). Based on our understanding of the dominance of the limbic brain when a person is remembering trauma, we might expect that verbal representation will be impossible (see Chapters 2 and 6). For some individuals, expression and meaning-making are more generally compromised, recognizable in those who habitually use a cognitive style of processing experience. For trauma clients this may arise from their intense fear of the physicality of any emotion, which in turn increases ANS activation. Full expression depends on words and feelings together.

There is a possible neurobiological explanation for this. It has been demonstrated that a brain structure called Broca's area, situated in the left cerebral cortex, is responsible for translating experience into language. This becomes underactive during exposure to traumatic material (van der Kolk [1996] 2007: 233; 2003: 187; Ogden et al. 2006: 237). It is not necessarily the case that such clients do not feel, however; they may know that they feel, but cannot communicate or process it (van der Kolk 2003: 187). We must assume that the body is more capable of knowing than can be put into words. This can leave people helpless, distanced from sources of human comfort and understanding. This speechless terror needs to be met on a different level, corresponding to those levels of the brain that are functioning (Heitzler 2009: 178).

> The nonverbal world of our shared communication is often an essential place to begin to make sense ... all of the associations, beliefs, and cognitions [of unresolved trauma] can be held within the spotlight of attention ... such that this shared experience can enable memory retrieval to begin.
>
> (Siegel 2012: 39-8)

The client is no longer alone with their trauma. The ubiquitous Gestalt enquiry, 'What's happening now?', is rendered useless in moments in which sensations are undifferentiated and words inaccessible. Rather, the methodology of phenomenological description is preferred for creating an embodied narrative.

To give an example, a client new to therapy could not identify or make meaning of physical sensations. I began by naming some observable body processes that accompanied states of distressing memory: 'I can see that you are pulling your arms tight in ... your breathing has become more shallow ... you turned your head', using statements rather than questions to create a narrative of how they organized themselves somatically in the moment. The client nodded silently in response to my interventions, as though they were able to observe and consider these phenomena themself, creating more distance from the experience. I understood this as a negotiation between my client and myself, increasing coherence in the relational field (BCPSG 2010: 195). My recognition led to their own, and moments of reflective awareness became possible. Over time I made my descriptions more precise as we learnt their body story together. I added my own resonant responses at times, such as: 'You are very still on the outside but I get the sense that there's a lot going on inside at the moment', so that they could experience their effect on me. We were working in a provisional space – the slow forming of coherence, integration and differentiation.

Another relational way to work with body process is to 'take on' the way the client embodies themselves. On the one hand, this offers up invaluable information when the therapist gains a first-hand map of how it feels to be inside the client's body, the residue of which will linger after the experiment. On the other hand, it communicates important relational messages to the client. I am not talking here about mimicry or even kindly imitation (Staemmler 2012: 97), but about showing the client that you want to know what it is like to be them, allowing them to 'feel felt'. To do this requires mindful attention and fine tuning, seeking the client's collaboration to get the tension in the back, the distribution of weight in relation to gravity, or the angle of the head 'just so'; it is surprising how it can be recognized once seen in you – mirror neurons at work. I am referring here to small aspects of experience rather than gross and intrusive observations, such as the clenching of hands in the lap. When the therapist offers feedback on their experience and understanding, the client in turn has an opportunity to 'try on' those words to see if they fit or not. This profound non-verbal confirmation has far-reaching implications for the safety and depth of the relationship.

Many of the experiments on developing body awareness throughout this book can be used in a collaborative manner with the people you work with. Simply suggesting that you spend a few moments together attending to your breath grounds you in a shared mindful field. I often offer back some detail of my somatic awareness, which can allow the client to own their phenomenology of the moment. This is especially helpful when something unexpected or unfamiliar emerges in my embodied awareness, and this leads me to be curious about its presence in the space between us: is this to do with me, or them, or both of us, in this moment? Because this work is so dependent on right brain processes, we can rely on our creativity to adapt to the situation. It is sometimes astonishing, when we listen with our embodied selves, to feel oneself drawn to a particular pain, for example, in a client that has not been spoken of; it is communicated through the energetic field. In these subtle ways the client guides us to the unknown figures, co-creating the experiments.

We are trying to find an entry point into a number of self- and relational functions, often outside of awareness. Among these are developing embodied self-awareness, establishing new learning through collaboration and negotiation relationally, the owning of experience that begins to form a new sense of self, reorganizing of traumatically held experience, and strengthening differentiation and coherence, alongside opening up the integrative capacity of language. Boadella (1987: 123) describes this integrative function as 'the fusion of the body-stream and the word-stream'. According to Wilkinson, we need to build a new narrative 'that is not so unbearable that it has to be split off again' (Wilkinson 2010: 11). Pennebaker (1997) reports that health and cognitive function also improve as a result of journal writing, which seems to involve complex integrative processes of verbalization, stepping back, reflecting and following the continuity of experience. Top-down interventions and practices have their place.

The more complex the layers and modalities of experiencing involved, the richer, more stable and more coherent the narrative will be. 'While language is increasingly incorporated into these [relational] encounters with development, the structure of the encounter itself may never be represented in words. It is simply enacted and grasped implicitly in its enacted form' (BCPSG 2010: 69). The emerging story begins to take shape as it is worked and reworked, held lightly over time, consistent with the hologrammatic process of Kepner's (1995)

Healing Tasks Model. Equally, the body may never reveal its story in a form that can be represented by words, and a different subjective meaning will arise from that.

Dropping in

Turn your focus inwards, and let it rest with whatever bodily sensation draws your attention, pleasant or unpleasant. Take a few moments to investigate your experience and try to find six adjectives to describe it. Investigate the qualities of tension, energy, pulsation, weight, space, depth. Use these ideas to begin to compile a list of words to describe sensations, aiming for 40 or more. You could use some of these words as prompts with clients to help them differentiate sensations for themselves.

The trauma therapist's hand needs to hover continually over the pause button, as it were; the skill of interrupting the client is part of stewarding arousal (see Chapter 10). This allows for close attention to the client's internal arousal as well as to co-regulatory processes together, the moment-to-moment process which carries the therapeutic leverage (Beebe and Lachman 2002: 218). It is easy to misinterpret a client's embodied communications when there are no words to accompany them; there is wisdom in stopping and listening afresh to what is unfolding. Someone I worked with appeared to be on the verge of freezing into a dissociative state; believing that she was reliving some terror, I worked diligently to invite her back into contact with me, to no avail. This happened again over several sessions until she was able to tell me that my efforts reminded her of people trying to force her do something. Her freezing was not directly connected to the past, but to a misattunement in the here-and-now process between us.

Touch

Touch in psychotherapy is deeply controversial, because it 'can leave open the possibility for grave misuse' (Kertay and Reviere 1998: 20). Few therapists are well trained in the practice of therapeutic touch, and different schools of thought become quite polarized and moralistic around the issue. It is true, nevertheless, that ethics evolve: '[s]ocietal consciousness changes; the position of psychotherapists in society changes; and research informs us of false data that have been translated into ethical pronouncements' (Smith 1998: 50). It is as indiscriminate a position to forbid touch in a psychotherapy setting as it is to hold a client's hand whenever they cry. After all, in the words of Staunton (2002: 75), 'There is no evidence to suggest that touch or physical contact with

clients increase the likelihood of acting out sexually, nor that distance or analytic rigour prevent it.'

When we place so much emphasis on the role of the body in working with
trauma it would be perverse not to give this most human form of communication some serious thought, ethical considerations notwithstanding. Issues
about the appropriateness of non-erotic touch, whose needs it serves, and the
giving and withdrawing of consent must be taken into account because they
form the ground from which touch might safely be used. Figurally, though, we
need to weigh up the potential therapeutic value in offering particular touch to
some individual clients against that of withholding it. Ogden et al. (2006: 201)
suggest three parameters for the use of touch in trauma therapy: it must be well
considered, boundaried and therapeutic.

Touch is one form of human connection which triggers the release of the
hormone oxytocin. Present in mothers and their babies during childbirth
and immediately afterwards, oxytocin is associated with love, attachment and
bonding, strengthening feelings of safety and well-being in relationships.
Oxytocin works in conjunction with other hormones, particularly vasopressin,
which maintains healthy states of arousal and excitement. We can consider
these two hormones operating in the relational window of tolerance, oxytocin
representing the safe state of parasympathetic arousal and vasopressin pushing more towards the edges, the safe emergency. We all have different base
levels of natural oxytocin, and the variation in this may account for differing
degrees of resilience among our clients as well as for ourselves.

We can use touch in a number of ways in trauma psychotherapy, including to heighten awareness, to offer the client a sense of ownership of their
body, to support a postural realignment or to bring comfort. Whether
or not comforting touch will foreclose on something that might be felt or
worked through more fully is contingent on the client's level of arousal in
the moment, and the intervention needs to be assessed accordingly. Those
clients who have experienced traumatic physical injury or violation urgently
need to learn the difference between healthy and dangerous touch, which
can help to separate past from present. They also need to be able to determine when to say 'yes' or 'no' or 'not now'. The use of self-touch by clients
in therapy sessions is accepted by some as a sort of compromise position.
For example, an experiment with skin boundaries and containment might
involve inviting the client to use their own hands to mindfully hold or rub
their limbs or body surfaces.

Touch is a communication between therapist and client, expanding the
capacity for contact (Kepner [1987] 1999: 76). Offered as an experiment, it creates an opportunity for reflective and pre-reflective dialogue. Kepner points
out that the goal of touch is 'what is *experienced* by the person being touched,
rather than the production of some predetermined change' (Kepner [1987] 1999:
77, original italics). It should be added that the therapist's phenomenology and
feedback are also valid in the dialogue. Finally, and importantly, touch is a
vehicle for increasing the client's experiential range, learning to make choices
about what is liked and helpful and what is not.

Special considerations in tolerating relationship

The Window of Tolerance Model challenges fixed gestalts about trauma and confounds creative adjustments by highlighting the price at which they have been earned. Particularly for clients whose experience has included severe relational traumas, the availability of the longed for but feared relationship may also be a cause of intense distress and grief. Casement calls this the pain of contrast, sometimes misconstrued as resistance to receiving positive experiences in therapy, which I recognize more commonly than might be assumed. This pain 'exposes the depth of early deprivation or the true nature of damaging experience in childhood', and is experienced as an acute shock (1990: 106). The pain of contrast brings the client's wounds directly into the therapeutic space.

For other reasons related often to the traumatic circumstances, some trauma clients hold kindness in great suspicion. Coercion by means of charm, kindly attention or generosity – which is more correctly labelled as grooming – may set the stage for mistrust of the therapist's kindness and compassion. The version of conditionality which rests upon giving something back similarly configures the relational possibilities in therapy. It is for the therapist to decide whether to make these dilemmas explicit, bearing in mind the effect on the shared mindful field.

A limitation of the Window of Tolerance Model can be seen in the following example. A particularly shame-prone client found my prompting to 'drop' disturbing images and return to their sense of safety to be an indication that they were doing something wrong. They had assumed that they had to try and conform to what they understood to be an 'ideal' state that I expected them to attain. Partly, my error was to be too enthusiastic in applying the model, but I additionally failed to appreciate that they weren't able yet to access resources, still at the level of the conceptual rather than of lived and felt experience. Their shame and anxiety triggered a fearful state that needed acutely fine attention.

It was not yet possible to call this person out of their trauma, but instead I brought my more resourced presence into it. I would come to sit close by them, offering either a blanket or a cushion, with a box of tissues, a glass of water and some essential oil close to hand. I stroked the back of their hand with the corner of the blanket, placed oil on a tissue for them to smell, as I told them how I could feel their fear of being hurt again, of the small and secret place they had taken themselves into, of their terror, and of how I resonated with these.

I used my body as a regulator, my breath, my timing, my energy field, my temperature, imagining that my client could be aware of these even without the use of direct touch. Communication was body to body. Listening with my body I sensed into what each next step might be, informed by what area of this person's experience seemed figural; this required a reliance on my ability to resonate, coupled with my client's subtle energetic communications. The pace of this phase of our work was agonizingly slow, needing to be reworked over many subsequent sessions.

Summary

Forming a relationship with trauma clients can be extremely complex, especially when they have been wounded relationally. The relational themes of their lives need to be understood within the therapeutic context, where they replay on an implicit level, the level at which much trauma is held. Non-verbal features of relating and connecting therefore play a significant part in establishing and maintaining the therapeutic alliance. Included in this are the ways in which we resonate energetically with others as a form of communication, and the part that this can play in the development of a mindful relational field. Within such a field, the trauma can be shared and reflected upon together, and a process of mutual regulation develops incrementally. The window of tolerance can be understood as a relational model for the intersubjective process and for the co-creation of the relationship.

Trauma narratives come into the therapy setting as fragments of largely speechless terror. Alexithymia, the inability to differentiate sensations and emotions or to make sense of them, is common in trauma clients; they cannot tell a coherent story that will connect them to us or to the world. Neurologically, the part of the cortex that is responsible for language, called Broca's area, is less active during reminders of trauma. This has significant implications for working with trauma clients, and directs therapists to interventions which start with the body. Creating narratives that describe the client's observable body process is a form of reflective dialogue with the body, as is the thoughtful use of touch, increasing awareness and the integrative possibility of language. The work is kept close to the client's phenomenology as well as the therapist's, building a containing relational space which confirms their experience and strengthens self-functions.

13 Transforming relational wounds

Because of its hologrammatic and recursive nature, Kepner's model takes into account the breaking through of the traumatic memories in the form of implicit memory at any stage of therapy. Almost inevitably, the trauma will come to life spontaneously within the therapy, either by means of a rupture or a relational enactment closely resembling a previous unfinished and traumatic situation. In this chapter these dynamics are explored and discussed, arguing that for clients with early and complex trauma histories they are actually a necessary part of working through the trauma. Ruptures are placed in the context of disorganized attachment, and the dysregulation that they cause is applied to the relational window of tolerance. Different approaches to processing trauma are also considered. To put this into context, the chapter opens with a consideration of the often disrupted attachment processes that accompany trauma. We close by considering what it means for a trauma client to become more integrated during the course of therapy, and return finally to Eve's story.

Disorganized attachment and complex trauma

The almost universal acceptance of attachment theory in western psychology is, according to Fanen, culture-bound. Based on the premise of the nuclear family, it doesn't account for other attachments, such as to 'birds, plants, spirit, ancestors, land' (Fanen 2022: 215). This reimagining of attachment is also taken up by Haines (2019: 143), who writes: 'We also need to belong in our communities. Our communities need to belong to the wider social fabric. There is a broader circle of belonging that affects attachment, a sense of security, and real choices for connection and interdependence.' A wider framing of attachment opens the door to making sense of both intergenerational trauma and intergenerational survival. Haines questions attachment even within some western cultures, for example when some communities are regularly targeted by the police (Haines 2019). This prompts us to think more sensitively about our own communities and how our environment might promote or hinder secure attachment. With this ground for our thinking, let us now return to the attachment paradigm western practitioners are familiar with, and think about it through the lens of trauma.

Attachment difficulties tend to go hand in hand with the debilitating effects of trauma. Developmental trauma (sometimes termed relational trauma) is always part of what shapes early attachment patterns (including 'secure attachment'), which in turn establish what Bowlby called 'internal working models'. 'Internal working models include procedural memories which organize the core self and its relative degree of vulnerability to destabilization' (Bromberg 2011: 99). Thus '[i]t is through an understanding of attachment disorders [*sic*] that we can most easily make sense of findings related to simple and complex or developmental post traumatic stress disorder' (de Zulueta 2008: 61).

Many psychotherapists assume that recovery from trauma at any age depends to a large extent on the availability of one or more secure key attachment relationships. Sadly, significant traumas often have a knock-on effect on those closest to the victim, who because of their own shock, distress and lack of understanding are unable to provide the necessary regulating milieu for recovery. Furthermore, where early developmental traumas have been significant, in later life the individual becomes more sensitized to interpreting subsequent experience as actual or impending repetition of the original trauma (Stolorow 2007: 11). It is these repeating attachment patterns that distinguish complex trauma from PTS.

The style known as disorganized or type 'D' attachment can be seen in people whose parents were experienced as frightening or frightened or were themselves disoriented and dysregulated, and is associated with abuse and neglect, sometimes across generations in families. Disorganized attachment can resemble the phenomenology of dissociation (Schore 2007, cited in Bromberg 2011: 28). Clinically, we notice disorganized attachment in adults with incoherent life stories and abrupt shifts in states of mind, suggesting that trauma is unresolved (Siegel 1999: 110). Three further features of disorganized attachment, according to Hughes (2009: 11), are an inability to rely on self or others in any consistent way; unpredictability in responding to stress; and attempts to rigidly control the events in their lives in order to create some sense of safety. In addition it is treated as almost synonymous with pathologizing diagnoses such as so-called borderline personality 'disorder', dissociative identity 'disorder' and sometimes bipolar 'disorder'. Countering this typology robustly, Stolorow comments: 'To attribute the affective chaos or schizoid withdrawal of patients who were abused as children to "fantasy" or to "borderline personality organization" is tantamount to blaming the victim and, in doing so, *reproduces features of the original trauma*' (Stolorow 2007: 11, my italics).

Disorganized attachment can be held up against its polarity of secure attachment, that safe base which allows for growth, differentiation, integration and connection. Many contemporary writers make the link between secure attachment and emotional regulation (see Siegel 1999, 2007; Beebe and Lachman 2002; Schore 2003a, 2003b; Gerhardt 2004; Wilkinson 2010). Disorganized clients tend to feel very unsafe, both internally and in relation to the field; as we have seen in Chapter 6, recovery is predicated on the felt sense of safety. My proposal that the initial therapeutic alliance be formed around attention to safety is the precursor to establishing experiential relational safety. 'Attunement to your patient's safety ... must be experienced from *within* the relationship, rather than by trying to emphatically "provide" it as a technical stance' (Bromberg 2006: 141, original italics). Siegel (2012: 20–6) confirms this: 'Security is not a feature of the [individual], but rather it describes the nature of an interpersonal connection.' Trauma therapy is not quick work; having *'long experience* of consistency and continuity in therapy becomes a route to a more coherent internal relationship [between dissociated parts]' (Richardson 2008: 71, my italics).

It appears to be *unresolved* trauma, rather than trauma itself, that signals disorganized attachment (Siegel 1999: 111). Hughes (2009: 58) observes that while attachment patterns tend to be stable, they do not have to be rigid. This gives rise to hope, then, that in the relative safety of the therapeutic relationship, traumas and losses can be resolved and attachment patterns reconstructed. Being part of a therapeutic dyad will inevitably 'reactivat[e] attachment needs and developmental strivings' (Richardson 2008: 67), and it is in this context that the pain of rupture can be felt and become available for healing.

Rupture and repair in trauma therapy

I contend that the effectiveness of therapy is contingent on the success of the interactive repair process after ruptures, and the new understanding that can arise from it. This process involves the loosening of fixed relational gestalts, some attenuation of unfinished business, and experience in the dialogic dimension of open communication. Lest it be presumed that therapeutic ruptures are problems to be solved, they are indeed inevitable, necessary and – if handled skilfully – potentially healing. We cannot learn how to regulate the real and present relationship without regulating within it, and ruptures represent opportunities to do so. They may be experienced as mutual dysregulation. There is no one way of managing ruptures, and there is a skill in being able to assess what to do about them, resting in part on intuitively understanding the meaning a client might make of them.

A rupture may be something as small as a moment of asynchrony between therapist and client – for example, talking over them. To someone with a traumatic relational history, this might variously be interpreted as a violation of personal space, as a sign of the therapist's disconfirmation, as reinforcing that they cannot make themselves heard, or trigger them into flashbacks of parental discord. For Bromberg (2011: 106), 'genuine mutuality brings noisiness ... any experience of disjunction between subjectivities that raises the level of affective disharmony'.

Working with ruptures requires a non-defensive position as far as possible, and the willingness to listen and recalibrate the meaning of what happened. You may wish earnestly that the rupture never took place, for they can be threatening to the continuity of the relationship, turning on a coin towards negative transference. Together you listen to what the event meant to the other, and in what ways it represents an enactment (see the section 'What's going on? Trauma in the room' below). If appropriate, you may choose to offer an apology for your part in the rupture, and enquire whether the other person is interested in hearing what your side of the story was, without overdisclosing.

> **Clinical vignette**
>
> *My previous client had used the last tissue in the box. A replacement was ready on the shelf, but I had neglected to open it and place it within reach of the next person. This happened to be someone who was very startled if I ever made an unannounced movement, especially in dissociative moments when she was less able to distinguish current reality. When they became tearful in the session and looked around for a tissue, my embarrassment at having forgotten the box of tissues caused me to leave my seat quickly and fetch it. Stunned, my client said 'You frighten me', and I could viscerally feel the session being sucked into a vortex. Of course my embarrassment was invited by 'knowing' my client's vulnerability to misattunement; the trap was set and we dropped right into it.*

We can use the example in the clinical vignette as a springboard for thinking about the relationship between the window of tolerance and mutual *dysregulation*. In Chapter 12, the Window of Tolerance Model was presented as a relational dynamic, the space of optimal arousal being co-created through mutual regulation. By the same token, moments of dysregulation, leading to either hyperarousal, hypoarousal or both, are co-created. This is not to suggest that all moments of dysregulation within the therapy setting are ruptures, but simply that the relationship is not yet sufficiently aligned for reliable regulation.

However, the degree to which either individual is responsible is variable, and to some extent irrelevant. So long as the therapist is able to recognize that they have a part in dysregulation, the regulation can proceed without risk of blaming the other. 'If the patient goes away from a session feeling bad about him- or herself, attributing negative thoughts or feelings to the therapist, this is an event in which the therapist plays a part' (Yontef 2005: 94). The emotions evoked by a rupture can be intense, including rage, fear, sadness, hurt and shame – for either party. There is a risk of escalating arousal if these are not recognized and reflected on together (Hughes 2009: 158).

Ruptures are a specifically relational kind of dysregulating or triggering event, and the repair process is also mutually regulated (Tronick 1998), both parties needing to engage in the recovery. 'Embedded within the patient's often vociferous communication of the dysregulated state is also a definite, yet seemingly inaudible, urgent appeal for interactive regulation' (Schore 2003b: 92). When ruptures do arise, the repair process may itself be overstimulating. It can come to represent the intrusion of the therapist in wanting to re-establish connection, when the client may prefer to withdraw a little in order to regulate

(Siegel 1999: 116). Regulation and dysregulation are both properties of the shared field.

Any kind of open communication risks an intimacy that is potentially overwhelming. As Jacobs (2012: 65) points out, 'Openness to dialogue ... becomes increasingly difficult as situations are more emotionally charged, and are all but impossible when one has been triggered into a traumatized state of mind.' Trauma victims have already experienced the catastrophic effects of massive disruption of the boundary between self and other, and will naturally find it difficult to stay present, especially when the potential conflict involves someone they depend on (Bromberg 2011: 82). Until the relational bond is strong enough, it may simply be enough to acknowledge the rupture non-defensively, apologize for your part in it and seek a stabilizing resource in the moment. The important factor is the therapist's ongoing willingness to initiate repair of perceived disruptions (Sapriel 2012: 110), guided by the other person's capacity to tolerate it.

Surviving ruptures

The fact that a therapeutic relationship can survive ruptures along the way makes therapy and the trauma more tolerable. 'The internalization of the relational bond is strengthened rather than disrupted by having to deal with an absence of perfect harmony, *provided the disharmony is reparable*' (Bromberg 2011: 107, my italics). The relationship can now withstand stress. 'Paradoxically, real security is only discovered when the therapist has "failed" the patient but, unlike the past traumatizing object, is able to empathically attend and respond to the patient's distress' (Harding 2009: 71). The therapist needs to have confidence that the client and the relationship can recover (Harding 2009: 27). Trauma clients are often highly sensitive to state shifts in others, alert to their safety with you *in this moment*. For example, a rupture occurred with one client when I used humour unexpectedly. 'We can never be entirely sure whether what we intend as helpful and therapeutic is actually a repetition of the wounding and counter-therapeutic' (Soth 2006).

The open communication which is the vehicle for repair is crucial because it helps each of you make sense of *one another*. The essential relational function of 'mentalization', the capacity to reflect on the experience of self and on the state of mind of the other, is closely related to the quality of attachments (Fonagy et al. 2004: 97). 'Clinically, the most interesting aspect of the intersubjective environment between patient and analyst is the mutual knowing of what is in the other's mind, as it concerns the current nature and state of their relationship' (BCPSG 2010: 7).

Ruptures and their repair involve confrontation with another subjectivity, increasingly differentiating self. 'It is [also] required of the therapist to "decenter" from the structures of his own subjectivity in order to understand those of his patient ... these elements may have been unnoticed or considered unimportant by us, but can be shown to have enormous significance to the patient' (Brandchaft and Stolorow 1994: 109). Further, to work effectively to resolve these moments, the therapist needs to listen to 'the immediate and residual effects of his own participation' (Bromberg [1998] 2001: 151). The next step, according to Brandchaft and Stolorow (1994: 105), is that the 'intersubjective field in which such behavior takes place should now be equally minutely studied'. It is by repetition of these processes that the client becomes able to decouple the trauma from the relationship.

What's going on? Trauma in the room

Generally speaking, in the early stages of therapy most of the crises that present are those day-to-day disruptive events which the traumatized person is as yet unable to negotiate on their own or to avoid. Surviving these together, without judgement for the messes they get into, prepares the ground for the emergence of crisis within the therapy. The therapist themselves becomes a bridge to the trauma. At some point, the therapeutic relationship gets into a mess, and needs to. Soth (2006) describes this evocatively as the wound entering the therapy: 'The wound [of trauma] gets experientially constellated in the therapeutic relationship', and this dynamic is referred to as an enactment. Enactments bring the work to the heart of the client's relational and traumatic wounds, speaking to their most intense, secret and shame-laden fears and longings. For example, a phobia of the therapist (see Chapter 6), with which many trauma clients enter therapy, includes a fear of emotional engagement as a defence against their longing for connection, and the therapist may thus be cast into the role of the disengaged other.

However, more than feeling cast in a certain role or otherwise pulled out of shape, an enactment is a situation in which a therapist is drawn, unaware, into repeating something of significance to the person they are working with. According to Philippson (2012: 89), 'the fixed patterns [self-states] rely on others to pick up and take on their parts in the interactions'. Thus therapeutic enactments involve both parties in the relationship:

> To insist that when patients feel endangered by a therapist their perceptions of him must be faulty ... constitutes a 'cordon sanitaire' around the therapist. It precludes the unhampered investigation of the patient's subjective reality, so that the persecutory experiences can be understood in greater depth, including the therapist's unwitting contribution to them.
>
> (Brandchaft and Stolorow 1994: 98)

In Kepner's model, enactments of this nature come under the umbrella of 'undoing'. This involves 'placing back into the interpersonal field those things now experienced as part of the self that were originally part of the interpersonal world but never experienced as such' (Kepner 1995: 110), which happens outside of awareness. Ultimately transformative, the pair first need to 'hang around' in, and live through, the mess (Bromberg 2011).

A central tenet of Bromberg's writing ([1998] 2001, 2006, 2011) is that during an enactment the therapy enters a *co-created dyadic dissociative process*, creating a shift from shared mindful states to shared dissociative states. Dyadic dissociation is a hallmark of an enactment. This process 'drains the interpersonal context of meaning. By unlinking the mind from the reflective perception of dyadic affective experience, a person is isolated from the danger of directly experiencing an other's "otherness"' (Bromberg 2011: 52). Neither therapist nor client is fully open to contact within the shared reflective space, although either one may think they are. For a time, the relationship comes under enormous pressure.

Bromberg usefully describes the phenomenology of how the therapist comes to lose their bearings and becomes unable to think about what is going on:

> He cannot even find what appears to be a useful way of engaging with his patient in the here and now because his patient's mind is feeling so unfamiliar. He then dissociates ... Is this bad therapy? Only if the analyst is content to be relationally unawake for too long.
>
> (Bromberg 2011: 110)

Eventually the dreaming therapist must awaken (Bromberg 2006), and the shared mindful and regulating field is restored. This then creates an opportunity to understand 'how the client experiences the therapy, and the therapist, *through* their character, *through* their wounding' (Soth and Eichhorn 2012: 15, original italics). There is an inherent paradox in these enactments, as Soth (2006) describes, in which the seemingly counter-therapeutic enactment and its transformation are actually two sides of the same coin. Stolorow (2007: 26), writing of his own experience of trauma, puts it beautifully: 'When my traumatized states could not find a relational home, I became deadened, and my world became dulled. When such a home became once again present, I came alive, and the vividness of my world returned.'

Clinical vignette

For the first year or more of our work together, I was able to use my knowledge of trauma to manage my own anxieties about being with Jocelyn. However, I became increasingly and irrationally concerned about her lack of relationality with me; she invariably turned away from me; she neither greeted me nor thanked me nor said goodbye at the end. Our relationship was often conflictual, but she seemed unable to hear of my side of it, even after these months of therapy. I could not recognize myself in her descriptions of me. Jocelyn seemed to want to know who I was and yet when I offered her more of myself she rejected me. If I showed her my felt response she thought I had too many issues of my own, like her mother, and if I didn't I became uninvolved. This process was unusually intense and increasingly impinged on my thoughts; it was something particular to Jocelyn and me. There were times when I felt as though she was playing mind games with me. It was all my fault and I duly felt that I was doing a bad job with Jocelyn. I was lost in wanting to increase contact with her, and became preoccupied with thoughts of needing to be seen as a human being by her.

It so happened that I needed to cancel a session at short notice when an elderly relative became ill. I took it as an opportunity to show myself as a human being, and told Jocelyn the real reason for my cancellation instead of cloaking it in something vague. Her response was that she hadn't wanted to come today anyway, which when I reflected later, pulled me up short. When she did not arrive for her next session I finally woke up, and consulted my supervisor. Jocelyn's relational history included chronic sexual abuse by her womanizing father, a man of dark charm, and a mother who was mentally unwell, in and out of hospital, always needy and lacking boundaries. Her mother, when she was not in thrall to her illness, repeatedly contradicted Jocelyn's subjectivity – 'You don't think that, you think this.' Little wonder, then, that Jocelyn presented in such a disorganized manner.

With the support of my supervisor I was able to decentre my preoccupation with Jocelyn's recognition of me, in order to recentre my recognition in her experiential world. My supervisor's challenge was: 'Why shouldn't she spend the whole session with her back to you if she wants?' At the beginning of our next session, Jocelyn made eye contact with me, a serious, pained expression in her that moved me greatly, a small and almost miraculous reorganization of our contact. Jocelyn seemed momentarily to be taking me in through her eyes, as I saw into her loss and longing for connection. Her life had been difficult, but she began to speak of it from a more integrated and resourced state. My implicit recognition of the intrusions and neglect of Jocelyn's early years, and my access to the effects of shame, objectification, separation, denial and dissociation, now gave us a 'shared' history. Our contact became more potent and vibrant thereafter.

Acts of triumph

Working through enactments provides the opportunity to make implicit levels of communication explicit, and to reorganize somatic creative adjustments. Trauma manifests itself not only through relational enactments but through the multiple and subtle ways in which the 'body keeps the score'. Because of unresolved attachments, the trauma, held in the body, remains for some considerable time unresolved or unprocessed. The body has unfinished business.

Kepner's account of the third stage of therapy – undoing, redoing and mourning – which this resolution correlates to, includes a comment that abreaction for the sake of it should be avoided (Kepner 1995: 113). He argues, however, that in order to experience themselves differently, the trauma client *may* need to engage in large, noisy and energetic expressive experiments, cautioning that the *'drama should be congruent with the readiness of the client to integrate the drama as a part of the evolving self'* (Kepner 1995: 114, my italics). It is helpful to recall here that recursive trauma responses are the result of overstimulation and a mass of stressful material that cannot be integrated by the nervous system of the victim. My criticisms of Kepner's thinking here are therefore that these expressive experiments do not necessarily increase the client's control over or awareness of the trauma in the body; they do not necessarily reorganize the somatic experience of the client, and they do not necessarily allow for slow and calibrated integration of the new experience. These criticisms should not suggest that there is no place for the release of expressive experiments, but caution that slow integration is preferable.

Compare this to the Sensorimotor approach, in which 'slivers' of traumatic memory are reactivated at the margins of the window of tolerance, now expanded sufficiently to increase capacity to feel without becoming dysregulated. These slivers can then be processed through the body, returning again and again to the resources available (Ogden et al. 2006: 243). This is achieved through phenomenological tracking – the stewarding of arousal – based on the client's increased ability to disengage from the content and meaning of the trauma, and instead attend mindfully to the physical components of the experience as they arise. This helps to uncouple the linkage between traumatically generated associations experienced somatically. It is interesting to note that the oscillation between traumatically charged material and resourced states resembles the rhythm of EMDR (Shapiro 1995), the 'technological' approach to trauma processing, in which successive periods of arousal associated with 'target' memories are triggered by bilateral stimulation, followed by periods of quiet and reflection. It is this oscillation that seems to support the integration of the brain, strengthening linkages between limbically mediated activation and the cortex.

The intention behind the processing of fragments of memory through the body relates to the theory of immobilized defences (Chapter 7), and the need to complete those defences that were truncated or aborted at the time the trauma took place: 'It is a basic tendency of the organism to complete any situation or transaction which for it is unfinished' (Perls et al. [1951] 1998: 77). Where trauma has interfered with and delayed this natural process, resources provide the ground for its restoration. '"When the implicit (procedural) memory is activated and completed somatically, an explicit narrative can be constructed; not the other way round"' (P.A. Levine, cited in Ogden et al. 2006: 248). Ogden et al. (2006) describe this active completion as the execution of 'acts of triumph' over the trauma.

From the frozen or collapsed state of immobilization, the client needs to find actions which will support the completion of the defence – pushing, turning, kicking, running. These may be very small but significant reorganizations of the range of choices available to the client. By tracking sensations as they rise and fall in the body, the client is encouraged to identify the emergence of impulses to move, and to allow the body to find the movement it needs. This translates to the undoing of inhibited or retroflected somatic impulses. Voluntary movements certainly play a part in this, but so do emerging involuntary movements. It requires an enormous amount of control over the body to trust in the possibility of surrendering to involuntary processes such as shaking, especially those associated with trauma. However, this is necessary because it pertains to unresolved autonomic arousal, orienting and defensive reactions (Ogden et al. 2006: 253).

These writers also suggest searching for 'peritraumatic' resources: those maybe even counter-intuitive instinctual defences that were available at the time of the trauma (Ogden et al. 2006: 244). One person had witnessed a bloody scene of domestic violence as a young child, and remembered that they had closed their eyes at the horror of it. This minute action, the only one possible in the extreme danger of the moment, felt enormously powerful to them, releasing some residual trauma. By encouraging them to repeat this action, the client was enabled to mindfully access a sequence of impulses, interspersed with moments of present orientation, that incrementally turned first their eyes and head, and then their whole body in the opposite direction, one in which they were free to walk away. The freedom that comes from this is beautifully captured in this quote from Kopp 'I shall take my sadness and as I can I will make it sing' (1972:159); this sadness may be interpreted as any suffering.

Dropping in

Consider some aspect of unfinished business in your own life. What is needed to help you find some resolution? Is there a need for interactive repair of some sort, or for you to reclaim a defensive function that for some reason has been unavailable to you thus far? What needs to be communicated that has yet to be confirmed in the context of a relationship? And what does your body need to do to release the fixed patterns? Write about your situation and your response to these questions.

Integration, narrative and earned attachment

The healing of splits with which we started, and which we have explored through the lens of dissociation in the relational field, is, as we have seen, a complex task. The lens has many facets: the implicit, making it explicit; the discontinuous, making it continuous; the disembodied, making it embodied; the timeless, making it present; the uncontainable, making it containable; the fragmented, making it coherent. The challenge of integration happens at multiple levels, including emotional, verbal, neural, narrative, cognitive and sensorimotor (Siegel 1999; Ogden et al. 2006: 300). Exclusion of any one of these modes of being would by definition not be fully integrative. We have come to see that both unresolved trauma and attachment issues can, through relational trauma-specific therapy, be resolved and the splits restored. As Boadella (1987: 123) says, '[t]herapy is a journey towards the joining of what was split, the coupling of broken images'.

What then, do we mean by integration at this stage of the therapeutic journey? We revisit Siegel's important contribution to the understanding of integration in psychotherapy. At its most simple is his definition of the linkage of differentiated parts (Siegel 2009: 165) as a polarity to dissociation, providing a fundamental dimension of health (Siegel 2012: 16-1). Integration might therefore be seen as a desirable outcome of trauma therapy. Siegel states that 'The maintenance of the differentiated qualities of the individual components of the system even while linking them is an essential aspect of integration' (Siegel 2012: 16-4). A feature of such linkage is thus that the 'whole is greater than the sum of the parts', speaking to the values of Gestalt therapy (Siegel 2012: 16-4). Beyond this rather technical description, however, for Siegel (1999: 321) integration is a process that creates coherence in the mind. In his inimitable style, he uses the word 'coherence' as an acrostic: connected, open, harmonious, engaged, receptive, emergent, noetic [a sense of knowing], compassionate and empathic (Siegel 2012: 16-5). After the confusion and messiness of trauma, we have arrived at a point of clarity where the mud can settle. This concept of coherence has relevance to attachment, trauma, memory and self.

One of several interlinked areas that Siegel is interested in is that of attachment. He contends that it is possible for attachment wounds to be healed, via the emergence of 'earned' autonomous attachment for adults (Siegel 2007: 201). For Hughes (2009: 56), also, attachment security can be attained, while at the same time the adult is able to function autonomously. Siegel suggests further that the creation in therapy of *a coherent narrative of self, even though it will necessarily be a painful one, is the organizing factor* in earned attachment. The original trauma narrative has been reorganized to include new, realistic and more consistent perspectives on identity, self and other. In a similar vein, Wilkinson argues that 'an emphasis on *co-constructing* narrative may play a vital part in assisting the patient not only in coming to terms with the reality of his or her internal world, but also in the process of mourning what was and what might have been' (Wilkinson 2010: 133, my italics). This enables a greater capacity to live with vitality in the present situation.

Narrative gives the trauma client authorship of their life, allowing them to adopt 'different perspectives on or versions of the experience of self' (Siegel 1999: 324), where previously the sense of power was placed in the field. Coherence of narrative may actually be what constitutes self, or rather having a sense of self, that is compatible with the Gestalt understanding of self in process, in contrast to self being more fixed. At the heart of this is being able to 'make sense' of their life, which in turn can alter their 'attachment status' as adults, including the possibility of raising children who thrive (Siegel 1999: 204). Through mindfulness the adult trauma victim is able to reflect on their relationships with others, communicate openly, empathize and repair ruptures.

The unfinished business of trauma can never be truly finished; trauma brands its imprint into the very fibres of its victim's being, and is at the heart of their narrative. But the trauma victim emerges from therapy into a different world, by virtue of the fact that they have changed and will continue to change. As Siegel (1999: 336) says, 'Creating coherence is a lifetime project. Integration is thus a process, not a final accomplishment. It is a verb, not a noun.' Traumatized people continue to create their own fields of reciprocal influence throughout their lives, and thus the ripples of our work may spread far.

Case study: Part 5

After a particularly difficult stage in her therapy, when Eve and I worked through a significant rupture, she realized that she could no longer stay in her job because of the harmful impact it was continuing to have on her. These are her words: 'I told him what I want, didn't make excuses, just told it straight ... it was a relief actually. I feel like I can see better, it's not about being strangled by it but about having choices. It releases something, I'm out of there.'

Despite her financial insecurity, Eve was able to tell herself that she had already survived something far worse than this, and that she and Freya would manage somehow. They moved into a smaller and cheaper flat, nearer to school so that Eve did not have to pay bus fares. Eve found she didn't miss her larger flat, saying that she had more sense of space inside her and that new possibilities were opening up. Eve felt safer inside and more in control of her life. She was vulnerable to setbacks, though, particularly when her mother had cancer treatment and she didn't find it easy to set limits on the help she offered.

Eve said the thing that made the most difference to her was my patience and calm, and that my honesty and openness helped her gain trust in me. She felt understood by me, which grew from how I confidently conveyed my understanding of trauma.

Eve's therapy came to an end more quickly than she had planned because she had run out of money. We continued to meet less frequently for a few months, and Eve learnt to rely on herself to manage triggers and her reactions. However, there was still some work that we were not able to address, and her phobia of pain remained, as did the occasional temptation to self-harm, which when I last saw her she was not acting on.

Summary

Our ways of being in relationship to others tend to reflect the dynamics of our early upbringing, and this has a connection with the development of disorganized attachment. Associated with complex trauma, disorganized attachment arises from the experience of being raised by caretakers who were either frightened or frightening, or themselves disorganized; an absence of safety is definitive of this relational tendency. It is an explanation for the transmission of trauma between generations in a family. This attachment style brings with it particular sensitivities which come to be enacted one way or another in the therapeutic relationship.

First, ruptures are an inevitable part of therapy, and have particular implications for working with trauma clients and in reconfiguring the disorganized relational ground on which they stand. For some, ruptures signal conflict and are thus minimized as a regulatory manoeuvre. For others the dialogic attitude of paying close attention to the relational dynamics of ruptures requires an intimacy which is extremely anxiety-provoking. Either way, for the client, therapeutic ruptures can be experienced as a threat to a relationship which they depend on. They have yet to discover the therapeutic value of restoring relationships that have gone off track.

A further way in which therapeutic relationships get into difficulty is when the relational wounds of the client are replicated in the here and now. These enactments happen outside awareness – a co-created dissociative process, according to Bromberg. Both parties become disoriented to the relational context and to the subjectivity of the other. However frightening and painful these episodes may be, they are necessary in order to make explicit that which has previously been dissociated from the client's awareness. The therapist has taken on a part which feels familiar to the client, creating what can be seen as a shared history, deepening understanding and enabling transformative shifts once the therapist has 'woken' from the dream state.

In so far as the body has been implicated in the trauma, the trauma also needs to be released from the body. Expressive techniques of classical Gestalt therapy can be used within the client's capacity to tolerate them. However, shuttling between activated slivers of memory at the margins of an expanded window of tolerance and more resourced states holds the potential of integrating the processing of trauma, leading to a more resolved outcome. The integrative capacity of the body is one mode, among several others, of accessing a more coherent sense of self, a narrative that includes different perspectives and the possibility of reaching 'earned' autonomous attachment as an adult.

Glossary

In addition to the terms defined below, readers unfamiliar with Gestalt concepts are recommended to turn to an excellent small book, *Gestalt Therapy: 100 Key Points and Techniques* by Dave Mann (2010).

aggress The ability to act as an agent in the world, to get one's needs met, to make contact.

assimilation A stage on the cycle of experience following contact, as the figure recedes, before the new figure emerges. It is a stage of integration of contact and novelty that is necessary before a new figure emerges.

awareness Related to **phenomenology** and **figure** formation, awareness is turning attention to something, often the perception of a sense, a moment of contact, patterns or emerging excitement.

awareness continuum The ongoing sequence of unrepeatable aware moments. The sense that one thing follows another, that the experience of life is not fixed but fluid and in constant process.

body; body/mind Body is inseparable from self. We exist not only through our thoughts, language and intention, but also through action, sensation and feeling. Body is a medium for contact, and expresses our way of being in the world. Gestalt works with the whole self, not simply the contents of thoughts and beliefs. The body is valued for its integrative potential; seen as the seat of inherent wisdom and authenticity. There is a reciprocal feedback loop between the trunk, limbs and organs of the body and the brain. Body and mind are reflections of one another. It is in this sense that body/mind is used; the mind is not confined to the brain as an organ.

confluence A **modification to contact** whereby the boundary between self and other is not distinguished and becomes blurred or merged.

contact Contact is not the same as togetherness or joining – rather it is the meeting of difference. Contact and withdrawal are two sides of a coin; withdrawal is contactful in a limited way. We cannot be in contact with the total field at any one time. Contact is the most active process in the cycle of experience, involving a combination of sensing, energetic engagement and inclination towards the other/environment. Gestalt therapists are interested in the quality and style of contact. The ability to make good contact is one way Gestalt therapists understand psychological health, as fluid, satisfying and receptive to novelty to support growth.

contact boundary The point in space and time where meeting occurs. In Gestalt **self** emerges in contact with the other at the boundary. The boundary can be disturbed *by an individual* in a number of ways, modifying contact. This has important implications for understanding reactions to trauma, in which there is a devastating reorganization of the boundary between self and other.

contact functions Elements of behaviour, usually observable, by which an individual reaches into the environment in order to support contact. They are differently available and developed in every individual. They include: movement, voice, seeing, hearing, feelings and bodily process (Joyce and Sills 2010: 59).

contact style The **phenomenology** of contact processes.

creative adjustment Responses to the demands of the other or of the environment in the best way available to ensure ongoing survival, regulation and relationship. Sometimes creative adjustments are compromises, especially when made at some disadvantage, such as those made early in life and in the face of powerful others.

creative indifference A relational position associated with the **Paradoxical Theory of Change**. The therapeutic creative stance of not being attached or invested in any particular outcome for the client, which according to the **phenomenological** approach is for the client to define.

cycle of experience Concerned with the formation of **figures**. The cycle, often illustrated as a wave, involves the following stages: sensation, awareness, mobilization, action, contact, satisfaction, assimilation and withdrawal. The figure arises from a ground known as the fertile void.

desensitization A **modification to contact** diminishing awareness of sensation at the beginning stage of figure formation. Desensitization can be seen in those removed from embodied life, sometimes to the extent of numbing or deadening.

dialogue One of the three pillars of Gestalt therapy, which reaches beyond everyday conversation, focusing on deep meeting, verbally and non-verbally, between people. Dialogue incorporates Buber's I–Thou and I–It of relatedness. For Gestalt therapists, relationship is co-created and emphasizes a dialogic attitude, aware of and open to the humanity of the other. Buber's four principles of dialogue are presence, confirmation, open communication and inclusion. Inclusion is similar to but uniquely different from empathy. It means leaning into the world of the other without losing one's own subjectivity.

egotism A **modification to contact** which limits contact by self-criticism, over-analysing and preoccupation with how one comes across. In a healthy sense, it supports reflexivity, self-regulation and self-reflection.

experimentation Allows clients to expand their range of available choices by becoming more fully who they are. Traditional 'staged' Gestalt experiments can involve challenge and sometimes confrontation. In contrast, experiments can be quite small, such as trying out 'I' language, or imagining a new behaviour. Experimentation creates the 'safe emergency' whereby the client can rehearse and adjust new ways of being. Experiments arise naturally from the dialogue, are co-created with the client and are calibrated according to the support available, so as not to be exposing or dysregulating. Experiments can develop missing polarities and resources, often by exaggerating or repeating an embodied communication, and can introduce playfulness into therapy.

field One of the three pillars of Gestalt theory. The term 'field' in Gestalt is used in reference to different things, and derives from two sources. First, Gestalt psychology refers to the perceptual field, an individualistic concept. By this interpretation, there can be no shared field. The second meaning is based in Lewin's field theory, and refers to what is sometimes known as the 'life space' of an individual, the terms 'environment' and 'situation' also being used interchangeably with field. A contemporary rendering of the concept of field rests on the interdependence of all species and the entire cosmos across time, and is therefore a systems approach. According to Lewinian theory, the behaviour of the individual is embedded in a context. This is a more integrative frame of reference. For the purposes of this book, we must also emphasize that the fluctuating internal physiological state of the individual is also part of the context to be taken into account. This concept is closely related to that of **self**.

figure What is being attended to now; the dynamic organization of experience. The emergence or formation of a figure is always set against a **ground**, from which it is indivisible and into which it recedes, like the relationship of a wave to water. There may be a number of dominant themes in any life at any one time, but only one is the figure which is selected from that ground in any one moment.

fixed gestalt A process whereby selfing (see **self**) gets stuck and is less responsive to change and outside influence. It is a rigid pattern repeated continuously in an individual's life, a more structural form of **creative adjustment**. This is a key concept in understanding trauma, in which responses become embedded and solidified in the structure of contacts, and cannot easily be updated according to current conditions.

gestalt A German word roughly translated as the configuration of something in its entirety. It relates to the holistic stance of Gestalt and to the need to complete inherent in the concept of unfinished business, key for trauma therapy.

ground An undifferentiated condition containing aspects of the field, historical and contemporary. It also consists of traces of experience and physiology which provide a context to the perception of the **figure**. A healthy relationship between figure and ground is always dynamic. Ground and **field** are not the same.

inclusion See **dialogue**.

mobilization A stage in the development of a **figure** in which energy is gathered in the interests of making good contact.

modification to contact The temporary or fixed adjustment to contacting according the current or historical **field**.

organismic self-regulation The biological organism's innate ability to return to a state of balance after disturbance. It is based on the principle that the body is able to restore itself to healthy functioning, which is seriously compromised in trauma.

Paradoxical Theory of Change A philosophical foundation of Gestalt therapy, Beisser's theory of change. This states that change occurs not when one tries to be different, but when one is able to be fully who one is. The theory informs and underpins much of the process and relational position of Gestalt therapy.

phenomenology One of the pillars of Gestalt therapy, which places emphasis on the study of the subjective experience of the client as they perceive and make sense of their world. It involves observation of experience and perception by both client and therapist, privileged over interpretive approaches. Phenomenology is interested in sensation as the basis of felt experience, an entry to embodiment. Phenomenology can be described as being 'experience-near'. The client comes to make their own meaning of experience.

polarities Dynamic and opposing properties, both of which need to be supported to achieve a state of equilibrium and form a complete gestalt. Such properties may be disowned or separated through denial of one pole while the other is emphasized more. Working therapeutically with polarities seeks to establish the 'middle ground'. The middle ground can be represented by a range of possibilities on a continuum between the poles.

retroflection The **modification to contact** of turning towards oneself, as opposed to expressiveness and spontaneity, e.g. holding in anger or sorrow.

response-ability The ability to make fluid and spontaneous responses in the moment rather than stereotyped or habitual ones.

safe emergency The safe emergency is a state of inner and relational safety, in which exploration, novelty and challenge can be tolerated by the client, without tipping them into a dysregulated state. This allows for choices, increased flexibility and the possibility of processing previously unbearable feelings and sensations. It is therefore a point of growth, change and integration.

self In Gestalt therapy self is a dynamic emergent process (selfing) rather than the essence of someone or something that is fixed. Self actively organizes and manages experience within the **field**, and is a function of that field. There is ongoing debate in the Gestalt community about the existence of a 'core self'. From a field perspective, self is sometimes referred to as 'organism', though this is more accurately understood as the biological organism.

References

Abramson, A. (2022) New frontiers in neuroscience: Recent discoveries about the biological underpinnings of human behavior are helping psychologists find new ways to improve people's lives, *American Psychiatric Association*, 53(1). https://www.apa.org/monitor/2022/01/special-frontiers-neuroscience (accessed 30 November 2023).

Alleyne, A. (2022) *The Burden of Heritage: Hauntings of Generational Trauma on Black Lives*. London: Karnac.

American Psychiatric Association (2000) *Diagnostic and Statistical Manual of Mental Disorders IV-TR*. Washington, DC: American Psychiatric Association.

Anagnostopoulou, L. (2015) Vertical Grounding: The body in the world and the self in the body, in G. Marlock and H. Weiss (eds) *The Handbook of Body Psychotherapy and Somatic Psychology*. Berkeley, CA: North Atlantic Books.

Appel-Opper, J. (2012) Relational living body psychotherapy, in C. Young (ed.) *About Relational Body Psychotherapy*. Galashiels: Body Psychotherapy Publications.

Armsworth, M.T., Stronk, K. and Carlson, C. (1999) Body image and self-perception in women with histories of incest, in J.M. Goodwin and R. Attias (eds) *Splintered Reflections: Images of the Body in Trauma*. New York: Basic Books.

Attias, R. and Goodwin, J. (1999) Body-image distortion and childhood sexual abuse, in J.M. Goodwin and R. Attias (eds) *Splintered Reflections: Images of the Body in Trauma*. New York: Basic Books.

Aves, W. (2022) 'Trauma informed care' left me more traumatized than ever, blog post, 12 July. https://www.psychiatryisdrivingmemad.co.uk/post/trauma-informed-care-left-me-more-traumatised-than-ever (accessed 18 May 2024).

Badouk Epstein, O. (2022) Primary shame: Needing you and the economy of affects, in O. Badouk Epstein (ed.) *Shame Matters: Attachment and Relational Perspectives for Psychotherapists*. Abingdon: Routledge.

Bakal, D. (1999) *Minding the Body: Clinical Uses of Somatic Awareness*. New York: Guilford.

Bednarek, S. (2022) Who needs to change? Reflections on the complex relationship between climate change, mental health and the profession of psychotherapy, in S. Wright (ed.) *The Change Process in Psychotherapy During Troubling Times*. Abingdon: Routledge.

Beebe, B. and Lachman, F.M. (2002) *Infant Research and Adult Treatment: Co-constructing Interactions*. Hillsdale, NJ: Analytic Press.

Beisser, A. (1970) The Paradoxical Theory of Change, in J. Fagan and I.L. Shepherd (eds) *Gestalt Therapy Now*. New York: Harper and Row.

Boadella, D. (1987) *Lifestreams*. London: Routledge, Kegan and Paul.

Bocian, B. (2009) From free association to connection, *Studies in Gestalt Therapy*, 3(2): 37–59.

Boon, S., Steele, K. and van der Hart, O. (2011) *Coping With Trauma-Related Dissociation*. New York: Norton.

Boston Change Process Study Group (2002) Non-interpretive mechanism in psychoanalytic therapy. The 'something more' than interpretation, *International Gestalt Journal*, 25(1): 37–71.

Boston Change Process Study Group (2010) *Change in Psychotherapy: A Unifying Paradigm*. New York: Norton.

Bowman, C. (2012) Reconsidering holism in Gestalt therapy: A bridge too far?, in T. Levine (ed.) *Gestalt Therapy: Advances in Theory and Practice*. London: Routledge.

Brandchaft, B. and Stolorow, R.D. (1994) The difficult patient, in R.D. Stolorow, G. Atwood and B. Brandchaft (eds) *The Intersubjective Perspective*. Lanham, MD: Rowman and Littlefield.

Bromberg, P. ([1998] 2001) *Standing in the Spaces: Essays on Clinical Process, Trauma and Dissociation*. New York: Psychology Press.

Bromberg, P. (2006) *Awakening the Dreamer: Clinical Journeys*. Mahwah, NJ: Analytic Press.

Bromberg, P. (2011) *The Shadow of the Tsunami: And the Growth of the Relational Mind*. New York: Routledge.

Brownell, P. (2009) Executive functions: A neuroscientific understanding of self-regulation, *Gestalt Review*, 13(1): 62–81.

Brownell, P. (2012) *Gestalt Therapy for Addictive and Self-Medicating Behaviors*. New York: Springer.

Capra, F. and Luisi, P.L. (2014) *The Systems View of Life: A Unifying Vision*. Cambridge: Cambridge University Press.

Carroll, R. (2009) Self-regulation – an evolving concept at the heart of body psychotherapy, in L. Hartley (ed.) *Contemporary Body Psychotherapy: The Chiron Approach*. London: Routledge.

Casement, P. (1990) *Further Learning from the Patient*. London: Routledge.

Chefetz, R. (2022) Attackments: Subjugation, shame and the attachment to painful affects and objects, in O. Badouk Epstein (ed.) *Shame Matters: Attachment and Relational Perspectives for Psychotherapists*. Abingdon: Routledge.

Chidiac, M.-A. (2023) Fields of power: The moderation of relational moments, *British Gestalt Journal*, 32(1): 8–20.

Clarkson, P. (1989) *Gestalt Counselling in Action*. London: Sage.

Clarkson, P. and Mackewn, J. (1993) *Fritz Perls*. London: Sage.

Clemmens, M.C. ([1997] 2005) *Getting Beyond Sobriety: Clinical Approaches to Long-term Sobriety*. Cambridge, MA: Gestalt Press.

Cohen, A. (2003) Gestalt therapy and post-traumatic stress disorder: The irony and the challenge, *Gestalt Review*, 7(1): 42–55.

Cook, A, n.d., Somatoform Dissociation. https://www.body-mind.co.uk/a_resources/book.html (accessed 23 May 2024).

Cozolino, L. (2002) *The Neuroscience of Psychotherapy: Building and Rebuilding the Human Brain*. New York: Norton.

Cozolino, L. (2006) *Interpersonal Neurobiology: Attachment and the Developing Social Brain*. New York: Norton.

Crompton, T. (2013) On love of nature and the nature of love, in S. Weintrobe (ed.) *Engaging with Climate Change: Psychoanalytic and Interdisciplinary Approaches*. Hove: Routledge.

Damasio, A. (2000) *The Feeling of What Happens: Body, Emotion and the Making of Consciousness*. London: Vintage Books.

Dana, D. (2021) *Anchored: How to Befriend your Nervous System Using Polyvagal Theory*. Boulder, CO: Sounds True.

D'Andrea, W., Sharma, R., Zelchoski, A.D. and Spinazzola, J. (2011) Physical health problems after single trauma exposure: When stress takes root in the body, *Journal of the American Psychiatric Nurses Association*, 17(6): 378–92.

Davidson, J.R.T. (2000) New strategies for the treatment of posttraumatic stress disorder, *Journal of Clinical Psychiatry*, 61(7): 3–4.

Davies, J. (2022) *Sedated: How Modern Capitalism Created our Mental Health Crisis.* London: Atlantic Books.

Davis, D.M. and Hayes, J.A. (2011) What are the benefits of mindfulness? A practice review of psychotherapy-related research, *Psychotherapy Theory Research Practice Training*, 48(2): 198–208.

De Zulueta, F. (2008) Developmental trauma in adults, in S. Benamer and K. White (eds) *Trauma and Attachment*. London: Karnac.

Delisle, G. (2011) *Personality Pathology: Developmental Perspectives*. London: Karnac.

Delisle, G. (2013) *Object Relations in Gestalt Therapy*. London: Karnac.

Denham-Vaughan, S. (2005) Will and grace, *British Gestalt Journal*, 14(1): 5–14.

Denham-Vaughan, S. and Chidiac, M.-A. (2013) SOS: A relational orientation towards social inclusion, *Mental Health and Social Inclusion*, 17(2): 100–7.

DeYoung, P.A. (2015) *Understanding and Treating Chronic Shame: A Relational/Neuro-biological Approach*. New York: Routledge.

Eliotson, J. (1835) *Human Physiology*. London: Longman.

Emsley, E., Smith, J.., Martin, D. and Lewis, N. (2022) Trauma-informed care in the UK: Where are we? A qualitative study of health policies and professional perspectives, *BMC Health Services Research*, 22(1). DOI:10.1186/s12913-022-08461-w.

Falconer, R. (2023) *The Others Within Us: Internal Family Systems, Porous Mind, and Spirit Possession*. Brisbane: Great Mystery Press.

Fanen, L. (2022) *Warp and Weft: Psycho-emotional Health, Politics and Experiences*. Donji Budacki, Croatia: Active Distribution.

Figgess, S. (2009) Gestalt and EMDR, *British Gestalt Journal*, 18(1): 34–41.

Fisher, J. (n.d.) Self harm and suicidality. Unpublished paper. https://janinafisher.com/wp-content/uploads/2023/03/selfharm.pdf (accessed 20 May 2024).

Fisher, J. (2001) Dissociative phenomena in the everyday lives of trauma survivors. Unpublished paper. https://janinafisher.com/wp-content/uploads/2023/03/dissociation.pdf (accessed 20 May 2024).

Fisher, J. (2017) *Healing the Fragmented Selves of Trauma Survivors: Overcoming Self-Alienation*. New York: Routledge.

Flannery, R.B. Jr (1987) From victim to survivor: A stress management approach in the treatment of learned helplessness, in B. van der Kolk (ed.) *Psychological Trauma*. Arlington, VA: American Psychiatric Publishing.

Fogel, A. (2009) *The Psychophysiology of Self-Awareness: Rediscovering the Lost Art of Body Sense*. New York: Norton.

Fonagy, P. (2002) Multiple voices versus meta-cognition, in V. Sinsaon (ed.) *Attachment, Trauma and Multiplicity: Working with Dissociative Identity Disorder*. Hove: Brunner-Routledge.

Fonagy, P., Gergely, G., Jurist, E.L. and Target, M. (2004) *Affect Regulation, Mentalization and the Development of the Self*. London: Karnac.

Frank, R. (2001) *Body of Awareness: A Somatic and Developmental Approach to Psychotherapy*. Highland, NY: Gestalt Press.

Frank, R. (2008) Somatic experience and emergent dysfunction, *Studies in Gestalt Therapy: Dialogical Bridges*, 2(2): 11–41.

Friedlander, S. (1918) *Schöpferische Indiffereze*. Munich: Georg Müller.

Frosh, S. (2012) Hauntings: Psychoanalysis and ghostly transmission, *American Imago: A Psychoanalytic Journal for the Arts and Sciences*, 69(2): 241–64. https://www.researchgate.net/publication/236744398 (accessed 14 July 2023).

Fuhr, R. (2005) Dialogue respondent in G. Yontef, Gestalt therapy theory of change, in A. Woldt and S. Toman (eds) *Gestalt Therapy: History, Theory and Practice*. Thousand Oaks, CA: Sage.

Fulton, P.R., Posner, M.I., Waldenfels, B. and Yontef, G. (2009) Attention, awareness, and mindfulness: A dialog, *Studies in Gestalt Therapy*, 3(2): 13–36.

Gerhardt, S. (2004) *Why Love Matters: How Affection Shapes a Baby's Brain*. Hove: Routledge.

Gilbert, P. (2010) *The Compassionate Mind: How to Use Compassion to Develop Happiness, Self-Acceptance and Well-Being*. London: Constable.

Goldstein, J. (2007) Emergence and psychological morphogenesis, in C. Piers, J.P. Muller and J. Brent (eds) *Self-organizing Complexity in Psychological Systems*. Lanham, MD: Aronson.

Goodwin, J.M. and Attias, R. (1999a) The body speaks, in J.M. Goodwin and R. Attias (eds) *Splintered Reflections: Images of the Body in Trauma*. New York: Basic Books.

Goodwin, J.M. and Attias, R. (1999b) Conversations with the body, in J.M. Goodwin and R. Attias (eds) *Splintered Reflections: Images of the Body in Trauma*. New York: Basic Books.

Grigsby, J. and Osuch, E. (2007) Neurodynamics, state, agency, and psychological functioning, in C. Piers, J.P. Muller and J. Brent (eds) *Self-organizing Complexity in Psychological Systems*. Lanham, MD: Aronson.

Haines, S. (2019) *The Politics of Trauma: Somatics, Healing and Social Justice*. Berkeley, CA: North Atlantic Books.

Harding, C. (2009) The ghost at the feast, in D. Mann and V. Cunningham (eds) *The Past in the Present: Therapy Enactments and the Return of Trauma*. Hove: Routledge.

Harman, R.L. (1982) Gestalt theory: Working at the contact boundaries, *Gestalt Journal*, 5(1): 39–48.

Harris, E.S. (2007) Working with forgiveness in Gestalt therapy, *Gestalt Review*, 11(2): 108–19.

Harris, N. (2011) Something in the air, *British Gestalt Journal*, 20(1): 21–8.

Hebb, D.O. (1949) *The Organization of Behavior*. New York: Wiley and Sons.

Heitzler, M. (2009) Towards an integrative model of trauma therapy, in L. Hartley (ed.) *Contemporary Body Psychotherapy: The Chiron Approach*. London: Routledge.

Herbert, C. (2006) Healing from complex trauma, in J. Corrigal, H. Payne and H. Wilkinson (eds) *About a Body: Working with the Embodied Mind in Psychotherapy*. Hove: Routledge.

Herbert, C. (2012) Posttraumatic stress disorder, in C. Feltham and I. Horton (eds) *Handbook of Counselling and Psychotherapy*. London: Sage.

Herman, J.L. (1992) *Trauma and Recovery: From Domestic Abuse to Political Terror*. London: Basic Books.

Hillman, J. (1996) *The Soul's Code: In Search of Character and Calling*. London: Bantam.

Hilton, R. (2012) Bioenergetics as a relational somatic therapy, in C. Young (ed.) *About Relational Body Psychotherapy*. Galashiels: Body Psychotherapy Publications.

Hoppenwasser, K. (2008) Being in rhythm: Dissociative attunement in therapeutic process, *Journal of Trauma and Dissociation*, 9(3): 349–67.

Howell, E. (2022) Foreword, in O. Badouk Epstein (ed.) *Shame Matters: Attachment and Relational Perspectives for Psychotherapists*. Abingdon: Routledge

Hughes, D.A. (2009) *Attachment Focussed Parenting*. New York: Norton.

Hycner, R. (1993) *Between Person and Person: Toward a Dialogical Psychotherapy*. Highland, NY: Gestalt Journal Press.

Hycner, R. and Jacobs, L. (1995) *The Healing Relationship in Gestalt Therapy: A Dialogic/Self Psychology Approach*. Highland, NY: Gestalt Journal Press.

Jacobs, L. (2003) Being a repeat, repeating being, *International Gestalt Journal*, 26(1): 38–45.

Jacobs, L. (2006) That which enables – support, *British Gestalt Journal*, 15(2): 10–19.

Jacobs, L. (2012) Critiquing projection: Supporting dialogue in a post-Cartesian world, in T. Levine (ed.) *Gestalt Therapy: Advances in Theory and Practice*. London: Routledge.

Johnson, D.H. (1995) *Bone, Breath and Gesture: Practices of Embodiment*. Berkeley, CA: North Atlantic Books.

Johnson, R. (2018) Queering/queerying the body: Sensation and curiosity in disrupting body norms, in C. Caldwell and B. Leighton, *Oppression and the Body: Roots, Resistance and Resolutions*. Berkeley, CA: North Atlantic Books.

Joyce, P. and Sills, C. (2010) *Skills in Gestalt Counselling and Psychotherapy*. London: Sage.

Juhan, D. (2003) *Job's Body: A Handbook for Bodywork*. Barrytown, NY: Station Hill Press.

Keenan, B. (1993) *An Evil Cradling*. London: Vintage.

Keleman, S. (1985) *Emotional Anatomy*. Berkeley, CA: Center Press.

Kennedy, D. (2003) The phenomenal field, *British Gestalt Journal*, 12(2): 76–87.

Kennedy, D. (2005) The lived body, *British Gestalt Journal*, 14(2): 109–17.

Kepner, E. ([1980] 2000) Gestalt group progress, in B. Feder and R. Ronal (eds) *Beyond the Hot Seat: Gestalt Approaches to Group*. Montclair, NJ: Beefeeder Press.

Kepner, J. ([1987] 1999) *Body Process: A Gestalt Approach to Working with the Body in Psychotherapy*. Cambridge, MA: Gestalt Institute of Cleveland Press.

Kepner, J. (1995) *Healing Tasks: Psychotherapy with Adult Survivors of Childhood Abuse*. San Francisco, CA: Jossey-Bass.

Kepner, J. (2002) *Energy and the Nervous System in Embodied Experience*. https://www.pathwaysforhealing.com/pdfs/Phenom%20of%20NS.pdf (accessed 18 May 2024).

Kepner, J. (2003) The embodied field, *British Gestalt Journal*, 12(1): 6–14.

Kertay, L. and Reviere, S.L. (1998) Touch in context, in E.W.L. Smith, P.R. Clance and S. Imes (eds) *Touch in Psychotherapy: Theory, Research, and Practice*. New York: Guilford.

King, A. (2012) 'More than words': Moments of meaning in relational body psychotherapy, in C. Young (ed.) *About Relational Body Psychotherapy*. Galashiels: Body Psychotherapy Publications.

Kolodny, R. (2004) Why awareness works, *British Gestalt Journal*, 13(2): 92–9.

Kopp, S. (1972) *If You Meet the Buddha on the Road, Kill Him!* London: Sheldon Press.

Kornfield, J. (1993/2002) *A Path with Heart*. London: Rider.

Kurtz, R. (2007) *Body-Centered Psychotherapy: The Hakomi Method*, revised edn. Mendocino, CA: LifeRhythm.

Laub, D. and Auerhahn, N.C. (1993) Knowing and not knowing massive trauma: Forms of traumatic memory, *International Journal of Psychoanalysis*, 74(2): 287–302.

LeDoux, J. (2002) *Synaptic Self: How Our Brains Become Who We Are*. New York: Penguin.

Lee, R.G. (1996) Shame and the Gestalt model, in R.G. Lee and G. Wheeler (eds) *The Voice of Shame: Silence and Connection in Psychotherapy*. San Francisco, CA: Jossey-Bass.

Lee, R.G. and Wheeler, G. (eds) (1996) *The Voice of Shame: Silence and Connection in Psychotherapy*. San Francisco, CA: Jossey-Bass.

Levin, J. and Levine, T. (2012) Gestalt in the New Age, in T. Levine (ed.) *Gestalt Therapy: Advances in Theory and Practice*. London: Routledge.

Levine, P.A. (1997) *Waking the Tiger: Healing Trauma*. Berkeley, CA: North Atlantic Books.

Levine, P.A. (2010) *In an Unspoken Voice: How the Body Releases Trauma and Restores Goodness*. Berkeley, CA: North Atlantic Books.

Lewin, K. (1997) *Resolving Social Conflicts and Field Theory in Social Science.* Washington, DC: American Psychological Association.

Lichtenberg, P. (2012) Culture change: Conversations concerning political/religious differences, in T. Levine (ed.) *Gestalt Therapy: Advances in Theory and Practice.* London: Routledge.

Lindblom, J. (2007) *Embodied Social Cognition.* London, Springer. https://link.springer.com/book/10.1007/978-3-319-20315-7 (accessed 18 May 2023).

Linehan, M. (1993) *Skills Training Manual for Treating Borderline Personality Disorder.* New York: Guilford.

Loewenstein, R.J. and Goodwin, J. (1999) Assessment and management of somatoform symptoms in traumatized patients, in J.M. Goodwin and R. Attias (eds) *Splintered Reflections: Images of the Body in Trauma.* New York: Basic Books.

Lyons-Ruth, K., Stern, D., Sander, L. et al. (1998) Implicit relational knowing: Its role in development and psychoanalytic treatment, *Infant Mental Health Journal,* 19(3): 282–9.

Mackenzie-Mavinga, I. (2009) *Black Issues in the Therapeutic Process.* Basingstoke: Palgrave Macmillan.

Mackewn, J. (1997) *Developing Gestalt Counselling.* London: Sage.

MacLean, P.D. (1990) *The Triune Brain in Evolution.* New York: Plenum.

Macy, J. (2009) The greening of the self, in L. Buzzel and C. Chalquist, C. (eds) *Ecotherapy: Healing with Nature in Mind.* San Francisco, CA: Sierra Club Books.

Mann, D. (2010) *Gestalt Therapy: 100 Key Points and Techniques.* Hove: Routledge.

Maté, G. (2022) *The Myth of Normal: Trauma, Illness and Healing in a Toxic Culture.* London: Vermillion, Kindle edition.

McConville, M. (1995) *Adolescence: Psychotherapy and the Emergent Self.* San Francisco, CA: Jossey-Bass.

McFarlane, A.C. ([1996] 2007) Resilience, vulnerability and the course of posttraumatic reactions, in B. van der Kolk, A.C. McFarlane and L. Weisaeth (eds) *Traumatic Stress: The Effects of Overwhelming Experience on Mind, Body, and Society.* New York: Guilford.

McGarvey, D. (2022) *The Social Distance Between Us: How Remote Politics Wrecked Britain.* London: Penguin.

McGilchrist, I. (2010) *The Master and His Emissary: The Divided Brain and the Making of the Western World.* New Haven, CT: Yale University Press.

Melnick, J. and Nevis, E. (1986) Power, choice and surprise, *Gestalt Journal,* 9(2): 43–51.

Melnick, J. and Nevis, S. (1997) Gestalt diagnosis and DSM IV, *British Gestalt Journal,* 6(2): 97–106.

Merleau-Ponty, M. ([1945] 2009) *The Phenomenology of Perception.* Abingdon: Routledge.

Miller, G.D. and Baldwin, D.C. (2000) Implications of the wounded-healer paradigm for the use of self in therapy, in M. Baldwin (ed.) *The Use of Self in Therapy.* Binghampton, NY: Haworth Press.

Mitchell, J., Bogenschutz, M., Lilienstein, A. et al. (2021) MDMA-assisted therapy for severe PTSD: A randomized, double-blind, placebo-controlled phase 3 study, *Nature Medicine,* 27(6): 1025–1033. https://www.nature.com/articles/s41591-021-01336-3 (accessed 29 November 2023).

Monson, C.M. and Friedman, M.J. (2006) Back to the future of understanding trauma, in V.M. Follette and J.I. Ruzek (eds) *Cognitive Behavioral Therapies for Trauma.* New York: Guilford.

Naranjo, C. (1993) *Gestalt Therapy: The Attitude and Practice of an Atheoretical Experimentalism.* Carmarthen: Crown House Publishing.

Nevis, E. (2001) Choices for the future, *Gestalt Review,* 5(3): 175–83.

Nhat Hanh, T. (2012) *Fear: Essential Wisdom for Getting Through the Storm.* London: Random House.

Nijenhuis, E. (2004) *Somatoform Dissociation: Phenomena, Measurement and Theoretical Issues.* New York: Norton.

Oaklander, V. (2000) Gestalt work with children: Working with anger and introjects, in E. Nevis (ed.) *Gestalt Therapy: Perspectives and Applications.* Cambridge, MA: Gestalt Press.

Office for Health Improvement and Disparities (2022) Guidance: Working Definition of Trauma Informed Care. https://www.gov.uk/government/publications/working-definition-of-trauma-informed-practice/working-definition-of-trauma-informed-practice (accessed 5 June 2024).

Ogden, P., Minton, K. and Pain, C. (2006) *Trauma and the Body: A Sensorimotor Approach to Psychotherapy.* New York: Norton.

Olsen, A. (2002) *Body and Earth.* Lebanon, NH: Middlebury College Press.

O'Neill, B. (2012) Gestalt family therapy: A field perspective, in T. Levine (ed.) *Gestalt Therapy: Advances in Theory and Practice.* London: Routledge.

Orange, D. (1995) *Emotional Understanding: Studies in Psychoanalytic Epistemology.* New York: Guilford.

Orange, D. (2010) *Thinking for Clinicians: Philosophical Resources for Contemporary Psychoanalysis and the Humanistic Psychotherapies.* New York: Routledge.

Panksepp, J. (1998) *Affective Neuroscience: The Foundations of Human and Animal Emotions.* New York: Oxford University Press.

Parlett. M. (1991) Reflections on field theory, *British Gestalt Journal*, 1(2): 68–91.

Parlett, M. (2005) Contemporary Gestalt therapy: Field theory, in A. Woldt and S. Toman (eds) *Gestalt Therapy: History, Theory and Practice.* Thousand Oaks, CA: Sage.

Parlett, M. (2011) Fields in practice: Letter to the editor, *British Gestalt Journal*, 20(2): 53–5.

Pennebaker, J.W. (1997) Writing about emotional experiences as a therapeutic process, *Psychological Science*, 8(3): 162–6.

Pennebaker, J.W. (2000) Psychological factors influencing the reporting of physical symptoms, in A.A. Stone, J.S. Turkkan, C.A. Bachrach et al. (eds) *The Science of Self Report.* Mahwah, NJ: Lawrence Erlbaum.

Perlman, L.A. and Saakvitne, K. (1995) *Trauma and the Therapist: Countertransference and Vicarious Trauma in Psychotherapy with Incest Survivors.* New York: Norton.

Perls, F. ([1947] 1992) *Ego, Hunger and Aggression: A Revision of Freud's Theory and Method.* Highland, NY: Gestalt Journal Press.

Perls, F. (1969) *Gestalt Therapy Verbatim.* Lafayette, CA: Real People Press.

Perls, L. (1992) *Living at the Boundary.* Goldsboro, ME: Gestalt Journal Press.

Perls, F., Hefferline, R. and Goodman, P. ([1951] 1998) *Gestalt Therapy: Excitement and Growth in the Human Personality.* London: Souvenir Press.

Perry, B. and Szalavitz, M. (2006) *The Boy Who Was Raised as a Dog: And Other Stories from a Child Psychiatrist's Notebook.* New York: Basic Books.

Perry, B. and Winfrey, O. (2021) *What Happened to You?: Conversations on Trauma, Resilience and Healing.* London: Bluebird.

Philippson, P. (2001) *Self in Relation.* Highland, NY: Gestalt Journal Press.

Philippson, P. (2005) Paradox: Strategic, naive and Gestalt, *International Gestalt Journal*, 28(2): 9–17.

Philippson, P. (2009) *The Emergent Self: An Existential-Gestalt Approach.* London: Karnac.

Philippson, P. (2012) Mind and matter: The implications of neuroscience research for Gestalt psychotherapy, in T. Levine (ed.) *Gestalt Therapy: Advances in Theory and Practice.* London: Routledge.

Piers, C. (2007) The language of complexity theory, in C. Piers, J.P. Muller and J. Brent (eds) *Self-organizing Complexity in Psychological Systems*. Lanham, MD: Aronson.

Polster, E. (1991) Tight therapeutic sequences, *British Gestalt Journal*, 1(2): 63–8.

Polster, E. (1993) *A Population of Selves: A Therapeutic Exploration of Personal Diversity*. San Francisco, CA: Jossey-Bass.

Polster, E. (2012) Flexibility in theory formation: Point and counterpoint, in T. Levine (ed.) *Gestalt Therapy: Advances in Theory and Practice*. London: Routledge.

Polster, E. and Polster, M. (1973) *Gestalt Therapy Integrated: Contours of Theory and Practice*. New York: Vintage.

Porges, S.W. (2009) Reciprocal influences between body and brain, in D. Fosha, D.J. Siegel and M. Solomon (eds) *The Healing Power of Emotion: Affective Neuroscience, Development and Clinical Practice*. New York: Norton.

Richardson, S. (2008) The hungry self, in S. Benamer and K. White (eds) *Trauma and Attachment*. London: Karnac.

Riggs, D.S., Cahill, S.P. and Foa, E.B. (2006) Prolonged exposure treatment of posttraumatic stress disorder, in V.M. Follette and J.I. Ruzek (eds) *Cognitive Behavioral Therapies for Trauma*. New York: Guilford.

Romanyshyn, R. (2007) *The Wounded Researcher: Research with Soul in Mind*. New Orleans, LA: Spring Journal Inc.

Ross, C. (1997) *Dissociative Identity Disorder: Diagnosis, Clinical Features and Treatment of Multiple Personality*. New York: Wiley.

Rothschild, B. (2000) *The Body Remembers: The Psychophysiology of Trauma and Trauma Treatment*. New York: Norton.

Rotter, J.B. (1954) *Social Learning and Clinical Psychology*. New York: Prentice Hall.

Ruzany, G. (2020) Signature movement, in M. Clemmens (ed.) *Embodied Relational Gestalt: Theories and Applications*. Abingdon: Routledge, Taylor and Francis.

Sachs, A. (2013) Intergenerational transmission of massive trauma, in J. Yellin and O. Badouk Epstein (eds) *Terror Without and Within: Attachment and Disintegration – Clinical Work on the Edge*. London: Karnac Books.

Sander, L. (2000) 'I sense that you sense that I sense …': Sander's recognition process and the specificity of relational moves in the psychotherapeutic setting, *Infant Mental Health Journal*, 21(1–2): 5–20.

Sapriel, L. (2012) Creating an embodied, authentic self: Integrating mindfulness with psychotherapy when working with trauma, in T. Levine (ed.) *Gestalt Therapy: Advances in Theory and Practice*. London: Routledge.

Scarry, E. (1985) *The Body in Pain*. New York: Oxford University Press.

Scheper-Hughes, N. and Bourgois, P. (eds) (2004) *Violence in War and Peace: An Anthology*. Malden, MA: Blackwell.

Schiable, M. (2009) Biodynamic massage as a body psychotherapy and as a tool in body psychotherapy, in L. Hartley (ed.) *Contemporary Body Psychotherapy: The Chiron Approach*. London: Routledge.

Schore, A. (2003a) *Affect Dysregulation and Disorders of the Self*. New York: Norton.

Schore, A. (2003b) *Affect Regulation and the Repair of the Self*. New York: Norton.

Schore, A. (2003c) Early relational trauma, disorganized attachment and the development of a predisposition to violence, in M. Solomon and D.J. Siegel (eds) *Healing Trauma: Attachment, Mind, Body and Brain*. New York: Norton.

Schultz-Venrath, U. (2022) Mentalizing shame, shamelessness and frendscham (shame by proxy) in groups, in O. Badouk Epstein (ed.) *Shame Matters: Attachment and Relational Perspectives for Psychotherapists*. Abingdon: Routledge.

Schwartz, R. (1995) *Internal Family Systems Therapy*. New York: Guilford.

Shapiro, F. (1995) *Eye Movement Desensitization and Reprocessing*. New York: Guilford.

Sheldrake, M. (2021) Can we grow the concept of ourselves?, in G. van Horn, R. Wall Kimmerer and J. Hausdoeffer (eds) *Kinship: Belonging in a World of Relations*, vol. 3: *Partners*. Libertyville, IL: Center for Humans and Nature Press.

Shields, D., Fuller, A., Resnicoff, M., Butcher, H.K. and Frisch, N. (2016) Human energy field: A concept analysis, *Journal of Holistic Nursing*, 35(4): 352–68.

Shub, N. (2000) Gestalt therapy over time: Integrating difficulty and diagnosis, in E. Nevis (ed.) *Gestalt Therapy: Perspectives and Applications*. New York: Gestalt Institute of Cleveland and Gardner Press Inc.

Siegel, D.J. (1999) *The Developing Mind: How Relationships and the Brain Interact to Shape Who We Are*. New York: Guilford.

Siegel, D.J. (2003) An interpersonal neurobiology of psychotherapy, in M. Solomon and D.J. Siegel (eds) *Healing Trauma*. New York: Norton.

Siegel, D.J. (2007) *The Mindful Brain: Reflection and Attunement in the Cultivation of Well-Being*. New York: Norton.

Siegel, D.J. (2009) Emotion as integration, in D. Fosha, D.J. Siegel and M.F. Solomon (eds) *The Healing Power of Emotion: Affective Neuroscience, Development and Clinical Practice*. New York: Norton.

Siegel, D.J. (2010) *The Mindful Therapist: A Clinician's Guide to Mindsight and Neural Integration*. New York: Norton.

Siegel, D.J. (2012) *Pocket Guide To Interpersonal Neurobiology*. New York: Norton.

Sills, F. (2011) *Foundations in Craniosacral Biodynamics: The Breath of Life and Fundamental Skills*. Berkeley, CA: North Atlantic Books.

Sinason, V. (2008) How do we help ourselves?, in S. Benamer and K. White (eds) *Trauma and Attachment*. London: Karnac.

Smith, E.W.L. (1998) A taxonomy and ethics of touch in psychotherapy, in E.W.L. Smith, P.R. Clance and S. Imes (eds) *Touch in Psychotherapy: Theory, Research and Practice*. New York: Guilford.

Snyder, C.R., Parenteau, S.C., Shorey, H.S., Kahle, K.E. and Berg, C. (2002) Hope as the underlying process in the psychotherapeutic change process, *International Gestalt Journal*, 25(2): 11–19.

Soloman, Z., Laror, N. and McFarlane, A.C. ([1996] 2007) Acute posttraumatic reactions in soldiers and civilians, in B. van der Kolk, A.C. McFarlane and L. Weisaeth (eds) *Traumatic Stress: The Effects of Overwhelming Experience on Mind, Body, and Society*. New York: Guilford.

Soth, M. (2006) How the 'wound' enters the room and the relationship, *Therapy Today*, December.

Soth, M. and Eichhorn, N. (2012) The relational turn, in C. Young (ed.) *About Relational Body Psychotherapy*. Galashiels: Body Psychotherapy Publications.

Spagnuolo Lobb, M. (2009) The therapeutic relationship in Gestalt therapy, in R. Hycner and L. Jacobs (eds) *Relational Approaches in Gestalt Therapy*. Santa Cruz, CA: Gestalt Press.

Spinelli, E. ([1989] 1998) *The Interpreted World: An Introduction to Phenomenological Psychology*. London: Sage.

Staemmler, F.-M. (2012) *Empathy in Psychotherapy: How Therapists and Clients Understand Each Other*. New York: Springer Publications.

Stauffer, K.A. (2010) *Anatomy and Physiology for Psychotherapists: Connecting Body and Soul*. New York: Norton.

Staunton, T. (2002) Sexuality and body psychotherapy, in T. Staunton (ed.) *Body Psychotherapy*. Hove: Brunner-Routledge.

Staunton, T. (2022) Holding the body in mind in times of transition, in S. Wright (ed.) *The Change Process in Psychotherapy in Troubling Times*. Abingdon: Routledge.

Stern, D. (1998) *The Interpersonal World of the Infant: A View From Psychoanalysis and Developmental Psychotherapy*. London: Karnac.

Stern, D. (2004) *The Present Moment in Psychotherapy and Everyday Life*. New York: Norton.

Stolorow, R.D. (2007) *Trauma and Human Existence: Autobiographical, Psychoanalytic and Philosophical Reflections*. New York: Analytic Press.

Stolorow, R.D., Brandchaft, B. and Atwood, G.E. (1987) *Psychoanalytic Treatment: An Intersubjective Approach*. Hillsdale, NJ: Analytic Press.

Stratford, C. and Braillier, K. (1979) Gestalt therapy with profoundly disturbed persons, *Gestalt Journal*, 2(1): 90–103.

Sweeney, E., Filson, B., Kennedy, A., Collinson, L. and Goddard, S. (2018) A paradigm shift: Relationships in trauma-informed mental health services, *BJPsych Advances*, 24(5): 319–33. https://www.cambridge.org/core/journals/bjpsych-advances/article/paradigm-shift-relationships-in-traumainformed-mental-health-services/B364B885715D321AF76C932F6B9D7BD0 (accessed 10 September 2023).

Taussig, M. (2004) Terror as usual: Walter Benjamin's theory of history as a state of siege, in N. Scheper-Hughes and P. Bourgois (eds) *Violence in War and Peace*. Malden, MA: Blackwell.

Taylor, M. (2013) On safe ground: Using sensorimotor approaches in trauma work, *British Gestalt Journal*, 22(2): 5–13.

Taylor, M. (2021) *Deepening Trauma Practice: A Gestalt Approach to Ecology and Ethics*. London: Open University Press.

Taylor, M. (2023) The ecological self: Narratives for changing times, *British Gestalt Journal*, 32(1): 39–48.

Terr, L. (1990) *Too Scared to Cry: How Trauma Affects Children . . . and Ultimately Us All*. New York: Basic Books.

Thomas, M. (2019) Shot hen harrier found on North Yorkshire grouse moor, RSPB website. https://community.rspb.org.uk/ourwork/b/investigations/posts/shot-hen-harrier-found-on-north-yorkshire-grouse-moor (accessed 29 November 2023).

Totton, N. and Priestman, A. (2012) Embodiment and relationship: Two halves of one whole, in C. Young (ed.) *About Relational Body Psychotherapy*. Galashiels: Body Psychotherapy Publications.

Tronick, E. (1998) Dyadically expanded states of consciousness and the process of therapeutic change, *Infant Mental Health Journal*, 19(3): 290–9.

Turner, S.W., McFarlane, A.C. and van der Kolk, B. ([1996] 2007) The therapeutic environment and new explorations in the treatment of posttraumatic stress disorder, in B. van der Kolk, A.C. McFarlane and L. Weisaeth (eds) *Traumatic Stress: The Effects of Overwhelming Experience on Mind, Body, and Society*. New York: Guilford.

Van der Hart, O., Nijenhuis, E. and Steele, K. (2006) *The Haunted Self: Structural Dissociation and the Treatment of Chronic Traumatization*. New York: Norton.

Van der Kolk, B. (1994) The body keeps the score: Memory and the emerging psychobiology of posttraumatic stress, *Harvard Review of Psychiatry*, 1(5): 253–65.

Van der Kolk, B. ([1996] 2007) The complexity of adaptation to trauma, in B. van der Kolk, A.C. McFarlane and L. Weisaeth (eds) *Traumatic Stress: The Effects of Overwhelming Experience on Mind, Body, and Society*. New York: Guilford.

Van der Kolk, B. (2000) Posttraumatic stress disorder and the nature of trauma, *Dialogues in Clinical Neuroscience*, 2(1): 7–22.

Van der Kolk, B. (2003) Posttraumatic stress disorder and the nature of trauma, in M. Solomon and D.J. Siegel (eds) *Healing Trauma: Attachment, Mind, Body and Brain*, 2nd edn. New York: Norton.

Van der Kolk, B. (2014) *The Body Keeps the Score: Mind, Brain and Body in the Transformation of Trauma*. London: Penguin.

Van der Kolk, B. and Greenberg, M.S. (1987) The psychobiology of the trauma response, in B. van der Kolk (ed.) *Psychological Trauma*. Arlington, VA: American Psychiatric Publishing.

Van der Kolk, B. and McFarlane, A.C. ([1996] 2007) The black hole of trauma, in B. van der Kolk, A.C. McFarlane and L. Weisaeth (eds) *Traumatic Stress: The Effects of Overwhelming Experience on Mind, Body, and Society*. New York: Guilford.

Van der Kolk, B., McFarlane, A.C. and van der Hart, O. ([1996] 2007a) A general approach to treatment of posttraumatic stress disorder, in B. van der Kolk, A.C. McFarlane and L. Weisaeth (eds) *Traumatic Stress: The Effects of Overwhelming Experience on Mind, Body, and Society*. New York: Guilford.

Van der Kolk, B., van der Hart, O. and Burbridge, J. (1995) *Approaches to the Treatment of PTSD*. http://www.trauma-pages.com/a/vanderk.php (accessed 15 September 2012).

Van der Kolk, B., van der Hart, O. and Marmar, C.R. ([1996] 2007b) Dissociation and information processing in posttraumatic stress disorder, in B. van der Kolk, A.C. McFarlane and L. Weisaeth (eds) *Traumatic Stress: The Effects of Overwhelming Experience on Mind, Body, and Society*. New York: Guilford.

Van der Kolk, B., Weisaeth, L. and van der Hart, O. ([1996] 2007c) History of trauma in psychiatry, in B. van der Kolk, A.C. McFarlane and L. Weisaeth (eds) *Traumatic Stress: The Effects of Overwhelming Experience on Mind, Body, and Society*. New York: Guilford.

Watters, E. (2010) *Crazy Like Us: The Globalization of the Western Mind*. London: Constable and Robinson.

Wheeler, G. ([1991] 1998) *Gestalt Reconsidered: A New Approach to Contact and Resistance*. Cambridge, MA: GIC Press.

Wheeler, G. (1996) Shame, guilt and co-dependency, in G. Wheeler and R. Lee (eds) *The Voice of Shame: Silence and Connection in Psychotherapy*. San Francisco, CA: Jossey-Bass.

Wheeler, G. (2000) *Beyond Individualism: Toward a New Understanding of Self, Relationship, and Experience*. Cambridge, MA: GIC Press.

Wilkinson, M. (2010) *Changing Minds in Therapy: Emotion, Attachment, Trauma and Neurobiology*. New York: Norton.

Woldt, A.L. and Toman, S.M. (eds) (2005) *Gestalt Therapy: History, Theory, and Practice*. Thousand Oaks, CA: Sage.

World Health Organization (WHO) (2022) *International Classification of Diseases (ICD 11)*, World Health Organization website. https://www.who.int/standards/classifications/classification-of-diseases (accessed 13 December 2023).

Yontef, G. (1993) *Awareness, Dialogue and Process: Essays on Gestalt Theory*. Highland, NY: Gestalt Journal Press.

Yontef, G. (1996) Shame and guilt in Gestalt therapy, in R.G. Lee and G. Wheeler (eds) *The Voice of Shame: Silence and Connection in Psychotherapy*. San Francisco, CA: Jossey-Bass.

Yontef, G. (2005) Gestalt therapy theory of change, in A. Woldt and S. Toman (eds) *Gestalt Therapy: History, Theory and Practice*. Thousand Oaks, CA: Sage.

Yunkaporta, T. (2020) *Sand Talk: How Indigenous Thinking Can Save the World*. New York: HarperOne.

Zinker, J. (1977) *Creative Process in Gestalt Therapy*. New York: Random House.

Index

Abandonment 140–1
Abuse *see* trauma
Abuser internalized *see* shame
ACES *see* trauma
Acceptance 43, 147, 149, 152, 157–8
Acts of triumph 214
Adjustment, creative *see* creative
    adjustments
Adverse Childhood Experiences (ACES)
    see trauma
Affective neuroscience *see* neuroscience
Agency 45, 116, 123–5,
Aggress, to 82, 219
Alienation xv, 121, 129, 132, 140
Alexithymia *see* language
Alleyne, Aileen 138, 151
Amygdala *see* brain
Anger 69, 126, 158–9, 173
Anxiety 5, 52, 97, 99, 107
Arousal 58–66, 68, 155, 166–7, 198, 203
    Autonomic Nervous System (ANS)
        60–1, 66–7
    energy 25–6, 59, 117–20, 193
    excitement 25, 59, 99, 107, 203
    hyper–arousal 18, 58, 71, 101
    hypo–arousal 71, 64–5, 134, 209
    moderation of 61, 120
    optimal 63, 79, 84, 198, 209
    parasympathetic 61, 66–7, 71, 116, 118
    sympathetic 61–2, 66–7, 71, 116, 118
    tolerance, window of 63 *see also*
        window of tolerance
Attachment 62, 107–8, 137, 149–50,
    206–8, 216
    cry 105
    defence against 155
    disorganized 206–8
    earned 208, 215
    secure 6, 23, 206–7
    shame of 144
    styles 150
    traumatic 141, 152
Attention 24, 29, 35–6, 47, 82
    concentration 85–6
    focus of 63, 78, 69, 184–5, 101, 189

shift in 62, 81, 102, 111, 158
Autonomic Nervous System (ANS)
    see arousal
Autonomy *see* agency
Avoidance 98
Awareness 13–4, 26–7, 78–87, 130,
    137–8, 141–3
    of body 52
    concentration 85–6
    continuum 79, 85, 171, 219
    of current experience 78–9, 84
    directed 82, 196
    dual *see also* time, 78, 110, 138, 175
    zones of 77–8, 82
Ayahuasca *see* pscychedelics

Beisser, Arnold 43–4, 50, 165, 169
Belonging, sense of 8, 110, 132, 140,
    147–8, 206
Betrayal *see* shame
Binaries *see* polarities
Blame *see also* shame 128, 152, 158,
    173, 184
    self–blame 116, 121, 153
    of victim 151
Body
    awareness of 52–3, 70
    dissociated 131–2, 139, 142
    embodiment 7, 16–7, 66, 83, 120
    as enemy 99, 120, 152, 154
    helpless 117–8
    history held in 133, 200, 202, 213
    impulse 71, 188, 214
    memory 78, 133, 214
    process 66, 142, 182, 200
    resonance 175, 196
    shameful 153
Body structure
    collapsed 71, 118–9, 214
    rigid 118, 192
Boston Change Process Study Group
    (BCPSG) 10, 45–6, 51, 196
Boundary
    contact boundary *see also* contact 3,
        12, 100, 116, 193–4

functions 99, 130
Bracketing, epoché *see* phenomenology
Brain 7–10, 47, 49–50, 86–7
  amygdala xix, 49, 103, 104
  brainstem 48, 61–2
  corpus callosum 49–50
  cortex 48–9, 60, 86, 103
  fear circuitry 10, 48, 103
  hemisphere, left, right 12, 134, 155, 201
  hippocampus 49, 103, 104, 134
  limbic system 48–9, 62, 86, 181, 199
  neural pathway 35, 47, 52, 103
  relational 50, 155, 177, 195, 198
  thalamus 49, 134
  triune 47, 49, 62
Breath, breathing 62, 67, 110–1, 119,
  125, 189
Bromberg, Phillip 16, 140, 142–3, 146–51,
  208
Brownall, Phillip 14, 16, 59, 60, 86

Calibration 65, 82
Capacity, therapeutic xvi, 1, 173, 175,
  186–7, 199
Capitalism xviii, 65
Chaos 1, 32–4, 64, 66, 153, 192
Change
  Integrated Model of 54, 80, 83–4, 165–6
  moments of 45
  Paradoxical Theory of 42
  relational aspects of 45, 169–70, 166
  therapist as agent of 45, 55, 167
Choice 1, 34–5, 41, 116, 137, 158
  field of 13, 16, 33, 50, 123
Climate 31, 32, 76, 108, 139, 176
Co–creation 152, 174
Coercion 170, 204
Cognitive Behavioural Therapy 4
Coherence 22–3, 52, 132, 135, 200–1, 216
Collapse, *see* defences
Colonialism 139, 176
Commodification xx–xxi
Compartmentalization *see* fragmentation
Compassion 67, 86, 116, 158–9
Complexity 31–2, 33, 37, 41, 66
  complex systems 59
Complex trauma *see* trauma
Concentration *see* awareness
Connection *see also* disconnection xix,
  10–11, 86, 110, 140–1, 198–9
Connectome *see* neuroimaging

Contact (Gestalt theory)
  boundary 3, 12, 100, 110, 116, 193–4
  cycle *see* cycle of experience
  functions 30, 62, 130, 198, 220, 222
  modifications of 66, 100, 130, 219, 220,
    222
Containment 34–5, 80, 118, 174, 189
Context xvi–xx, 11, 27–8, 77, 93, 152
Continuity 79, 132, 176, 201, 208
  of self 1–3, 110, 115, 148
  of time 26, 131
Control 44, 76, 148, 150–1, 156
  locus of control 121–3, 148
  loss of sense of 115
  restoring sense of 22, 35–6,
  voluntary 8, 13, 50, 116, 119
Corpus callosum *see* brain
Cortex *see* brain
Cortisol *see* neurochemicals
Co–transference *see* transference
Cozolino, Louis 13, 101, 103, 134, 155
Creative adjustment 28, 116, 132, 135,
  146, 220
Creative indifference 169–70, 220
Creativity 28, 43, 65, 110, 220
Crisis 59, 122, 129, 211
Culture 26–7, 65, 94, 107, 176, 206
Cycle of experience 25, 46, 59, 84, 116,
  220

Damasio, Antonio 134, 181
Danger *see* fear
Defences 105, 147
  see also creative adjustments
  aborted 71, 214
  attach 105
  collapse 62, 48
  fight, flight 62, 105
  freeze 62
  immobilized, passive 105, 115, 121,
    141, 148, 192
  mobilized, active 48, 105, 116, 192, 214
  submit 136, 153
  survival instinct 48, 105, 116, 192, 214
Delisle, Giles 16, 69, 76–7, 174
Denial 132
  cultural 42, 104, 132, 156
  self–denial 45, 120, 121, 147, 151
Depersonalization *see* dissociation
Derealization *see* dissociation
Developmental trauma *see* trauma

Diagnosis xviii, 80
Dialectical Behavioural Therapy 4
Dialogue (Gestalt theory)
 see Gestalt
 inner 131
Differentiation 13, 77–8, 116, 201
Disconnection see also connection 107,
 137, 147, 154, 176, 199
Disorder xviii, 3, 41, 207
Dissociation 129–31, 187
 co–consciousness 137
 collective 139
 depersonalization 131
 derealization 131
 function of 132
 healthy everyday 132
 neurobiology of 9, 71, 132, 134
 part selves and 134
 relational 140–1, 177, 212
 somatoform 133, 139
 spirit possession 138
 Structural Dissociation Model 135
 Unattached Burdens 138
Distance 35, 43, 80, 131, 140–1
Domestic violence see trauma
Dorsal vagal see Poly Vagal Theory

Eating, distressed 3, 36, 133
Egotism 80, 220
Embodiment 7, 14, 16–7, 83, 182, 186
Emergence 26, 37, 102, 214
Empathy 141, 181
Enactment see repetition
Endorphins see neurochemicals
Energy see arousal
 fields 190, 193, 204
Environment 23, 47–8, 58–9, 93, 133, 165
Ethics 202
Excitement see arousal
Executive function 60
Experiments 10, 140, 200, 203
 embodied 67, 82, 87, 117, 180, 194
 reflective 29, 109, 188, 202, 146, 172
Expert position xviii, 8, 45, 165–6, 170, 173
Explicit memory see memory
Exposure techniques 4, 6, 68, 104, 135,
 200
External locus of control
 see locus of control
Eye Movement Desensitization and
 Reprocessing (EMDR) 5, 35, 214

Failure, sense of see shame
Family xviii, 110, 132, 156, 206
Fanen, Lisa xviii, 64, 93–5, 107, 206
Fear 97
 circuits 103
 conditioning 103
 phobias 98
 threat, danger 27, 30–2, 66–7, 98–9,
  101–5, 116–8
 triggers 98–9, 103, 153
 unintegrated 101
Field (Gestalt theory)
 contemporaneous 27, 31, 45, 104,
  130, 221
 current 77
 historical 27, 140, 222
 legal 1, 156
 political 1, 94, 108, 139
 relational 13, 22, 122–4, 141, 177, 215
 shared mindful 85, 201, 204, 212
 situation 8, 11, 26, 105, 197–8
 social, societal 1, 94–5, 101, 115, 139
Fight response see defences
Flight response see defences
Figure (Gestalt theory) 24
 formation 25–8, 59–60, 85, 116, 221
 see also ground
 trauma 34–5
Fisher, Janina 70, 143, 154, 167
Fixed gestalt see Gestalt
Flashbacks see intrusions
Flexibility 1, 47, 104, 166
Flow 36, 62, 79, 95, 125, 193
Fluids, fluidity 13, 33, 51, 116, 130–1, 143
Fogel, Alan 52, 61, 181, 185, 197–8
Forgiveness 158
Fragmentation x viii, 2, 95, 132, 134–5,
 137
 splitting xvi, 31, 130, 137
Freeze see defences

Gender xviii, 176
Generalization xviii, 9, 77, 111, 120
Genocide139
Gestalt
 dialogue 31, 124, 166, 193, 203, 220
 empty chair technique 13
 experimentation 5, 35, 220
 field theory see also field 11, 221
 fixed 24, 47, 116, 151, 201, 221,
 meaning 23

organismic self–regulation *see also*
   regulation 29–30, 32, 59, 196, 222,
phenomenology *see also*
   phenomenology 11, 79–81, 83–4, 94,
   203, 222
   relational 61, 171
   theory 12, 25, 59, 80, 157
   values 14, 42, 137
Grading 36, 65
Ground (Gestalt theory) *see also* figure
   24
   restructuring 27, 33, 35, 37
   structure of 21, 26, 29, 34
Grounding 37, 69, 85, 110, 166, 189
Growth xx–xxi, 9, 22, 42, 47, 50–1
Guilt *see also* shame 149, 155

Hakomi method 5
Hebb's axiom 47, 103
Healing Tasks Model 14–5, 41, 54–5, 79,
   83, 157
   see also Kepner
   safety 15
   self–functions 15, 54, 83,
   support 15, 83
   undoing, redoing and mourning 15, 55,
   83, 157, 211, 213
Heart rate variability 67
Helplessness 115–23, 147–8, 170,
   see also defences
   collapse 48, 62, 78, 105, 115, 123,
   139
   freeze 28, 62, 66, 78, 148
Hemisphere *see* brain
Here–and–now *see* time
Herman, Judith Lewis 4, 106, 121, 125,
   129, 149
Hippocampus *see* brain
Holism 11, 159
Hope xxi, 30, 45, 198, 208
   hopelessness 45, 148
   placebo effect and 45
Horizontalism 80, 169
Humiliation *see* shame
Husserl, Edmund 79
Hyperarousal
   see arousal
Hypoarousal
   see arousal
Hypervigilance
   see trauma

Identity xv, 30, 130–1, 151, 216
Identification xviii, xix, 121
Ideology xvii
Immobilization *see* defence
Impasse 50, 117, 185
Implicit memory
   see memory
Impulse 71, 77, 118–20, 125
Indigenous, traditional, 93
   thinking 77, 93
   world view 77
Individualism, individualistic 8, 26, 109,
   125
Insomnia 28
Integration xvi–xvii, 2, 32–3, 523, 143,
   215
Integrated Model of Change *see* change
Internal Family Systems 137–8
Internal locus of control
   see control
Interoception 67, 181
Intersubjectivity 181, 190, 210
Intimacy 23, 99, 173, 190, 210
Intrusion 41, 140, 147, 192, 209
   flashbacks 4–5, 27, 78, 97, 185
   intrusive thoughts 121
   nightmares 27, 40, 44, 97, 184

Jacobs, Lynne 35, 61, 78, 123, 166, 210
Janet, Pierre 5, 105
Johnson, Don Hanlon 7, 67
Justice, injustice 115, 148
   see also social justice

Kepner, James 14–5, 27, 30, 52
   see also Healing Tasks Model
   and arousal 63, 68, 213
   and body adaptation 81, 117
   and embodiment 117, 124, 182, 199
   and energy 81, 130, 194
   and shame 148, 155
   and touch 203
Ketamine *see* psychedelics

Language xviii, 80, 122, 124, 192–3,
   199–20
Levine, Peter 4, 185
Limbic brain
   see Triune brain
Locus of control
   see control

McGarvey, Darren 104, 122
Maté, Gabor xix, xx, 7, 81, 133
MDMA
  see psychedelics
Medical model xvi, 8, 94
Meditation
  see mindfulness
Memory 13, 68, 98, 130, 167
  explicit 86
  implicit 46, 53, 86, 214
  state dependent 99
  traumatic 4, 36, 40, 74–5, 131, 214
  unprocessed 76
Memory states
  affective 46
Mentalization 22, 177, 210
Merleau–Ponty, Maurice 81
Mind 7, 50, 138,
Mindfulness 84–7, 190
  and the brain 86–7
  compassion 86
  concentration *see* awareness
  directed awareness as 190
  limitations 85
  and regulation 85–6
  shared mindful field 85, 201, 204, 212
  training
Minority, minorities xviii, xix, 151, 153,
  176
Mirror neurons 181–2, 195, 201,
Misattunement 16, 146, 149, 171, 202
Mobilization
  see defences
Modelling 174–5
Modification of contact 130, 222
Modulation *see* grading
Moral injury 183
Movement 22, 25, 51, 71–2, 117, 119–20
  rhythmic 69, 125
Muscle
  contraction 72, 119, 193
  smooth 61
  tension 71, 119
  tone 6, 69, 71, 118–9, 167, 198

Narrative 37, 97, 124, 152, 193, 215
Neglect
  see trauma
Nervous system
  see arousal
Neural pathways

see neuron
Neurobiology
  see neuroscience
Neuroception 62
Neurochemicals
  adrenaline 6
  analgesic effects of 71, 133–4
  cortisol 6, 104
  endorphins 134, 155
  neurotransmitter 9, 104
  opiates 106, 120, 133
  oxytocin 63, 203
  stress 58
  vasopressin 203
Neurodiversity xviii, xix, 130
Neuroimaging 9, 86
  Connectome 9, 48
  fMRI scanning 9–10
Neuron 9, 47, 61
  neuronal growth 47
  neuro–imaging 9 neural networks 13,
    134, 181, 199
  neural plasticity 47, 103
Neuroscience 18, 46–50, 102, 134
  affective 10
  biology, neuro 5, 16, 102, 165
  limitations of 8
  principles of 8
Neurotransmitter
  see neurochemicals

Objectification 120, 166
Ogden, Pat 5, 49, 63, 105
Open communication (Gestalt theory) 9,
  208, 210, 220
Oppression 94, 98, 109, 115, 120–1, 156
Orange, Donna 83, 147, 154, 185, 199
Organism 29, 59–60, 123
Organism/environment system 46, 59, 93,
  140
Organismic self–regulation *see*
  regulation
Organization 23, 60
  of experience 24, 79
  re–organization 30
  self–organization 23, 29, 60
Orientation
  to danger 23, 171–2
  orienting response 102
Overwhelm 1, 64, 66, 99, 123
Oxytocin *see* neurochemicals

Pacing *see* grading, calibration
Pain of contrast 204
Panic *see* fear
Panksepp, Jaak 103, 155
Paradoxical Theory of Change 42–4
  see also change
  self–functions associated with 43
Parlett, Malcolm 11, 35, 132
Parts *see* dissociation
Pathology 135
Pathologization xviii, 97, 196, 207
Perception 24, 27–8, 62, 101, 111
Perls, Fritz
  influence of 5, 42
  life and interests of 23, 44, 84–5
  theories of 12–3, 28, 34, 66, 170
Perspective 16, 85, 93–4, 122, 150
Phenomenology 11, 79–81, 83–4, 94, 222
  bracketing, epoché 80
  description 68, 80–1, 198, 200
  horizontalism 80
  observation 53, 68, 80, 88, 130
  therapist's 203, 212
  tracking 5, 53, 81, 130, 143, 214
Philippson, Peter 50–1, 54–5, 134–5
Phobias *see also* fear 98
  of feeling 99
  of therapy 211
Physiology 32, 59
Polarities *see also* fragmentation
Polyvagal Theory 61–3
  dorsal vagal system 62
  social engagement system 61–2, 105
  vagal brake 61–2, 67,
  ventral vagal system 62, 64, 66, 109
Porges, Stephen 61–2, 101
Post Traumatic Stress (PTS) xx, 3, 42,
    58, 97
  disorder xviii, 207
Post traumatic growth xx
Poverty xviii
Power 17, 42, 95, 107
  personal 17, 107, 121–3
  systems xv, 42, 95, 120–1, 124
  therapist xviii, 17, 165–6, 170
Presence 11, 140–2, 165, 174, 185
Present moment *see also* time 13, 79, 82,
    84, 86, 172
Privilege 94, 109, 176
Processing 13, 46, 52–3, 78, 198, 214
Psychedelics xix–xx

Psychoeducation 159
Psylocibin *see* psychedelics

Race xviii, 138–9
Rape *see* trauma
Reactivity 46, 108
Reductionism xvi, xvii, 10
Reflection 46, 151, 166, 214
Refugees, climate, 108
Regulation 59, 146
  dyadic 85, 111, 149, 166
  dysregulation 85, 155, 167, 208–10
  mutual 196, 198, 209
  organismic self–regulation 29–30, 32,
    59, 196, 222
  regulatory processes 68–9
Relationship, relational
  attitude 42, 55
  brain 50
  field 13, 122, 124, 141, 149, 177
  history 45, 166, 171, 208
  rupture and repair 16, 146, 208–10
  style 29, 147, 150
  therapeutic 13, 158, 182–3, 211
  trust xvii, 7, 43, 108, 182, 199
  turn 13
Repetition of trauma
  compulsion 106
  enactment 138, 207
  reliving 105, 210
Resilience xviii, 3, 84–5, 203
  of therapist 190
Resistance
  physical 110, 125
  psychological 50, 95, 117, 185
Rescue, rescuer 94, 117, 172, 185
Resonance 170, 188, 193–5
Resources 21, 34–7
  access to 9, 66, 94, 109
  external environmental 29, 188
  internal 52, 188
  part selves as 137
  and privilege 94
  safety 109
  somatic 182, 184, 189, 199
  therapist 109, 175, 179, 185–6
Responsibility 41, 94, 122, 151–3, 166–7
Retraumatization *see* trauma
Retroflection see contact,
    modifications of
Rhythm, rhythmic movement 69, 125

Rigidity 31–4, 64, 118, 192
Risk 4, 107, 109, 139, 209
Rothschild, Babette 78, 103, 175
Rupture and repair *see* relationship

Safety *see also* resources 23, 62, 103,
   107–11, 125
  safe emergency 33, 44, 66, 198, 203,
   222
  safe place 109
  therapist representing 110, 171–2,
   208
Sander, Louis 23, 195
Schore, Allan 50, 153, 155
Self
  self–agency 45, 125
  self care 41
  coherence of 132, 135
  continuity of sense of 1–3, 110, 115,
   148
  self–disgust 147
  embodied 52, 133, 181, 185, 201
  fragmented 134, 142
  as function of field 11, 222
  self–functions *see also* Healing Tasks
   Model 40, 59, 66, 131
  self–harm 28, 59, 154–5
  self– identity, identification xviii, xix,
   30, 121, 151
  and integration 32, 41, 52
  self–medication 133
  and mirror neurons 181–2
  part selves *see* dissociation
  self–organization of *see also*
   organization 23, 29, 60
  as process 14, 80, 116, 131, 135
  self–regulation *see also* regulation 3,
   59, 85, 122, 167, 196
  self–states 115, 130, 132, 134–5, 137,
   174
  self–support 116, 196
  of therapist 165, 169, 172, 174–7
Sensorimotor therapy 5, 63, 174, 179,
   214
Sexual violence *see* trauma
Shame 120, 146–159, 185
  betrayal 140
  blame, self–blame 116, 121, 151, 153
  of body 153
  collective 156
  failure sense of 5, 116, 148, 156

  field dynamics 155
  guilt 149, 155
  and helplessness 120–1
  humiliation 147, 156
  internalized abuser 152
  and interpersonal trauma 149
  physiology of 155
  polarities of 157
  processes 147, 151
  regulatory function of 155
  and survivor guilt 149
  worthlessness, sense of 152
Shock, inescapable 2, 28, 97, 105, 156,
   207
Siegel, Daniel 16, 47, 190
  and attachment 198, 207–8, 215–6
  and complex systems 32
  and integration 141
  and mindfulness 85–7
  and mirror neurons 181
  and the window of tolerance 63
Silence xviii, 71, 153, 157
Situation *see also* field 11, 12, 26
Slavery 139
Social engagement system
  see poly vagal theory
Social justice xvi
Somatization 4, 8, 36, 46, 97, 133, 214
SOS model 11
  and revision 12
Spirit, spirit possession *see* dissociation
Splits, splitting
  see fragmentation
  see polarities
  healing of 13, 52, 143, 215
Stabilization *see* trauma
State dependence *see* memory
Stauffer, Kathryn 60–2, 66
Stewardship 166, 171
Stimulus 58–9, 69–70
Stress 6, 30, 47, 52, 58, 104–5
  chemicals *see* neurochemicals
Stuckness 47, 50, 117
Structural Dissociation Model
  see dissociation
Submission
  see collapse defence
Suicide, suicidality 137
  see also self–harm
Survival
  see defences

Tai–chi 50
Technique in trauma therapy 10
Terror
　see fear
Thalamus *see* brain
Threat
　see fear
Theory of causality 13
Therapist
　as change agent 44, 165–7
　embodiment of 17, 182, 185–6, 188
　as organiser of experience 174
　personal trauma of 174
　power of 17, 165–6, 169–70
　presence 174, 176–7, 185, 187
　as regulator of arousal 174, 204
　self of 180
　and window of tolerance 186
Time 74
　contemporaneity of, as field principle
　　51, 79
　continuity of experience 131
　dual awareness 78, 110, 138, 175
　fields of 76
　future 50, 76, 85, 88
　here–and–now 76, 175
　past, ongoingness of 74
　perspectives on current reality 74,
　　79–80, 130, 170, 176
　present 74–84, 86
Tipping point 33, 65
Tolerance
　see arousal
Touch 202
Tracking
　see phenomenology
Trafficking xvi, 108
Triggers 98
Triune brain *see also* brain 47–9
Transference 138, 171–4, 208
　co–transference 94, 172
　vicarious trauma 173, 182–6
Transformation xx–xxi
Trauma
　abuse 34, 149, 156, 207
　Adverse Childhood Experiences
　　(ACES) xvii–xviii
　brain adaptations to 6, 104
　childhood xviii, 14, 104, 131–2, 140
　cognitive effects of 155
　collective 1, 22, 139, 156

complex 3–4, 51, 122, 135, 144, 193,
　206–7
definitions 2
developmental 51, 207
domestic violence 12, 104, 107, 156,
　215
hypervigilance 74, 82, 101, 121, 155
illness following 7, 10, 81, 153,
informed practice xvii
interpersonal 2, 30, 120, 149
neglect xviii, 50, 195, 207
neurobiology of *see* neurobiology
as organizing principle 24, 97, 101,
　155
phases of therapy *see* Healing Tasks
　Model
physical assault 11, 132, 152
post traumatic growth xx
post–traumatic stress disorder PTS/D
　3, 58, 97, 131, 207
processing of 52–3, 55, 198, 214
rape 54, 105–6, 198, 214
responsive approach xvii
retraumatization 8, 44, 75
sexual trauma xviii, 75
single event 3
as social construct 95
stabilization 4
symptoms 3–4, 27, 32, 34, 78
transgenerational 27, 185
unresolved 22
vicarious *see* transference
war 104
Trust *see* relationship

Unattached burdens *see* dissociation
Unfinished business 23, 27, 158, 208, 213,
　216
Unformulated trauma xviii, 22, 34, 46,
　129, 139

Vagus
　see polyvagal theory
van der Kolk, Bessel 4–7, 34, 58, 152,
　199–200
Vasopressin *see* neurochemicals
Verbalization *see* language
Vicarious traumatization *see*
　transference
Victim, victimhood 17, 28, 107, 120, 149,
　151

Violence 99–100, 119
  domestic *see* trauma
  systemic, structural xviii, 54
Vitality 23, 36, 63, 65, 216
Vulnerability 98–9, 141, 157, 182

Western mindset 8, 93, 95, 130, 138, 206–7
Wheeler, Gordon 11, 13, 25, 156
Whiteness 95, 153
Wilkinson, Margaret 47, 49–50, 181,
  201, 216

Window of tolerance 63–6, 76, 82, 106,
  130, 167
  Window of Tolerance Model 63–4, 76,
  95, 167, 186, 198
  see also arousal
  see also Siegel, Daniel
Witness 1, 34, 133, 177, 187

Yoga 144
Yontef, Gary 29–31, 76, 209
Yunkaporta, Tyson 77, 93, 137